Language and
Language Disturbances

Language and Language Disturbances

Aphasic Symptom Complexes and their Significance
for Medicine and Theory of Language

by

KURT GOLDSTEIN, M.D.

New York City

GRUNE & STRATTON

New York · 1948

Printed at
WAVERLY PRESS
Baltimore, U. S. A.

CONTENTS

ACKNOWLEDGMENTS

This book is the fruit of studies extended over many years, carried out in collaboration with many co-workers and assistants. To all of them I am indebted for their help. I think especially with indeed nostalgic gratitude of my late friend, A. Gelb, my collaborator over so many years at a period when many of my basic ideas developed. I want to thank Dr. Martin Scheerer who worked with me for years in America and Miss Marianne Simmel who was of great assistance to me in the examination of patients.

I feel grateful toward many hospitals in Germany and America for the opportunity to examine patients. I should like to mention especially Montefiore Hospital, New York, where, after coming to this country, I found a new opportunity to resume my interrupted research under the auspices of the Harry H. Strauss Neurological Fund, and further, the Psychiatric Institute, New York, the Boston Dispensary, Tufts Medical School, Boston City Hospital, especially Dr. D. Denny-Brown, the Morrisania Hospital, Dr. N. Savitsky and the Metropolitan Hospital, New York.

Mention must be made of various publishers for the use of certain test and illustrative material, and acknowledgment is given at the pertinent points in the text.

I am pleased to have the opportunity to thank Mrs. Angelika W. Frick and Mr. Paul Rosenthal as well as Mr. Irving Cohen for their friendly interest and generosity in furthering my research. I am particularly indebted to the Dazian Foundation for Medical Research, New York, for its grant which was of decisive assistance in enabling me to finish the book.

I had several occasions to thank the Rockefeller Foundation for continued support of my studies in general. I want to acknowledge my deep appreciation again particularly for the fund granted for my research in speech disturbances.

K. G.

PREFACE

THE PURPOSE of this book is to present those speech disturbances observed in lesions of the brain cortex in a form useful both for practical and theoretic purposes in the clinic. Such a presentation should aid in the examination of patients and establish that body of facts which is always necessary as a sound basis for therapy: for operation, if necessary, and for systematic retraining.

It will be obvious that such an intention can be fulfilled only by consideration of facts and theories belonging to realms of knowledge somewhat removed from practical medicine. We shall have to consider problems of psychology, even of linguistics, and thus the presentation may become useful to the psychologist and philosopher of language also. They may find stimulation from pathologic material, and our interpretation of it may help them with problems in their own fields.

The organismic point of view, from which the phenomena of defective language are considered here, makes it necessary to discuss the basis of this standpoint, in at least its essential aspects. Its usefulness in the understanding of such a complex phenomenon as language and its disturbances can add valuable facts and interpretations to the theory underlying this viewpoint—a theory till now scarcely used for our present purpose. Thus, general biology may gain from our discussion.

It may be surprising that so much uncertainty and discussion exists in a field of research to which so many excellent scholars have contributed, and in which the literature, both book and periodical, is so extensive. When one considers the presentation of the subject in the usual textbooks, however, the current lack of concord becomes less remarkable. According to most of them, the distinction of various forms of aphasia and their definite localization appear to be well established. The presentation largely confines itself to a description of the phenomena which is adequate in these two respects. But the discussion of biologic and psychologic understanding of the changes in language, as far as it is presented at all, is based on theories upon which the various authors do not at all agree, and such an agreement is not considered essential for the problems of the clinic.

Indeed, if one tries to bring the findings in an individual case into relation to these descriptions in the textbooks, one usually meets with considerable difficulties. Cases considered as belonging to the same form of aphasia differ enormously as to their symptoms, and it is rare that one seems to fit the descriptions. The actual localization found in postmortems frequently—in apparently very similar cases—differs greatly as to locality and intensity of the lesion.

ix

In the clinical textbooks, not much attention was paid to this discrepancy; for gross clinical decisions the given distinctions appeared to be sufficient. The problems involved become obvious, however, when one digresses from the textbooks and delves into the presentations of the subject in the surveying manuals and, moreover, in the descriptions of individual cases in the literature. Here one is confronted with confusion in both theory and phenomena observed. The main reason for this confusion is that there is hardly one field of psychopathology in which the standpoint of the author concerning the problems involved is so personal as here, and determines to such a degree both examination and report of facts.

This state of affairs becomes understandable if one takes into consideration the many relations speech, normal as well as pathologic, has to medical and nonmedical problems and the widely differing special interests individual scientists take in one or the other of these relations. The realm of interest expands from gross anatomic localization of lesions in the individual case to the most complex biologic, psychologic, even philosophic interpretation of phenomena. Correspondingly, the protocols of the various authors are so divergent that one would hardly believe that we are dealing with the same subject.

A simplification of the examination was induced by the concept of localization, and for a long time the dominating point of view was description of findings with such schematic distinctions as cortical or subcortical, motor or sensory aphasia, etc. Many of the resulting protocols laid down in the literature are thus of very little value. They produce a misconception of the facts because they neglect a finer analysis of symptoms or analyze them from a theoretic point of view which leads to the overlooking of many of the phenomena. Theoretic bias has hindered investigation and reporting of many phenomena because these were not considered essential (see reference 105, p. 19). On the other hand, description of the phenomena after careful analysis in more psychologic or philosophic terms made it difficult for authors unfamiliar with these points of view to understand the material.

This divergence in viewpoint and reporting of facts would not be so disastrous if each of the procedures taken would serve its purpose, i.e., if the material gained with a particular point of view could be considered as sufficient for understanding the problems arising from it. This may apply when the only concern is gross distinction of various forms in the clinic and their localization for the diagnosis of a brain tumor or medical treatment of an aphasic patient with a vascular lesion. Here localization and determination of the underlying condition is more important than a finer analysis of the speech defect. But any attempt to make localization somewhat more precise, and to understand why in some cases our local diagnosis based on the symptomatology is wrong—and the literature contains a great number of such cases—needs consideration of factors which cannot be acquired by this clinical aspect alone (see 96, p. 8).

This becomes still more evident if one is interested in the question of spontaneous restitution and retraining of lost capacities. Here only a detailed analysis of the individual defect, with the aid of psychology, even philosophy of speech, will furnish a reasonable basis for management. On the other hand, a clear evaluation of the results gained with psychologic methods requires consideration of the relation of speech disturbance to our concept of brain function in general, to the premorbid constitution of the individual, to the personality as a whole, to the modification of all these factors by pathology, to the patient's capacities outside of speech, whether they are undisturbed or damaged, etc., and finally to the situation in which the individual has to live.

From the foregoing it will be evident that it is impossible to consider knowledge gained from separate viewpoints separately; one cannot restrict oneself to such narrowly acquired material even for such special purposes as retraining. The various facts elucidate each other. Even a simple examination presupposes some sort of theoretic concept and still more so does retraining. In scarcely any field of medicine are theory and practice so closely related, and support and correct each other to such a degree as in the field of speech disturbances. Our presentation of data thus involves a difficulty which finds its expression in the fact that, with the increase in knowledge and criticism, a comprehensive presentation of the total field has become progressively rarer in the literature. Although in the last decades of the nineteenth and the first decade of this century many systematic presentations comprising the whole field were published, the subsequent literature has been considerably less productive. To my knowledge, the last thirty to forty years have seen only a few publications which cover the whole field (H. Head; Weisenburg and McBride; Nielsen; Wilson; and my own presentation of the subject).

Since my first publication in 1905, I have tried several times to develop a comprehensive summary, but was always aware of the enormous difficulties involved in a systematic presentation of the facts. As long as I followed the distinction of the classic authors such a presentation was possible at least to a certain degree but it never seemed really satisfying. Experience showed that I must free myself from any definite theory and investigate patients in a way as unbiased from any of them as possible. The more cases I examined—and I think the number goes into the thousands—and the more published case material I studied, the more I realized that one can do justice to the underlying problems only by considering them from the broad point of view mentioned before.

Such an approach to the problem of aphasia may appear so difficult, particularly considering the education, skill, and time of the physician, that it may appear scarcely applicable. Of course if gross brain localization is the only consideration such careful case studies may not be necessary. But if we are more ambitious and want to understand the phenomena, there seems to me no other way out of the dilemma: either to give up any classification, or to take the considerable effort which such an attack on the problems incurs. Usually such an extensive study, demanding as it does so much knowledge and application of methods outside of the usual medical field, is rejected as not medical, not physiologic, not empiric, and depreciated as "philosophic."

In reply to such an objection I would like to refer to the general remarks made in my book, "The Organism" (p. 507), on this point. I came to the conclusion that the function of the organism could be understood only if we include that point of view usually called philosophic. When we approach the material with as unbiased an attitude as possible, and allow ourselves to be guided by the material itself and employ that method which the factual material dictates, the necessity of considerations customarily called philosophic may become apparent. The way in which these considerations have evolved from the material must show, indeed, that they actually belong to it. I should like to repeat the hope expressed in this previous volume: that it will be realized how irrelevant and little pertinent to reality are such lines of demarcation which are usually couched in the contradistinctive terms, "empiric research" and "philosophic reasoning."

KURT GOLDSTEIN, M.D.

New York City
July, 1948

Part One
THE ORIGIN OF APHASIC CONDITIONS

CHAPTER I

The Problem of the Origin of Symptoms in Brain Damage

FROM the point of view expressed in the Preface, it becomes clear that we cannot start with a systematic presentation of definite clinical pictures. Practical as well as theoretic considerations indicate the *individual symptom complex* as the center of interest. We consider the symptoms as due to disturbances of special functions which we wish to eliminate as much as possible, or, if this is not possible, to help the patient find an adjustment to his defect.

Such an attempt presupposes a knowledge of the relationship between the aphasic symptoms and definite functional disturbances. Thus, we are first of all confronted with the general theoretic problem of whether and how far we are justified in assuming such a relationship: *Are symptoms, i.e., modifications of behavior, the direct expression of a definite disturbance of function, or are there other factors involved which at least contribute to the production of symptoms?* In the latter case, we would be unable to draw from a symptom the simple conclusion that a definite disturbance of function exists, and we could not expect to help the patient by an attempt to improve what we assume to be a defective function.

Anyone who has tried to retrain aphasic patients knows how often such direct procedures show only moderate success. One important cause is the overlooking of the fact that the same symptom may be produced in totally different ways. Not all deviations of behavior are directly related to the underlying defect, but some are the expression of protective mechanisms which the organism utilizes against the disastrous effect of the defect (see p. 12). Only a careful analysis of each symptom and of the total situation in which it occurs will enable us to distinguish the origin of symptoms—a distinction of the greatest significance in deciding which symptoms one

1

should try to eliminate. Thus the question of origin is of paramount significance. Many mistakes in interpretation and in theoretic speculation could have been avoided in the past by this consideration. From the results in this respect alone, the problem of localization and spontaneous restitution in aphasia also can be attacked reasonably.

Our statements concerning a patient's condition either clinical or anatomic are based on the phenomena observed, i. e., the symptoms (p. 3). Symptoms do not always simply come to the fore by themselves. We have to apply definite methods to reveal them. There can be no doubt on this point as far as anatomic changes are concerned, but the same is true for neurologic and mental symptoms. There are only a few modifications of behavior we can observe directly and these may not always aid us in recognizing the defect. The patient does not speak or his speech is impaired, but a variety of causes may be operative here; only if we expose him to definite conditions may we be able to see the real cause. The same is true with defects in understanding, reading, etc. Thus the symptoms which we find in an individual patient are at least partly determined by our procedure or methods of investigation. Analysis of the structure of the methods will often also give us an insight into the structure of the disturbance of the patient.

The usual method of recording does not reveal the symptoms in any way of practical value. If the results are viewed as so many pluses or minuses, as often is the case, no real insight is gained as to what the patient can still do and what he can no longer do. A plus, that is, a performance correct de facto, may be attained in a quite incorrect, i.e., abnormal way, and we may not be able to see this in the result. The patient's pathology may actually consist in this abnormal procedure. In such cases the disturbance may be perfectly camouflaged. One will then be surprised to find, on a subsequent occasion, complete failure in the same or in a closely similar performance, namely, when the situation does not permit the patient to take a roundabout way.

As an instance, a patient had lost the concept of number; he could not even tell whether seven is greater than four. One would assume that he was not able to calculate. Nevertheless, he performed calculations quite accurately, that is, he got correct sums, products, etc. He could do this because he knew the correct answers by heart from the period before his disability, or had memorized them since. Now, these correct solutions do not effect unequivocal information about whether or not numbers are really understood.

As with the correct answer (the plus), the negative result (the minus) is also ambiguous. Factual failure in a task does not necessarily mean that the ability to perform it is lost. The patient's failure to act, to do anything at all, may spring from his feeling of apprehension, of uneasiness about the result he might reach; he is afraid that a wrong result will get him into a catastrophic situation (see p. 10). Only very searching observation of every factor in connection with the total situation in which the patient's reactions occur can give us information about his real performance status.

Besides these general aspects which have to be taken into consideration in an attempt to reveal the symptoms, we must be aware of the fact that the symptoms we observe in damage of the central nervous system are not at all simply manifestations of changes in definite function and structure, but can be due to the influence of other more general factors. From this point of view analysis of the symptoms causes us to distinguish between the *following groups of symptoms according to their origin:*

First, symptoms which represent direct sequelae of the impairment of the substratum. They are *defects of performance.* These are the *negative symptoms* of Hughlings Jackson.

Second, symptoms due to the effect of *separation* of an undamaged area from a damaged one. These are the *positive* symptoms of Jackson which we shall call *"indirect"* symptoms (symptoms due to "isolation").

Third, symptoms which are due to the *effect* which the pathologic process in the damaged area exerts *on other parts of the nervous system,* for instance by irritation of the immediate neighborhood. We shall call these *"depending"* or *"secondary"* symptoms.

Fourth, symptoms which represent *protective* mechanisms against the effect of the defect on the total personality. They serve to avoid "catastrophic conditions."

A. DIRECT SYMPTOMS

(1) *Symptoms Due to Dedifferentiation of Function*

It was long believed that any performance could be lost or impaired, and that the type of defect depended simply on the location of the lesion in the cortex. To a certain degree this is true. A lesion of the posterior central convolution produces sensory loss; a lesion of the anterior central convolution, disturbance of movement; a lesion of a particular part of the left third frontal convolution, language difficulties, etc.

But this simple relationship falls short if we consider the disturbances more carefully. In lesion of a "sensory" or "motor" area, the relevant performances do not drop out uniformly. The lesion produces effects according to a characteristic selective process. The sequelae of a cerebral lesion rarely take the form of a simple loss of performance; more commonly the defect shows itself in modifications which the performances undergo. These modifications are a result of a systematic disintegration of the function involved (Hughlings Jackson). As I was able to demonstrate, the structure of this disintegration—or, as I like to call it, dedifferentiation— invariably exhibits the same features, whatever region is involved, be it the spinal cord, the subcortical apparatus, or the cortex, and regardless of whether reflexes, motility, speech, thinking, or feeling is concerned (105*, p. 13). I speak in this respect of disturbance of the basic function of the central nervous system (cf. 105, p. 116) which leads to a change of the performance according to definite rules. Usually an attempt is made to trace the symptoms to a mass of separate functions. The new point of view tries to understand symptoms in a more unified fashion. It will be useful for our future discussion to outline these *general rules of disintegration*. In a rather broad way they may be formulated as follows:

All direct damage of the brain cortex causes a *rise of the threshold* and retardation of excitation. The receptivity of the patient is reduced; it takes him much longer to react. This manifests itself in the fact that patients may succeed perfectly in a task when given sufficiently long exposures, but fail in the same task with brief exposures; for instance understanding may be disturbed if one speaks too quickly to the patient, perception when he is examined by the tachistoscope, etc. Thus the tachistoscope has become an important instrument for revealing reduced function. (cf. 108, p. 99)

Prolongation of time of stimulation does not always bring about improvement of performance. The patient may perceive if the visual stimulus is strong enough, but after a time he may cease to see the object in spite of continued stimulation. After a certain time the stimulus may appear again. It seems that the threshold changes during stimulation (*lability of threshold*). This alteration of the threshold through stimulation which is due to the disturbance of the "equalization" process by the brain damage (See 105, p. 106) may concern—depending on the part of the cortex damaged—different performance fields, including speech. Stimulation of one part of a damaged performance field may influence the performance in other parts of the same field. A patient may be able to read silently with understanding but not if he has to read aloud (see p. 125), etc. (due to reduction of energy, see 105, p. 132).

If excitation takes place despite the obstacle imposed by the raised threshold it may *spread abnormally and last an abnormally long time*. This is also due to the disturbance of the process of equalization by the damage. (See 105, p. 132.) For example, the patient may be unable to locate the precise point stimulated on his skin. On the other hand, there is a long aftersensation. A word grasped by an aphasic with great difficulty sticks and influences subsequent performances, "perseverates." (Concerning the origin of "perseveration" and ways to avoid it, cf. later, p. 16).

A further characteristic effect of the damage is that performances of the organism are *determined* to a much greater extent than normally *by external factors* (cf. 105, p. 154). Normally, reactions are determined by processes within the individual *and* by the outer world stimuli. As a result of loss of structure, patients are deprived of functions and prior experiences; then external stimuli acquire an exaggerated importance. The resulting distractibility of the patient will strike the inexperienced observer as inability to concentrate. In a similar way a patient, under other conditions, may be abnormally fixated to a performance and appear "abnormally"

---

*Such numbers throughout refer to those in the general bibliography, p. 347.

attentive. It would be quite wrong to dispose of his condition under the general designation, "disturbance of attention" (see p. 212).

Modification of the patient's performance shows the effects of a *blurring of the sharp boundaries between "figure" and "ground"* (cf. 105, p. 109, 151). When we look at a picture we see and understand at once what is figure and what is background. The terms figure and ground can be applied not only to visual but to all performances. Figure and background can be discriminated as readily in speaking, thinking, feeling, etc. As examples of this figure-ground phenomenon, if one raises an arm vertically, the execution of this movement requires, as one can feel in oneself and observe in others, a rather definite position of the rest of the body. The raised arm is the figure, the rest of the body is the background. A word becomes meaningful from the context in which it appears; the meaning of a thought is conditioned by a vast contextual background—the individual's educational experience, social status, and so on.

Habitually we ignore the background of a performance and pay attention only to the figure. But figure and background are intimately interconnected. Neither of them can be properly evaluated without the other. Correspondingly, every change of background will produce a change of figure.

Figure-ground performances have their counterpart in processes of the nervous system. In any function of the organism the excitation in the nervous system is distributed in such a way that the process in a circumscribed area differs as to form and intensity from the state prevailing in the rest of the nervous system. The proces in the circumscribed area corresponds to what we call performance, designated by the term *"figure"*; the process in the rest of the nervous system we term the *"background,"* or, more briefly, *"ground."* In normal performances the figure and ground processes are in a definite relation. *All damage in the nervous system*, especially in the brain cortex, *disturbs this normal relation.* The sharp differentiation of figure from background suffers, inducing a general leveling or intermingling of figure and background. This is sometimes carried to the point of inversion, where the figure becomes background and the background figure. Many symptoms become understandable from this point of view. We expect the "figure" as reaction to a definite stimulus, and the patient may answer with the "background": instead of yes, the patient may say no; instead of black, white; instead of the demanded series of numbers, the series of the days of the week, etc.

The expression of dedifferentiation of function in impairment of abstract attitude.

There is one expression of dedifferentiation which we should consider especially because it is of greatest importance for understanding aphasic phenomena; it concerns dedifferentiation of attitudes in the form of *impairment of abstract attitude* (see p. 56). The patients might be divided into *two groups in which this attitude is or is not impaired.* Impairment does not mean simply a disturbance of mental capacity in general, but involves a disturbance in a qualitative way. Almost all performance fields are impaired to some extent, and examination and retraining promise much less success in patients of this kind. This "personality" change is to be found especially in cases of lesion of the frontal lobes, but it may also be observed to some extent in cases of lesion of other parts of the cortex (particularly in patients with lesions of the left hemisphere). The use of the term "abstract attitude" will be comprehensible in the light of the following explanation.

We can distinguish normally two different kinds of attitudes which we call the concrete and the abstract.   In the concrete attitude we are given over passively and bound to the immediate experience of unique objects or situations. Our thinking and acting are determined by the immediate claims made by the particular aspect of the object or situation.   For instance, we act concretely when we enter a room in darkness and push the button for light.   If, however, we desist from pushing the button, reflecting that by pushing the button we might awaken someone asleep in the room, then we are acting abstractively.   We transcend the immediately given specific aspect of sense impressions, we detach ourselves from the latter and consider the situation from a conceptual point of view and react accordingly. Our actions are determined not so much by the objects before us as by the way we think about them; the individual thing becomes a mere accidental example or representative of a "category."   Therefore, we also call this attitude the categorical or conceptual attitude.   The abstract attitude is basic for the following potentialities:

1. Assuming a mental set voluntarily, taking initiative, even beginning a performance on demand.

2. Shifting voluntarily from one aspect of a situation to another, making a choice.

3. Keeping in mind simultaneously various aspects of a situation; reacting to two stimuli which do not belong intrinsically together.

4. Grasping the essential of a given whole, breaking up a given whole into parts, isolating them voluntarily, and combining them to wholes.

5. Abstracting common properties, planning ahead ideationally, assuming an attitude toward the "merely possible," and thinking or performing symbolically.

6. Detaching the ego from the outer world.

In all these potentialities, the patients are more or less impaired.

During all activity the concrete attitude is dominant, but abstraction is required for beginning an activity, and if the course of action is interfered with or disturbed, to correct disturbances and to continue properly the activity in question.

Patients with impairment of abstract attitude may not appear to deviate grossly from normals in everyday behavior, because many routine tasks do not require the abstract attitude once these tasks have been learned. However, on observation of the patients in a variety of situations it becomes evident that they do not react even then like normal individuals. They appear more stereotyped and reserved.   They lack initiative and spontaneity.   Tasks which demand choice or shifting particularly reveal the defect. The above mentioned list of conditions has been compiled from analysis of the behavior of a great number of patients in various everyday and test situations; needless to say, such conditions can give rise to considerable personal difficulties.

It has been said that the defect of the patients consists in an inability to cope with new situations while retaining the ability to proceed in an abstract way as far as old experiences are concerned. As a matter of fact the patients fail equally in familiar situations and in new ones if they demand the abstract attitude. On the other hand, they can successfully cope with new tasks if the abstract attitude is not required. This is very important. If the defect would consist in an incapacity to handle new situations the patients never would be able to learn anything and the attempts to retrain them would be futile. Indeed, patients are more likely to fail in new situations than in old ones because the former frequently demand new sets, that is, the abstract attitude.

Abstract behavior is about the same as what Henry Head has called symbolic behavior in relation to speech.

Patients with impairment of abstraction differ also from normals in respect to the concrete activities of which alone they are capable. These activities show a more *passive, compulsive character; they are more stereotyped and rigid* (see p. 6).

In order to avoid misunderstanding, it must be emphasized that the process of dedifferentiation does not entirely destroy the ability to generate ideas and thoughts. What is affected and modified is the way in which thoughts and ideas are dealt with. Thoughts do arise, but can become effective only in a concrete way. Just as the patient cannot deal with objects in a conceptual frame of reference, so he can deal with ideas only as with things that belong to an object or situation. Concepts, meanings, categories other than situational means-end relations, are not within his scope.

It should be stressed further that we must differentiate various degrees of both abstract and concrete behavior. There are *various degrees of abstract behavior*, according to the degree of complexity which the performance in question involves. For instance, the highest degree of abstraction is required for the conscious and volitional act of directing any performance whatsoever, and for the act of accounting for these to oneself or to others; a less abstract degree for conceptual behavior is involved if unaccompanied by awareness of one's own doing, etc.

The gradation applies just as well to *concrete behavior*. The most concrete way of dealing with situations or things is when the individual is impressed by one property exclusively, experiences only this one and reacts to it; an example would be the reaction to only one color, or to the form of an object or its practical use. A less concrete approach is indicated when the subject embraces in his scope the total configuration of an object or situation, and is not determined in his response by only one impressive particularity.

A few examples taken from observation may illustrate the failures of these patients. A patient may be able to count if the examiner begins the series, "starts him off," but he cannot begin himself. Once interrupted he cannot continue. He has to begin again at the beginning. He has difficulty in stopping at an arbitrary point upon demand and tries to continue until definitely interfered with. He is unable to shift from reciting one series (e.g., numbers) to another series (e.g., days of the week), though he can recite each by itself. He can follow and even take part in a conversation on a familiar topic or the immediate situation, but if the conversation shifts to another topic—in itself equally familiar to the patient—he cannot follow and is completely at a loss (see p. 271). He may react successfully in a simple reaction test but cannot react differentially to two stimuli. He may be able to read a word at a time and at other times to spell it, but when asked to read and immediately afterwards to spell it he cannot do so. He may succeed in throwing a ball into boxes placed nearer or farther away, without being able to tell which box is farther away or which one is nearer. He may be able to orient himself in a complicated building which has become familiar to him but cannot say anything about even the simplest relations of rooms or floors to each other. He has the greatest difficulty in pretending. He fails on performances which are meaningful only with relation to future expectations or occurrences. If the patient with impairment of abstract attitude acquires certain materials by rote-learning, these new acquisitions lack stability. Only repeated experiences of the usefulness of these connections in concrete situations will stabilize them.

The behavior of patients may show further abnormalities by the *secondary effect which impairment of abstraction has on the learned activities*. Normally, these develop automatically, but there is a *definite dependence of the automatisms upon the abstract setting*. This is often overlooked. Pathology has taught us that patients with loss of abstract attitude in time lose to some extent the automatisms they have learned previously, and have great difficulty in acquiring new ones. It is important to consider this in the retraining of patients with a defect in abstraction (see p. 342).

What we have said in general concerns language in particular. We can distinguish *language belonging to the abstract attitude*, and *concrete language*. We shall have more to say concerning this later (see p. 25). This distinction is basic for understanding *aphasic symptomatology*.

(2) *Symptoms Due to Separation of an Undamaged Area from a Damaged One*

By such separation, or, as I call it, *"isolation,"* the function of the undamaged area is modified in a definite way (cf. 105, p. 133, et seq.). (Here we are dealing with the secondary positive symptoms of Jackson.) It is reasonable to assume that in the normal nervous system each part functions in interrelation with the whole, or at least with more extensive fields. Performances in a given field are therefore also conditioned by the functioning in other fields. Loss of certain performances, through damage of their substrata, brings about modification of other depending performances. Innumerable examples from pathology could be adduced to this cause: the appearance of exaggerated or abnormal reflexes, in the field of speech logorrhea, in sensory aphasia, etc., are cases in point.

B. Indirect or Depending Symptoms

The distinction between negative (or direct) and positive (or secondary) symptoms does not account fully for the complexity of the origin of symptoms in a circumscribed defect. There are secondary symptoms which are not an expression of isolation, but are produced by an effect of the changes in the damaged area on other parts of the nervous system. Frequently, patients improve after operation for a scar or tumor, even with respect to those symptoms which we believed were the result of damage to the substratum by the scar or tumor. More recent experiences, especially the results of removal of large sections of the frontal lobes damaged by a scar, have emphasized the fact that some symptoms may be produced not by the pathologic process itself but rather by its *influence upon other parts of the cortex*. We call symptoms produced in this way *indirect* symptoms.

The problem here involved has been raised time and again in the lengthy discussions about localization that were more in vogue two decades ago (see particularly Monakow and this author). Considerable evidence was collected at that time showing that the clinical picture depended not only upon the location of the lesion, but also upon the nature of the disease and the different effects which the various pathologic processes had on the function of other parts of the brain not directly affected. It was always assumed that some symptoms were due in part to *irritation* from the lesion indirectly affecting the immediate neighborhood or parts located farther away in the nervous system.

A disturbing indirect effect may be produced by a scar in the following way. The part of the brain where the primary lesion is located may be in functional relation with another part, and the two may represent a functional unit. In this case, impairment of either part puts the whole apparatus out of function (by "diaschisis"). The defective part disturbs the function of the other part, "inhibits" its function. Excision of the affected part may eliminate the disturbing factor and restore the function of the other part, at least to a certain degree. There are many examples from pathology by which the existence of such a mechanism could be proved. As mentioned on another occasion (see 105, p. 48), a partial defect of a functional unit may disturb the functioning of the whole organism more than a total defect of a field. Thus, for example, the difference in vision in hemianopsia and hemiamblyopia (see 105, p. 47) becomes explainable. Naturally, the existence of such a mechanism can be assumed only if we can prove that the part indirectly disturbed in its function is an essential part of the whole apparatus, and if we have other evidence that the injured part is essential for the performance in question (see p. 45).

From this point of view it becomes understandable that, under certain conditions, excision of a scar may help in regaining some performances disturbed before.

These distinctions have a definite bearing on our therapeutic procedure in the case of patients with brain lesions, especially of those who have scars as remnants of old injuries. If we can assume that we are dealing with secondary symptoms, we cannot expect surgical procedure to improve the condition; no procedure can eliminate isolation. If symptoms can be considered as indirect in the sense adopted above, operation certainly will be indicated. It may not always be easy to make a definite decision; nevertheless we must analyze the symptoms very carefully from this point of view.

C. Symptoms Due to Catastrophic Conditions

The fourth group of symptoms involves expression of *catastrophic conditions* and the tendency of the organism to *avoid them*. In order to understand this, some introductory remarks are necessary.

If patients with severe brain damage are observed without prejudice, one will frequently find considerable variation in performance. Similar tasks will sometimes be properly performed, sometimes not.

The common tendency has been to refer these variations to disturbances of attention or interest, to abnormal fatigue or exhaustion, etc.—in short, to disturbances of so-called general functions. This explanation remains hypothetic, because it has never been possible to demonstrate the independent existence of these supposed disturbances. Painstaking observation, as a matter of fact, discloses that attention, interest, memory, fatigue, etc., vary as much as the performances vary. They are sometimes good, sometimes bad. We have here the same problem as before: Why is the patient in one situation attentive, interested, etc., and in another inattentive, uninterested, tired, etc.?

The clue can be found through careful observation of the patient's behavior as a whole, in both the situation where he is able to perform a task, and in that where he fails. We shall find, then, that his behavior as a whole varies fundamentally. Here is a man with a lesion of the frontal lobe, to whom we present a problem in simple arithmetic. He is unable to solve it. But simply noting and recording the fact that he is unable to perform a simple multiplication would be an exceedingly inadequate account of the patient's reaction. Just looking at him, we can see a great deal more than this arithmetical failure. If he fails, he fumbles; a moment before amiable, he is now sullen, evasive, exhibits temper, or even becomes aggressive. It takes some time before it is possible to continue the examination. Because the patient is so disturbed in his whole behavior, we call situations of this kind *catastrophic situations*.

In the face of a task which he can perform, the same patient behaves in the opposite way. He looks animated and pleased, is steady and collected, interested, cooperative; he is "all there." One might infer from this contrast in behavior that the patient's reaction as a whole is simply his reaction to the experiencing of adequacy or inadequacy to the task. But the fact that the reaction-complex does not follow the performance or nonperformance, but occurs simultaneously with it, speaks against such an explanation. A further argument against it is that often the patients have no idea why they have been agitated, angry, or resistant.

As a matter of fact, the contrasting behavior is to be regarded as a manifestation of the capacity of the organism as a whole for success or failure in a task set for it.

This behavior contrast is not grounded purely psychically, and thus cannot be understood from a psychologic point of view alone. It can be grasped only from the *biologic point of view*, which has been dealt with at length on another occasion, and which can only be alluded to here (see 105, p. 35 ff.).

We are justified in assuming that the organism has a somewhat constant structure and somewhat constant functions. If an individual is confronted with tasks to which he is equal, he will not only perform them, but show objectively and subjectively the picture of harmonious functioning, the picture of order. The acts performed in such a situation will appear to us as performances of which this individual is normally capable, which suit this individual. Subjectively, they are experienced as activity in a mood of contentment and satisfaction.

It is very important to bear in mind that all new stimuli affect the condition of the organism (usually called the threshold) with the consequence that the recurrence of the same stimulus may elicit a response different from the previous one. This would supposedly lead to disorderly behavior of the organism. Actually, no such consequence occurs. We observe that processes in the organism have a relative constancy. I have explained elsewhere that this relative constancy can be maintained only under the condition that each change produced by a stimulus is *equalized* again within a certain time, so that the organism regains that "average" state which corresponds to its "nature," which is "adequate" to it.   However, if such is the case, the same environmental events can produce the same change, can lead to the same effect and to the same experience, which is necessary for the maintenance of the organism, its "existence."   This kind of coming to terms of the organism with the environment is due to the effect of the "equalization" process (see 105, p. 106).

The preservation of such a constancy requires a determinate environment, a definite kind of "milieu."   Only such events or processes in the external world as make such equalization possible fit into the milieu of the organism and take effect as stimuli.   Other changes in the environment are ineffective.   We know that each organism is unreceptive to certain environmental events.   If these are very powerful, however, they do force themselves upon the organism.   They do not produce orderly harmonious responses, but rather disorderly, disharmonious, defective performances, climaxing in *catastrophies* with all their concomitants, particularly anxiety. Since all damage to the brain involves an impairment of structure and thus of performance, *the equalization process is consequently upset*.   This results in a condition in which normal stimuli, i.e., the stimuli coming from the familiar environment, induce catastrophic reactions in the patient.   This is the reason for the *disordered behavior and anxiety* which we observe so frequently in our patients.   Moreover, in such catastrophic situations not only the specific performances are bad, but attention, memory, and the so-called general functions will also be affected.

The sick man has a strong urge to meet all demands as well as possible; his existence is bound up with such an endeavor to an even higher degree than the healthy man's.   Therefore, it is still more important for him not to be exposed to catastrophic situations.   There is a danger that the after-effects of these situations may deprive him, for a varying length of time, even of such power of performance as he would otherwise have.   Thus, he can exist only when he finds a new milieu adapted to his changed structure. The very endeavor to find such a milieu in which he can avoid catastrophic situations produces a definite behavior pattern.   Symptoms which may appear to result from the existing pathology are often only the *expression of the patient's flight from catastrophic situations* by means of building such a protective pattern.

There are different ways in which the patient evades the threat of catastrophe.   One of these is *complete self exclusion* from the world.   This is resorted to when almost every stimulus is felt as a precursor of catastrophe.   In the extreme cases, the only solution is—loss of consciousness.

If we go back now to the patient whose performance we described (see p. 12), we find that he remained in an "adequate milieu" as long as he was confronted with tasks to which he was equal.   But, when faced with a task to which he was not equal—

even if it were only, as instanced, an elementary arithmetic problem—he invariably fell into a state of violent trembling and finally even into a brief state of unconsciousness. In this case, a "catastrophic reaction," of the severest type, a reaction leading to unconsciousness, could be experimentally produced. When the patient was asked, after he had regained his normal condition, what had been the matter with him and what had been demanded of him, he would not be able to give any information whatsoever.

Lapsing into unconsciousness is of course hardly a suitable means for avoiding catastrophic situations, since it cuts off contact with all situations. The organism will, therefore, commonly seek protection in another way, namely, by seeking out situations which promise a minimum of irritating stimuli. The patient seeks tranquillity, and avoids company. But entirely tranquil situations cannot always be found, nor are they ever a complete protection from disturbances. Upsetting stimuli may arise in any situation, and then coming, so to speak, out of the blue, they fall upon the patient with the redoubled force of the unexpected.

Least of all is he able to meet anything unexpected. It is of the essence of his changed condition that every readjustment becomes painfully difficult. We observe time and again that patients will start violently upon being suddenly addressed. Nor is it even necessary that what is said to them should contain anything irritating. What acts upon them as an irritant is the mere fact that the stimulus comes from a situation not belonging to their present milieu. Under this condition, the patient may be unable to perform a demanded task, e.g., to answer to a simple question, which he may perform well when the task is related to the present condition. Many defects thus become understandable.

To avoid such sudden irritations, the patient seeks to surround himself with a protective fence that will prevent impinging stimuli from entering. He may build such a fence by constantly busying himself with doing something. Concentration upon a particular activity which he is able to perform without difficulty makes him relatively impervious to the undesired and dreaded stimulation from the outside. These activities need not have any great value in themselves; their usefulness to the patient consists in their protective character.

The trend to avoid catastrophic conditions may express itself in an "abhorrence of a vacuum." Let us say that we offer an aphasic a blank sheet of paper and ask him to write something on it. Even when he is specifically instructed to write in the middle of the sheet he will start as close as possible to the margin and squeeze his writing into the narrowest compass, as if afraid to venture into the open space of the paper. Any attempt to correct this procedure throws him into instant confusion. Another patient is unable to write unless a line is ruled on the paper. If it is not done for him, he may do it himself. He does not need the line because he has been accustomed to write on ruled paper, nor for aligning his letters properly. He needs the line as *something to take hold of in order to get started at all*. Another patient can read what is written on a sheet of paper only after the words are underlined. I write a letter on the blackboard, he is unable to read it. Now he takes the chalk and draws a line under it and immediately says, "That is an 'a.' "

These examples are important not only in respect to the specific physiognomy of the patient's pathology, but also for a correct recognition of the patient's performances in different fields and for his treatment. In the case of the patient who needs a starting line for writing, the condition may easily be misinterpreted as agraphia.

Another refuge for our patient is an *excessive orderliness*. As director of a large institute for brain injuries, I had the opportunity of keeping patients under observation for ten years and more.   It was our aim to place these patients in a setting as nearly normal as was practicable.   Among other things, each inmate was supposed to look after his personal belongings in the same way as would a well man.   Nothing was more illuminating than the wardrobes of these men and the meticulous way in which the innumerable odds and ends, the accumulation of ten years' residence, were always disposed.   Everything had its appointed place, and, moreover, had to occupy that place in a very definite way.   Looking more closely, one discovered a quite utilitarian motive behind this formal geometry, namely, bringing each article within the patient's reach with a minimum of effort on his part.   Seen in this light, it was not surprising to find the most rigid orderliness in the severest cases.

Some other examples may illustrate this "obsessive" orderliness.   While sitting and talking to a patient of this sort, I place some objects at random on the table.   If he becomes aware of them, he will at once proceed to arrange them in some order. Or again, a patient has just written something for me on a sheet of paper.   The examination is concluded.   "That is all," I say, make a quick note, and drop the pencil on the sheet of paper, which happens to be lying aslant.   The patient takes up the pencil, straightens the paper carefully so as to bring its side parallel with the side of the table, and then as carefully places the pencil parallel with the margin of the paper. I change the pencil to an oblique position.   This game can be kept up for some time. In fact, if the patient is made to desist, being told that the pencil should be left in the oblique position, he will obey with signs of visible discomfort.

One other characteristic peculiarity is that these patients are often utterly *unaware of their deviation from the normal,* and of their own state prior to the development of the cerebral injury.   This symptom was first described a long time ago by Anton, in connection with visual disturbance. Later, the phenomenon was observed in relation to a wide range of brain lesions.   This unawareness is strikingly displayed when the patients speak to the physician of their troubles; it is astonishing how infrequently and how little such patients complain of the paralysis or the hemianoptic defect, of disturbances of speech, of recognition, of acting, etc.   This becomes exceedingly impressive when the existing defect tends toward totality, such as complete blindness, complete loss of speech.

Now, it is important to note that what happens here is not simply that the patient is subjectively unaware of this defect, but that objectively he is compensated in his attitude and behavior so that the defect causes no difficulty of moment.   It must, however, be remembered here that such adequate behavior presupposes that the patient's milieu is free from potentially upsetting stimuli.   Adequate behavior indicates that the patient has found a milieu suitable to his altered state, one to which he can adjust himself. Closer examination shows that in order to readjust itself to the world, the injured organism has withdrawn from numerous points of contact. This new "order" he has attained is concurrent with a shrinkage of his environment.

I shall not go into the particulars here of how this adaptation is achieved, but two very important general facts which may be observed in that process should be mentioned.

First, the *degree of readjustment is directly related to the severity of the defect.* When the defect completely blocks any activity, the readjustment—as far as the achievement of a new order is concerned—may be even better than in cases of lesser disturbance. When, for example, sight is entirely gone, the patient compensates far more thoroughly than in the case of only impaired vision. In cases of one-sided paralysis, the patient will make more effective use of his other side in inverse proportion to the degree of function remaining on the injured side. This readjustment accomplished, he loses the realization of being paralyzed at all. Generalizing, we may say that *alterations are shut out from the consciousness of the organism when they would seriously impair any of its essential functions.* If, for example, total blindness remained permanently present to the patient's consciousness, he would be placed in the impossible situation of facing visual demands that he could never meet; his only possible response would be the catastrophic reaction. The organism so threatened will spontaneously reach a new equilibrium through readjustment to a nonvisual world. This involves, of course, a drastic shrinkage of one's world, and thus, at first, a profound disturbance of the organism and restriction of its function range. It will, therefore, not be resorted to as long as the injured function can be made use of after a fashion. Thus we find patients with partially impaired vision using their eyes but realizing that they do not see well. And here results the paradox that we may find less disturbance of general behavior and subjective feeling in cases of total loss of some function than in cases in which this function is only partially disturbed.

One example may illustrate the point. A patient who had been shot through the chiasm opticum was at first totally blind. As long as this lasted, he was not conscious of being blind. He used to talk of visual things like any seeing person; he was quiet, his behavior was orderly, and one could see that he managed to get along without difficulty in the hospital environment. Later, his injury improved and he regained sight to a certain degree. Now he became upset; he sought to orient himself by means of sight, but failed, owing to its imperfection. Thus, he was less well adapted to his world than he had been when blind. Now, for the first time, he spoke of something not being right with his vision, and this previously quite reasonably contented man dropped into a state of depression. "What's to become of me if I can't see?" he would cry.

A second important fact is that the readaptations in question are effected *without entering the patient's consciousness.* A patient of mine suffering from visual agnosia could not recognize a single letter visually, yet he could make out the significance of words. We ascertained that he accomplished this by way of kinesthetic experiences, gained through tracing the letters with movements of his eyes. In this connection, we are interested only in the fact that this patient was not at all conscious of any difference between this method of reading and his previous normal way of reading, and, further, that his substitute method—developed to a high degree of perfection —had evolved quite spontaneously.

The modification of general behavior which we have been considering finds its most pregnant expression in persons having major defects, but in principle we find the same in patients who have only minor defects. This way of looking at these things is not only of theoretic but also of practical importance. We have seen that the patient's capacity is determined to a high degree by the tasks set for him by the milieu, and that the adequacy of the latter depends not the least on the possibility to avoid catastrophic situations. We find, further, that a patient will sometimes endure a defect in such a way as to reach better performances in another direction and thus improve his chance of readjustment. In cases *where the pathology cannot be removed*, the task of the physician will therefore be to *secure the best possible milieu for the patient and to decide how much of his defect a patient may be able to bear without being too much disturbed in general*. The physician will have to decide which of his patient's symptoms are to be eliminated and which are to be retained. It is needless to explain how important the decision is for any treatment.

D. Symptoms Due to Fatigue and Perseveration

Fatigue and perseveration are phenomena very often observed in patients with damage of the brain, and are a great hindrance in examination and in determination of the symptoms related to the defect in the brain. Usually, these phenomena are considered as special defects due to the brain damage, and one tries to avoid their influence by shortening the duration of the examination and intercalating rest periods. There is no doubt that the disturbing influence of these phenomena can be reduced by this procedure. However, observation of the behavior of patients during examinations which are continued over a long time has taught me that the entrance of fatigue is not at all simply related to the duration of the examination, but depends to a large extent upon the particular character of the demanded performances. The degree of difficulty which the task represents to the patient is a paramount factor in whether fatigue occurs or not. If, in continuous activity, a later demanded task is easier to perform than the task in the first period of work, then the paradoxical situation may occur that (under such condition, in continuation of activity), fatigue may even decrease.   Indeed, the relation of fatigue to the difficulty of the task will come to the fore only if one considers the task in respect to the capacity of the specific individual.   The same task does not represent the same degree of difficulty for every individual, this holding particularly true for a patient. In an attempt to find the cause for difficult tasks producing earlier and stronger fatigue than easy ones, I came to the result: that *fatigue is more likely to occur the more the task is suited to bring the patient into a catastrophic condition* (see 110).

Certainly, some fatigue occurs in all individuals in all activities continued long enough.   We observe in all continued activities, first, improvement of performance as an effect of learning and adjustment.   Then, activity persists in about the same way for a certain time.   The curve shows a plateau as expression of acquired adjustment and of the organism's capacity to cope with the task.   After a certain time, the curve declines.   The decline consists not simply in a decrease of performance: first we see a fluctuation between low and about normal performances, then no performance reaches the normal level any more, until finally it goes down to a more or less low level.

These deviations from the norm observed in fatigue concern not only the objective phenomena but also the subjective feelings.   The individual feels discomfort, uncertainty, distress.   Subjective and objective fatigue sometimes may occur independent of each other.   Under certain conditions, somebody may get exhausted without being aware of it.   Such observations and the fact that subjective fatigue cannot be measured exactly have tended to result in the omission of subjective fatigue from research and consideration merely of objective findings.   This is unjustified.   Objective fatigue can, without doubt, be influenced by the presence or absence of the feeling of being fatigued.   It was a particularly careful study of the subjective phenomena which revealed that fatigue is not simply impossibility or unwillingness to act but a *behavior characteristic* for a special situation, namely, *the situation of stress.*   Not all cessation of activity means fatigue.   It can belong to a situation as a necessary part; then, it can be accompanied by agreeable feelings, as, for instance, in a pause belonging to a task or in a condition of contemplation.   However, if decrease of performance is paralleled by emotional distress, a feeling of discomfort, insecurity, or danger, we are dealing with fatigue.   Fatigue is related to distress; it is behavior in distress.   Hence, it becomes understandable why fatigue is so frequent and outspoken in patients who easily become distressed because of the impairment of their capacity to cope with many normal tasks (see the curves of fatigue in brain injured patients, 108, p. 115–132).

The relation of entrance of fatigue to the situation of distress shows itself by the similarity of the modification of behavior which we observe under both conditions.   A patient in fatigue shows symptoms similar to those of an individual in a catastrophic condition: irregularity of performance, variability, appearance of performances corresponding to a lower level (the more "simple" ones), abnormal sticking to a performance the patient is able to fulfill, e.g., rigidity, perseveration. He shows further in enforced continuation of performances the general reactions so characteristic for distress: yielding or aggressiveness; and subjectively, discomfort, insecurity, anxiety.

Hence, it becomes evident that tasks produce fatigue *because the difficulty or impossibility to fulfill a task produces distress*. The more the patient is exposed to such tasks, the more the phenomena characteristic for fatigue come to the fore; the more tasks which he can fulfill are demanded from him, the less he becomes fatigued, even if these are in the course of prolonged examination. This result is of *greatest significance for any examination*. The more we take it into consideration, i.e., the more we avoid the entrance of distress, the longer we are able to examine a patient in one session and thus to reveal the modifications of his behavior due to his damage. What holds true for examination is true also for training. Success in training is to a high degree dependent upon the consideration of the causes for entrance of distress and, hence, of fatigue.

We have mentioned that in a condition of fatigue, *perseveration* occurs. We consider perseveration as a means utilized by the organism to avoid catastrophe (see p. 12). As a matter of fact, it becomes apparent if a task is *particularly* difficult or the patient was exposed directly before to such tasks. In the latter case, he may perseverate even in "easy" tasks. The preceding difficult task made it impossible for the equalization process to "take place in an adequate way." Therefore, the new task touches the organism in an abnormal condition, and thus it may be unable to solve even "easy" tasks.

From what we have said, it is evident that *perseveration like fatigue can be eliminated at least to a certain degree* by arranging the examination in such a manner that it avoids the frequent menace or entrance of catastrophe.

CHAPTER II

The Organismic Approach to Brain Pathology in General

THE SURVEY regarding the factors determining the configuration of symptoms in brain damage has shown that symptoms are only partly the direct results of the damage. It has further become evident that, to a greater or lesser degree, the symptoms are an expression of the organism's struggle with the defect in its attempt to adjust itself in spite of some interference by the defect. The symptoms become understandable only from the organismic point of view which has become increasingly accepted in the different fields of biology in the last decades.

This approach goes back to Geoffrey de Saint Hilaire and Cuvier. As Cuvier has shown, the German poet Goethe played a considerable role in its development by pointing out the significance of morphology in the understanding of nature. The two great French natural scientists denied that there are accidental things in organisms and stressed the mutual dependence of all functions. Cuvier spoke the famous words: "Give me the feather of a bird of unknown and extinct species and I shall describe to you its whole structure." This point of view became paramount for comparative and paleontologic research. In recent times, these ideas were advocated in biology particularly by the English physiologist, J. B. S. Haldane, and by others.

In embryology, Coghill has shown that development could be understood as a total pattern determined by interaction between the organism as a whole and the environment. In psychology, with the increasing interest in the structure of personality, the concept of the organism as a whole gained an increasing appreciation (see particularly Allport, Kantor, Lashley, Tolman and others). In the field of physiology, I should like to point particularly to Herrick's and Cannon's work.

My own concept of the function of the organism was based on analysis of a great number of physiologic and psychologic phenomena—normal and pathologic—in man. I came to the conclusion that the basic motive of organismic life is the *trend of the organism to actualize itself*, its "nature," its capacities, *as well as possible* (see 105, p. 197). I have tried to formulate the rules which govern behavior of the normal organism and guarantee self-actualization.

The same rules—indeed somewhat modified in definite ways—determine behavior of the sick organism. *Pathologic behavior is behavior of functions of parts of the organism isolated from the whole.* Only if one takes this into consideration, i.e., the modification which functions suffer by *"isolation,"* will he gain insight into the structure of pathologic behavior and be able to use pathologic experiences for understanding normal behavior. The simple drawing of a conclusion from pathologic findings on normal behavior is doomed to failure in the same way as is an attempt to understand organismic behavior by simple synthesis of the phenomena acquired by the analytic method. Both procedures must fail because they overlook the *"fallacy of isolation"* (see 107, p. 224 ff.).

CHAPTER III

The Organismic Approach to Aphasia

THE organismic concept underlies the following presentation of the aphasic phenomena. According to the general trend of organismic behavior, the aphasic patient tries to achieve a condition which allows him to react as well as possible to the tasks arising from the environment. If he is successful in this endeavor, at least to such a degree that he can fulfill those performances which are "essential" to his nature, he will be in a new order, will avoid catastrophic occurrences, and be able to use his remaining capacities. From this point of view, it follows that every *individual speech-performance is understandable only from the aspect of its relation to the function of the total organism in its endeavor to realize itself as much as possible in the given situation.*

The organismic approach to aphasia deviates essentially from the so-called classic theory of aphasia which is based on an "atomistic" concept of the organism. In the second half of the last century when the interest in aphasia rose among physicians, the atomistic approach was widespread in biology, neurology and psychology; thus a corresponding theory of aphasia seemed justified—this the more so as normal psychology, even philosophy of speech, had absorbed certain of the physicians' ideas based on this atomistic approach (see, e.g., Erdmann).

The atomistic theory found its expression in brain physiology in the assumption of separate brain centers, those in which perception takes place, images and after-effects are deposited, and those which direct the motor actions. These centers were considered connected with other parts of the brain which should be responsible for recognition of objects, thinking, etc. The symptoms observed in lesions of the cortex, according to this theory, were the effect of damage of these centers or their connections. The atomistic concept of language regards language as based on images of words, motor and sensory, which are connected in various ways with each other, and with other images corresponding to objects, thoughts and feelings. Speaking and understanding is reproduction of these images. They develop by conditioning instigated by the needs of communication between men. Language is nothing but a conventional tool derived from expressive movements which appear in connection with emotional processes and develop into language. From this concept it was easy (or at least seemed to be) to describe the disturbances of speech in a systematic way as resulting

21

from defects in building or reproducing and understanding word images, due to circumscript lesions in the brain. From this point of view the various aphasia schemata originated.

This approach decisively influenced research in aphasia for decades. Even after Jackson, Pierre Marie, this author and others had criticized this concept, and particularly Head had loosed his whole sarcasm on the "diagram makers," the presentation of the subject in the textbooks did not change. Indeed, some of the classic authors were such excellent observers, as, e.g., Wernicke, that in spite of their theoretic bias they could not fail to notice that it was not possible to explain all cases in this simple way. It was particularly the facts with which they were faced in the "transcortical" aphasias on the one hand and the so-called "conduction aphasia" ("Leitungsaphasie") on the other, which induced them to enlarge the original simple schema. But the new facts did not change the basic concept. They tended to assume a new center, the "Begriffszentrum" (center of conceptualization), and a center for the "Wortbegriff" (concept of words) (Wernicke). But these supplements to the original schema were too theoretic and too much ad hoc to be really useful solutions. However, at least it was recognized that besides the word-image other factors are significant for normal language, and destruction of other factors for the origin of aphasia.

From these new facts grew the new organismic theory of aphasia, together with the criticism of the theory of images. Of course, the first theory of aphasia, based on the organismic point of view, was much older. Hughlings Jackson, in the middle of the last century, had stressed with emphasis that speech was not any unrelated succession of words. Speech is "propositions." The value of the word can be judged only from its use in a special connection. Loss of speech in aphasia is loss of power to propositionize. The patients have not lost words, but the words are not available for the higher service of propositional expressions, i.e., for some special purpose of the individual. Aphasia, for Jackson, is one expression of a defect of a basic mental function, similar to what I later called abstract attitude. These ideas of Jackson's surmounted so much the level of the concepts of the time that they scarcely found attention and did not influence the further development of the theory of aphasia. Contrarily, the atomistic theory became more and more dominant, particularly after the famous discussion in the British Association for the Advancement of Science, London, 1868, in which Jackson and Broca presented their respective theories and from which Broca emerged victorious.

The significance of the ideas of Jackson, however, gained recognition when Pick and Head, after new and unbiased observations, raised criticism against the classic theory and when from new facts a new viewpoint grew, similar to the one Jackson had inaugurated.

As for myself, when I began to be interested in the problem of aphasia I was influenced by my teacher, C. Wernicke. It was Storch who revealed to me the points where Wernicke's theory could not be upheld. My further studies led me to attack particularly the theories of images and of localization (see p. 45).

A. THE PURPOSE OF LANGUAGE AND THE PROBLEM OF MEANING

Applying my point of view to the study of the nature of language and its disturbances, I came to the following conclusion: *Language is a means of the individual to come to terms with the outer world and to realize himself.* It is the special purpose of language to facilitate man's coming to terms with his fellows (see further on this point, p. 94). Our way of speaking becomes understandable only if we always take into consideration the special relation of the speaking person to the environment in the given situation. This is valid in the same way concerning the defective speech which patients present.

I recognized (87) the great significance of Pierre Marie's ideas which had much in common with my own. I agreed particularly with his criticism of the role images were assumed to play by most of the contemporary authors. My own concept arose from the application of the organismic approach to the interpretation of aphasic phenomena. This approach, which has proved so fruitful to me for understanding a great number of pathologic neurologic phenomena, induced a careful consideration of each individual aphasic phenomenon in relation to the total organism.

The first result of the new approach was the new interpretation of amnesic aphasia which inaugurated a change in the concept of aphasia in principle. Amnesic aphasia, consisting (according to the general conception) of a dissociation between object- and word-images, was one of the strong pillars of the classic theory. It became evident by the analysis of Gelb and myself that we are not dealing with impairment of word-images or difficulty in evoking them, but that the difficulty in finding words—as names for objects—was the consequence of a change of the total personality, specifically of an impairment of the so-called categorical or abstract attitude. Thus, the problem of meaning assumed a central importance in the interpretation of aphasic symptoms.

This analysis was so important because it showed that at least one common form of aphasia is not due to a memory defect but is related to a defect in a higher mental function, a definite capacity.

The difference of abstract attitude and concrete behavior becomes particularly evident in language and its disturbances because the effect of abstract attitude on performances presents itself here in a characteristic way. Thus, it is understandable that the general concept of abstract and concrete behavior originated particularly from the analysis of aphasic symptoms.

The idea of the central role which disturbance of meaning plays in the development of aphasic phenomena corresponds particularly to the interpretation of the symptoms by Head. It became further important for theoretic discussions of the problem by L. Binswanger (13), A. Kronfeld (170) and others. It did not at all find general acceptance among the physicians occupied with aphasic patients, but, contrarily, met great opposition.

The authors who emphasized this factor of meaning in the discussion of aphasia often made the mistake of not carefully enough considering the facts observed in aphasic patients and not doing justice to the disturbances of what we call the instrumentalities of speech (see p. 25) which represent a large part of the symptoms observed in patients. The problem of speech disturbances cannot be settled simply with stress on the significance of meaning. In this respect, the criticism directed against Head and Binswanger was correct. Unfortunately, it did not do justice to the valuable element in this new theory, and thus was not so constructive as it could have been. From misunderstanding the tendency of the new approach, unproductive discussions originated and the fruitful nucleus which this new concept contained was overlooked. As far as the opposition concerned myself, I cannot consider it justified at all. However highly I evaluated the significance of the phenomenon of meaning for understanding aphasic symptoms, I never neglected the disturbances of instrumentalities. I stressed, for example, their significance in opposition to the explanations of Head who, indeed, had not done justice to them (see 96).

It was particularly my interpretation of amnesic aphasia which gave rise to criticism which I shall discuss on a later occasion when we shall deal with this form of aphasia (see p. 63).

As long as research in aphasia tried to understand the phenomena in an atomistic, simply structural way, there was little possibility of finding any relation to the concept of meaning. Only a functional interpretation of the phenomena observed in brain damage in general, and of speech in particular —physiologically as well as psychologically—could give the basis for a correct utilization of the facts and theories of this concept of meaning. I therefore placed the problem of meaning into the foreground because it had been, until then, so greatly neglected, and I found that a correct interpretation of meaning is absolutely prerequisite for interpretation of some aphasic symptoms (see p. 61). The problem of the relation between meaning and instrumentalities, almost generally neglected in the theory of normal speech and in research of aphasia, came increasingly into the center of my interest.   I saw that insight into this relation alone could help us to understand the modification of language in loss of meaning and the effect of loss of instrumentalities on the non-language performances and so also on the phenomenon of meaning.   (We shall come back later to the problem of meaning.   I refer particularly to the discussion, p. 61.)

B. CONCRETE AND ABSTRACT LANGUAGE

There should be distinguished—indeed somewhat abstractly—*two types of language* and correspondingly *two groups of aphasic symptom complexes:*

1. *Concrete language* which belongs to concrete behavior.   It consists of speech automatisms, of the "instrumentalities of speech": of sounds, words, series of words, sentences, one form of naming (see p. 61) and of understanding of language in familiar situations for which it has been conditioned, and finally of emotional utterances.   In pathology, it presents itself in somewhat isolated defects of speaking, understanding, etc., of so-called pure forms of aphasia and central aphasia.   Because of the difference of the relationship of emotional and nonemotional language to the personality, there is a difference of impairment of both in aphasia (see p. 59).

2. *Abstract language* which belongs to abstract attitude: volitional, propositional, rational language.   It is disturbed somewhat isolatedly if abstract attitude is impaired; further, in slight damage of instrumentalities which may leave intact other speech functions but disturbs the highly complex performance of voluntary actions (see p. 6).   Because the various speech performances as voluntary speech, conversational speech, speaking of isolated words or of series, repetition, naming of objects, reading, etc., are in a different degree dependent on the abstract attitude, the various performances may be damaged in different degrees.

Everyday language is a combination of both types of language; in a conversation, first automatisms may occur, then appearance of words may be determined by abstract attitude.   That form of language is used which permits the individual best to come to terms with the given situation in the trend to realize himself, particularly to express what he wants to express in the moment.   If one of the two forms of language is particularly disturbed by pathology, the individual tries to overcome the defect by increased use of the other form.   Thus, a complex clinical picture may appear in a damage of the first or second type which can be understood only by careful analysis of each utterance and the circumstances in which it occurs.

This distinction of different forms of speech disturbances does not correspond to the different symptom complexes which usually are distinguished

and according to which aphasic patients are examined. One speaks of
disturbances of understanding, speaking, repetition, finding words, etc.
Performances belonging to one or the other of these categories may represent—considered from the before-mentioned point of view—quite different
performances under different circumstances. Therefore, in most cases, the
usual terminology (see p. 148) does not fit the actual findings based on such
an analysis.

C. The Disturbances of Language Due to Pathology

If we consider the symptom complexes which patients with aphasia
present from the viewpoint of which performances the patients are able to
fulfill, which not, we are apt to be confronted with a rather confusing
picture.

An attempt has been made to explain the differences in performances
through the different localizations of the lesion in the brain (e.g., Henschen,
Kleist and others). There is no doubt that the special localization of the
lesion plays a role in the shape of the symptomatology (see p. 45), but the
assumption that defects in such special performances as pronunciation of
sounds, words, series, etc., are due to lesions of different localities does not
correspond to the facts, and is not compatible with the modern concept of
localization (see p. 45). The determination of the locality does not bring
us real insight into the nature of the differences and certainly does not give
any clue as to the procedure in retraining.

(1) The Significance of Images for Disturbed and Normal Language

The theory of different localization of different performances appears in
the classic theory of aphasia as localization of images and their destruction
in aphasics. It was particularly Bastian who ascribed great significance to
images and localized the effect of their destruction in definite speech centers
in the brain. This concept corresponded to the general ideas of psychology
at that time. According to these, mental contents are composed of images
or their after-effects.

Nobody has doubted and will doubt that there are images. The question
is: What role do they play in thinking and in language? I should like to
refer only to some authors who are in opposition to the assumption that
images are basic for thinking and language: In Germany, O. Kulpe; in
France, A. Binet; in the United States, Woodworth and others denied the
significance of images for thinking. They stressed that not only imageless
thinking exists but that the process of thinking differs in principle from the
use of images. Selz, who gave a careful analysis of the thought processes,
came to the conclusion that images follow the thoughts, are evoked by them.

Images have no meaning, are not signs for anything. The meaning which they may carry comes to them from interpretation, which could be proved experimentally. For Stout, "mental imagery clusters around a word and supports it in its function but the image is more a part of the sign than a representation of the meaning." As we mentioned before, some physicians came to the same conclusion from their experience with patients, for example, Jackson, Pierre Marie, Head, Goldstein (see p. 87).

From a survey of the literature, in addition to my own experiences and observations of normals and patients, I would say: To avoid misunderstanding it is necessary to define what is meant by the term "image." The word is used in the literature with two different meanings: on the one hand, it signifies *anatomic-physiologic processes*, so-called residuals; on the other hand, *conscious experiences*. The material after-effects of previous stimulations are assumed to influence our performances, though we are not aware of this. There is no doubt that such an influence exists and that it is based on material processes. What is doubtful is whether it takes place in the form of circumscribed processes corresponding to isolated images and whether a circumscribed lesion of the brain can destroy it. The greatest difficulty concerning this assumption is that we have no means to prove it. We can say something about the after-effects of nervous processes only by testing the conscious experience. There is no doubt that these experiences can be preserved in spite of speech defects. One can have images of words but not be able to use them in language (see p. 28). One erroneous tendency was that of considering words and language as identical.

One can try to examine a person's capacity to have images by special tests which can be fulfilled only on the basis of visual images. But results from all these tests are ambiguous. Such tests have the disadvantage of demanding especially voluntary action (see later, p. 60), which is often disturbed in patients. Thus, the inability to awake images, due to a defect of voluntary action, can be mistaken for a lack of images, which lack may not exist. But even if we were able to make sure whether an individual is able to evoke images or not, under the condition of the experiment, we would not be justified in assuming that he uses them or is able to use them in ordinary life. In the use of images in language there seems to be a great difference between the behavior in the learning situation, and the situation of speaking a language. Whether the first sounds or words of the child are learned with use of sensory images is at least doubtful. The child learns first by motor activities. If later he tries to perfectuate pronunciation of sounds, words, etc., he may correct his language performances by evoking images. Particularly in learning the written language images play a role. The child may, in writing, copy visual images. There exist individual differences in children in this respect. Which role auditory images play is not at all as clear as it is often assumed. I think they are overestimated in their significance for speaking (see p. 83).

In very familiar language performances, grown-up persons as a rule have neither visual nor auditory nor motor images. The first ones, if present at all, are poor and indefinite in most instances. And though auditory images may become manifest in an individually different strength during our speaking, they are not at all basic for it. The same holds true for motor images.

We observe appearance of images particularly if there is any difficulty in speech performance. If we do not know how to speak a word we may try different motor actions and accept that which we recognize as correct, or we may elicit a visual image of the word and read it, or we may evoke an auditory image. Anyone who has learned a foreign language can confirm this statement. Different opinions in this direction show that individual differences exist, often due to the particular way the person was taught in his acquisition of the foreign language. But on the other hand, each of these individuals has had the experience of abandoning the use of images in his language performances as his language becomes more fluent.

This becomes evident in observations of aphasic patients, among whom frequent experience has shown the use of images. With difficulty in pronunciation or writing, they may utter or write words which reveal that they are performed with use of visual images. They show mistakes which a normal individual would make if he would proceed in this way. The same may happen in the thinking of patients. However, this does not at all prove that the same individuals used images in their healthy days. An observation of Minkowski, whom we shall consider in other connection (see p. 144), is particularly instructive in this respect. His patient, suffering from motor aphasia, relearned speech by using visual images of words. The patient was unusually gifted visually. He could voluntarily produce visual images and had a very good visual memory. Although this helped him greatly in relearning the lost speech, it could not be proved that visual images of words normally played any role in his speaking. The patient *denied* expressly that such was the case previous to his insult (p. 60).

This and similar observations show definitely that *aphasia is not just loss of images.* But frequently we may be unable to prove that the patient has images by asking him to tell us about them. He may not be able to fulfill this task because of his impairment of voluntary attitude (see p. 16). Such experiences, among others, must induce us to distinguish between images under *voluntary* and under *involuntary conditions*, a distinction which is often neglected, but which is of great significance for all studies about images in aphasic patients. The patient (who may or may not have images) may be unable to evoke images voluntarily, but can use them involuntarily when the situation forces him to proceed in an abnormal manner.   Under these conditions, the images arise and enter the performance—which only in this way may become possible.   This distinction has some bearing on our use of images in retraining (see p. 328).

From my experience, I thus come to the following result concerning the significance of images for language and its disturbances:

Images in the sense of experiences may accompany language performances in an individually different degree, but they are not essential for language. They come to the fore particularly if any difficulty in normal language procedure arises and can then be used voluntarily or involuntarily for covering the defect.

Images in the sense of anatomic-physiologic processes are important for some normal language performances as memory effects, and so the damage of such processes may be one factor to be considered in the origin of aphasic symptoms.   But there is no reason to assume that aphasia is the effect of loss of images due to damage of circumscribed brain processes.   We shall discuss later which role this damage plays in the development of some aphasic pictures (see p. 45).

(2) *The Aphasic Symptom Complexes as Expression of Dedifferentiation of Language Due to Pathology*

According to our general viewpoint we are inclined to *understand the symptomatology* as expression of *dedifferentiation of language due to pathology*. Dedifferentiation of language will follow the same rules which determine dedifferentiation of performances in general.   We can assume that in brain damages those performances are lost first which are more differentiated while the less differentiated ones are preserved longer or are the only ones retained.   The problem is as to which are the more differentiated performances.   We can try to answer this question in two ways.   We can proceed empirically and try to find out which performances are disturbed first in a progressive lesion and, in turn, which come back first in recovery, and which later.   If our assumption is correct, there must be some regularity in progressive and regressive lesions.   There is not much material published which could serve as basis to prove our assumption and furnish us with knowledge suited for our decision.   This is understandable.   In order to be useful for this purpose, the examination of cases must be undertaken in a way which takes such a viewpoint into consideration.   Usually this has not been the case.   As far as material is available, it seems to fit such an interpretation quite well.

Another method which may bring us success in respect to our question is the use of analysis of the structure of the different speech performances.

Hence, it is only natural to see if we can learn something regarding our problem from the theory of normal language.

D. What Can We Learn from Research on Normal Language for the Interpretation of Aphasic Symptoms?

(1) *Significance of Research in Psychology of Language*

An attempt at elucidation from research in *normal psychology* is somewhat disappointing. If we do not take into account the research which attacked the problem of speech from the behavioristic viewpoint and which is not of much use for our problems, "it is," as E. L. Hatton expresses it correctly, "surprising how little attention has been devoted to language by psychologists." Thus, it is understandable that the problem of aphasia is scarcely touched in the literature of psychology. In the psychologic textbooks, the ideas are usually reviewed *without criticism* as they are developed in the medical literature. We can gain real profit only from research in *child psychology*, e.g., from W. Stern's and Piaget's work.

It is especially surprising that *Gestalt psychology* contributed so little to research on aphasia. Gestalt psychology is a wholistic approach similar to the new orientation in the field of aphasia. It developed at about the same time as the organismic approach in neurology. It repulsed association-psychology and stressed emphatically that the so-called part-processes can be understood only from the whole. "There are contents," wrote M. Wertheimer, "in which what is happening in the whole cannot be deduced from the characteristics of the separate pieces, but conversely, what happens to parts is determined by the laws of the inner structure of its whole." This idea was not a philosophic preconception but a description of observable phenomena. The terms *parts, whole, inner structure, determination,* are directly taken from factual experience.

This becomes evident for instance, if we consider a melody which, for the atomistic approach, consists of a series of definite elements, the tones. Mach and Ehrenfels had stressed that a melody is recognized also after it has been transposed into a different key, i.e. when no tone is identical with the first presentation of the melody. As a sum of elements, the object has changed completely. In spite of that, our experience remains the same. According to Ehrenfels, this finds its explanation in the fact that besides the experience of tones we have the experience of something else, which he called "Gestaltqualitaet" (Gestalt quality). Others considered the melody experience as due to an experience of the relations between the tones or, more generally, to a "synthetic function," or, in a more anatomic version, the effect of the function of "higher brain centers." Wertheimer denied the existence of the experience of tones under this condition: "What the melody gives me is not built up (by some added aids) secondarily out of the sounds of the individual parts, but what takes place in the individual parts radically depends upon the whole. . . ."

According to Wertheimer, the condition of the whole decisively determines what we see and hear in one part of this whole. One would think that from this point there is only one step to the organismic approach to language and language disturbances.

The general point of view of Gestalt psychology and the elaboration of many a special problem has fertilized brain pathology in general, but this theory has scarcely influenced the progress in our concept of aphasia. I know only some short remarks of Wertheimer and Poetzl which could be considered as contributions of Gestalt psychology to the theory of aphasia. These authors tried to explain one form of alexia as due to a defect in perception of visual Gestalten. This explanation was never worked out in detail.

We cannot discuss here the reason for this neglect of language by Gestalt psychology. It is related to the difference between the Gestalt psychologic approach and the organismic approach which I discussed on another occasion (see 105, p. 368 ff).

(2) Significance of Research in Philosophy of Language

More than from psychology, we may profit from *philosophy of language and from linguistics*, particularly from the new development of these disciplines, even though, until now, they have not influenced to any considerable degree the interpretation of aphasic symptoms. It was essentially A. Pick who stressed the significance of linguistics for our purpose. His explanations were not very fruitful because they were too theoretic and did not apply directly enough to the problems with which the clinician is confronted in aphasic patients. It was particularly unfortunate that Pick was not able to bring out the second volume of his book, "Agramnatismus," in which probably the implications of his studies for aphasia would have come more to the fore. Besides this book of Pick's, publications particularly of Isserlin, Lotmar and Binswanger, should be cited here, and in addition a recent study of R. Jacobson which is of great significance.

It is my conviction that *philosophy of language and linguistics* on the one side, and research in aphasia on the other, could profit much from each other, much more than has previously been the case. Therefore I should like to stress here some theories and results of this research.

It may be useful to consider first the development of these fields of science. It was not so long ago that it was considered possible to understand language (particularly the production of sounds) from a mechanistic, atomistic point of view. The immense progress of natural science in the last century could not fail to influence this discipline also. Even with the greater recognition of the mental character of human speech and the stressing of the significance of psychology as basis of linguistics, as, for example, by Paul, the mechanistic approach was not abandoned. This is not surprising when we consider that, for Paul, psychology was Herbart's theory of "Mechanik des Vorstellungslebens" (mechanic of the movement of images). A real change in the interpretation of language did not develop before a new analysis of language led to the viewing of this phenomenon in relation to the behavior of the individual in general.

This new approach to philosophy of language was prepared by G. Herder (140) and W. von Humboldt (149). For Herder, all language had its point of departure in feelings and expressions, in cries, sounds. But he denied that these utterances represent the whole of human language which is characterized by "reflexion." This capacity, intrinsic for man and separating him from all animals, enables him to abstract characteristics from the complexity of impressions, to fix them, and to recognize them again in their peculiarity, i.e., to build concepts. The agent for accomplishing this is the word. Through this capacity, sounds become language. This factor was stressed to an even greater degree in W. v. Humboldt's theory of language. According to him, the essence of language cannot be grasped as long as one considers it a mere collection of words. Words appear as separate entities only in an abstract consideration. They are nothing but a dead product of our bungling scientific analysis. Language is not a static phenomenon, not "ergos," as he says, but a dynamic process—"energeia." Words are not symbols for objects and events, but symbols for the concepts which we build of them; they mirror the kind and direction of our view of the world. The languages differ not simply as to sounds or signs but they represent various attitudes towards the world, various fundamental types of world perspectives (Weltansichten). For a long time, Herder's and Humboldt's ideas found little consideration. They appeared to the positivistically minded linguists of nineteenth century metaphysical speculations in a similar way as did H. Jackson's ideas about aphasia to the physicians of this time. The concept of Herder and Humboldt was resumed much later with great emphasis by E. Cassirer and furthered by presenting it in the frame of a general theory of knowledge. In his book, "Philosophie der symbolischen Formen," language takes a paramount place, and the new theory of language is illustrated by a great number of facts taken from voluminous material collected in research in different languages. Careful study of this book of E. Cassirer promises to be of great advantage to our studies of aphasia, so much the more so as the author himself tries to utilize the observations of aphasic patients in the development of his ideas about the structure of normal language.

(3) Significance of Research in Linguistics

Parallel to the mentioned development of philosophy of language, from research in the field of linguistics there originated a similar theory which considers meaning as an essential factor even for the understanding of structure and development of the "elements" of language—the sounds. This new theory of linguistics, "phonology" is particularly significant for us because it inaugurated a new interpretation of the structure of sounds, sound complexes, sound relations in words, etc., phenomena which we find frequently disturbed in aphasic patients. It presents a step forward from the analysis of artificially isolated phenomena to their interpretation from the viewpoint of the relation of each of them to the total organism. In this general attitude it is similar to our organismic approach. To characterize the general tendency of this new approach in linguistics, the following should be stated: It stresses the *systematic character of language; each phenomenon can be understood only from its position within the system.*

There are "systèmes de sons (phonèmes), systèmes de formes, et de mots (morphèmes et sematèmes) . . . chaque son doit dépendre de l'autre" (Viggo Broendal). Instead of the study of structure of isolated sounds, their relation to language as a system became increasingly important in research. Not the sounds but the phonemes* became the paramount phenomena of language, "les éléments constitutifs du language" (Trubetzkoy). To mention a few of the men who developed this point of view I should like to name particularly Saussure (Cours de linguistique générale, Geneva 1922), Trubetzkoy, and recently, Roman Jakobson. For research in aphasia, Jakobson's publication is particularly important.

The older phonetics studied movements of the vocal cord, the palate, the tongue, lips, etc., the effect of resonance in the cavities of mouth, pharynx, and, following the procedure of atomistic physiology, it tried to determine by the dissecting method the possibilities offered by anatomic-physiologic structures. However significant the results gained in this way may have been for some problems, they have proved insufficient for understanding the problems of phonetics themselves and have contributed little to the explanation of the defects in aphasia. From the units of speech distinguished in this way, speech cannot be reconstructed or can be only with the help of new hypotheses which frequently have been in contradiction to the original concepts. Here we meet the same situation which must be faced in general in the attempt to understand organismic behavior from the facts gained by the dissecting method (see 105, p. 67).

Not all movements which may appear possible if one considers the muscles of a limb separated by the dissecting method occur in the actions of the organism. Only a selected number is to be observed normally. These are the ones which are of significance for the self realization of the organism. I have called the selected phenomena—because they correspond to the "normal" performances—"ausgezeichnete," or *preferred*, performances (see 105, p. 340). Analysis of a great number of various pathologic phenomena has shown that pathology consists of a narrowing of the preferred realm which brings about a definite diminution of performances. *What is preserved, and what not, is determined by what is more usable for self realization of the organism—in spite of the defect.* What is valid in general applies particularly to language.

The new theory in linguistics takes a similar stand regarding sounds, as does the organismic approach in general. It originates (like the latter) in the assumption that not all possible innervations of the "speech muscles"

* The smallest units in language which have a distinctive significance in representation of definite objects, events, feelings. See p. 34.

appear in language in sounds, words, sentences, etc., not all possible sounds are used as basis of understanding. Only definite motor and sensory phenomena appear in language, and the selection is determined by their suitability to represent in a distinct way the intention of the speaker— expressed in our terminology, those which are suited to serve best as means for self realization of the individual.

From this aspect one has tried to determine the smallest units in language which have a distinctive significance in representation of definite objects, events, feelings. Those units are termed phonemes. By various combinations of sounds, simple and more complex units, complex phonemes, are built. Variations of the material, variations of pronunciation, differences in flexions of the word (syntactical variations), and variations in the order in which the words are placed (grammatical variations) give a great number of possibilities for expressing man's behavior in language.

All languages have in common some phonemes which correspond to the common reactions of all human beings. Each language, on the other hand, possesses its own system of phonemes, a definite phonematic pattern (Bloomfield).

The choice of the sounds or sound combinations as phonemes is determined by a number of different factors. To discuss the complex problem involved here would necessitate delving deeply into the research of phylogenetic and ontogenetic development and comparative theory of language. To be brief, let us consider only some factors which determine the choice of sounds as phonemes to demonstrate the origin of phonemes in principle.

The phonematic value of a sound complex may, for example, be determined by the intrinsic adequacy between a sound or a sound combination in a word and the "referent," as, for instance, in the onomatopoeic origin of some phonemes. In other cases, physiognomic experience plays a role. Coincidence or even voluntary selection, as in technical words, sometimes determines whether a sound or sound complex becomes a phoneme. Among the possible sounds or sound complexes, those are selected which allow at best for a *definite distinction* from others. This guarantees the relation between a sound complex and a certain meaning.

The modified language of patients is also a systematic whole of phonemes; what remains is not an at random collection of phonemes; the individual performances can be understood only as expression of dedifferentiation of the normal system. We do not know much about this from examination of aphasic patients, and considerable work needs to be done on this problem.

(4) *Significance of Studies on the Development of Language in Children*

We can expect from the study of development of language in childhood to gain some insight into the ways of dedifferentiation of language in aphasia.

From the point of view that development is increasing integration and pathology is disintegration, and the assumption that disintegration goes through similar steps (except in reverse) as the increasing organization in children, these studies should prove productive.

Attempts to draw on this material for the understanding of pathologic modifications of language have been undertaken several times. The work of Froeschels should be cited particularly, and the recent paper of Roman Jacobson, whose explanations I shall follow frequently. One must be cautious, it is true, in this comparison. As I have stressed repeatedly, it should never be forgotten that language is embedded in the total personality and that the distinctions between the personality of children and that of adults may produce essential differences. Therefore, retraining of aphasic patients cannot simply be a replica of the procedure in teaching or correcting language in children. We shall be able to use the studies of children better the more we take this point into consideration; i.e., consider the development of sounds, words, etc., always in relation to the general development of the personality of the child, his mind, attitudes, desires, etc.

Particularly the careful studies of Antoine Grégoire have proved that the sounds *appear* in childhood *in a definite sequence* (L'apprentissage du language). But this is correct only if one eliminates the "Lallperiode" (babble talk period) which has often erroneously been considered as the "first step" in the development of language. Babbling contains sounds which never appear in later language, which do not exist in the language of the people around the child. The child needs great effort later to learn sounds which he has uttered in the babble period apparently without any difficulty, e.g., the palatal consonants, sibilants and liquidae (157, p. 10). Finally, and of great importance, the infant loses nearly all the sounds which he has uttered in the babble period. There is frequently a gap between the "Lallperiod" and the development of language; for a certain time the child is mute (Meumann, p. 202). "The infant repeats these sounds persistently," says Jacobson; "he must have acquired the motor and sensory images," but in spite of this he loses the capacity to produce them. Here is an example of the general rule that *fixation in memory is not at all simply dependent upon repetition.* Only those repeated events which are embedded in meaningful relation to the total organism are kept in memory. The first utterances of the infant are not kept in memory because they do not possess such relation. This is understandable from the fact that the higher mental processes, which are a presupposition for building such relations, are not yet developed. The sounds in the babbling period are produced by movements which—like the other movements of the infant in this period of development—occur by use of the "machinery" without any other intention than the pleasure of using one's own possibilities, a trend which governs organismic life. Thus, they correspond to all possibilities in which the concerned muscles can be used. The infant produces, says A. Grégoire, all thinkable sounds. Because there is no relation to higher mental processes, no intention and no control by environment, the combinations are on a "chance" level.

If we omit the sound formation in this early period, the rule of Grégoire is correct that the sounds in infancy appear in a definite succession. Because there is no clear-cut division between the two periods, and the child begins to "speak" at a time when he still babbles, this may not be so evident. If we deny that movements in the babble talk period are predecessors of language, this should not be interpreted as meaning that we do not attribute to them any significance at all in the development of speech. The infant acquires some mastery of the concerned muscles which later helps him to build the sounds for "real" language.

The most characteristic difference between the sounds in babbling and in speech is that in the first condition the activities are occurring without relation to the outer world, while *real language from the beginning shows this relation*. The sound in language has always some, if also very "primitive" meaning; it has a phonematic value, represents a definite attitude of the individual toward the world. Thus, the infant answers with sounds if addressed by words, tries to imitate what he hears—though in an imperfect way; he tries to adjust his talking to the words, gestures, etc., of the people around him. The repetition of words observable in this period is distinguished from repetition in the babbling period by the fact that it does not show an echolalic imitation of the same sound complexes but rather permanent changes which are determined by the progress in motor and sensory perfection which the infant reaches. We observe a similar difference between repetition and echolalic imitation in aphasic patients (see p. 303).

Whatever language we consider, we observe, in the acquisition of the sounds, the same sequence in time. Roman Jakobson has confirmed this known phenomenon by comparing the following languages: Swedish, Norwegian, Danish, Slavic, Russian, Polish, Czech, Serbocroatic, Bulgarian, Indian, German, Dutch, Estonian, Japanese.

This observation of constancy in the sequence of the occurrence of sounds indicates that we are dealing with a fundamental phenomenon characteristic for man. *Can we expect that disintegration will show the same steps in opposite direction?* This question can be answered only if we know the cause of this constancy and if the same rules are valid for disintegration of language as apply in building it up.

The *sequence in acquisition of sounds* in infancy is assumed to follow the law of Fr. Schultze, i.e., the law of minimal expenditure of energy; that sound is acquired earlier which needs less effort to be produced. Of course, we have no reason to assume that this law is not valid in this field. However, it is not so simple to apply it to the problem in which we are interested. In order to determine which sound should be favored according to this law, we should know which sound is more simply produced than another under the given condition.

We are confronted here with a special example of a general biologic problem (see 105, p. 2): what characterizes an *easy* performance, what distinguishes it from a more difficult one? One assumes usually that a motor performance is more difficult if it is executed by a greater number of muscles. Such is not the case in this general form. Certainly the possibility to execute a performance finds its limitation in the apparatus at its disposal, i.e., the size and configuration of muscles or muscle groups by which an action is to be performed. But analysis of the anatomic-physiologic phenomena in isolation can never determine whether a performance is more or less difficult. Besides the mentioned factor, the energy expenditure is determined by difficulties the organism must overcome in performing a definite task in a definite situation. Such difficulties appear as obstacles in the outer world and in the apparatus itself. As to the latter, repeated performance facilitates action. But the main factor is the attitude in which an action has to be performed. Thus, for instance, voluntary action needs more energy than the same action incited by definite outer world stimuli. Automatic action may need less energy, but to set this in operation may demand again a particular amount of energy. Concrete reactions need less energy, in general, than reactions which presuppose abstract attitude. However, very familiar actions of the latter kind may need less energy than an unfamiliar concrete reaction, and so on. Thus, one sees that a number of factors determine whether a definite performance is more or less difficult to execute.

Roman Jacobson has voiced opposition to the application of Schultze's law to our problem by stressing the fact mentioned before that the child in the babbling period easily produces "complicated" sounds which later he is not able to produce at all, or only with great effort. Thus, one could be forced to ascribe to the child in this period a greater energy in sound production than in his later life. I think this argument is not quite pertinent, and the facts stressed by Jacobson do not speak against the validity of Schultze's law. The "same" phenomenon may, under certain conditions, in a definite state of development, need a totally different amount of energy to be produced than in another stage of development and under other conditions. If one analyzes the phenomena in relation to what the organism is doing, one may find that what appeared as a greater conplexity is a pseudo-complexity—in reality, a simpler phenomenon. The utterances in the babble period are pseudo-complex. They are, in reality, "simple" when judged according to the ability of the organism; they represent a figure-ground process of lowest degree.   What is produced at the moment may follow the law of least effort in the innervation of the various muscles.   The sound production in real language needs greater effort on the part of the individual, the sounds representing sharp figure-ground formations according to the special purpose they have.   The sound productions in the two periods are such different performances that they cannot be compared simply in relation to the law of least expenditure.

This is valid also when we consider the occurrence of different sounds in the development of language during childhood.   A consideration of this is of particular interest for us because it may give us some hints for understanding the facts observed in patients—why patients lose some sounds more than others, or regain some easier than others.

The first sound the infant utters is the vowel "a" (approximately as in "ah"); usually about the same time, the first consonant "m", appears. The "a" is advanced by opening the mouth, the "m" by closing it.   There was much discussion about the cause of the appearance of these two sounds. I think it becomes understandable from the organismic point of view.   The first sounds show the characteristics of the performances in general in the early state of development: they do not occur as isolated movements, but are parts of activities comprising more or less the total organism.   *The first sounds are expressions of the two reaction types of the organism, the turning-toward tendency and the trend to withdrawal* (see 105, p. 187).

"A" is an expression of the tendency of the organism to turn toward the stimulus object in the outer world, an experience of the beginning contact with the world.   This character of the "a" becomes evident by the fact that it occurs concomitantly with other movements which belong to the same attitude: opening of the eyes, extension of the arms, more or less turning of the whole body toward the outer world.   All these movements are, as I have explained on another occasion (105, p. 134), "extension performances."

The "m" corresponds to the opposite reactions—those which belong to the attitude of withdrawal.   It is accompanied by other movements which belong to this attitude, such as closing the eyes, wrinkling of the muscles of the forehead.   It is a flexion movement, it has, as do all flexion movements, a more voluntary character (see 105, p. 482).   It is more closely related to the personality, indicates more a turning of the organism towards itself, with that withdrawal from the outer world, and hence becomes suited to represent something objective, separated from the ego.   In contrast to this "objecting," "abstracting" character of the flexion movements, the extension movements belong to the concrete emotionally directed activities.

They occur more involuntarily, represent more passive submission of the organism to the world.

This explanation shows that already the development of the first sounds points to the relation of our speech utterances to the conditions of the total organism and the importance of the factor of attitude of the total organism in each speech performance.

Sounds, from their first appearance, show also the characteristics which make movements usable as material for building phonemes: *distinctness and discernibility*. This is reached by *using extreme movements* and *those which represent utter contrasts*, as extreme flexion and extension. Both factors show their significance in the development of language. The movements by which we produce "a" and "m" represent extreme movements.

Contrasting movements represent an important principle in development. "U" occurs in contrast to "a" as to narrowness, in contrast to "o" as to roundness; "t" occurs in contrast to "p", etc. Contrasting mouth and nasal consonants appear concomitantly as, for example, "p" and "m," or, a little later, labials and dentals ("p" and "t"), etc. Contrasting movements belong together. This becomes evident in the fact that at an early stage, when they are not definitely related to particular phonemes, they are easily confounded with each other. This is one origin of characteristic mistakes of the child. It is interesting in relation to similar experiences in aphasics that confounding occurs more easily in speaking than in understanding. Passy reports (according to Jakobson) the case of a little French girl who used the word "tosson" both for "garçon" (boy) and "cochon" (pig), but protested against anybody else using the word "cochon" for boy and "garçon" for pig. Children are often able to understand words without being able to speak them. However, this should not be generalized. It depends apparently on whether the grasped sounds—even if they are absolutely "alike"—are sufficiently differentiated from one another and related to different meanings. If such is not the case, the child does not "understand." Differentiation in speaking is more difficult indeed, than in hearing. We observe corresponding experiences in aphasics who show a greater defect in speaking than in understanding (see p. 231).

The development in contrasts, and hence confounding of contrasting performances, does not concern only the sounds but also more complicated speech performances. Words with contrasting significance are often mixed up by children, for example, "yes" and "no," "tomorrow" and "yesterday," "down" and "up," "cold" and "warm," etc. We are interested in this phenomenon because we find the same in aphasic patients.

There was much discussion about this "Gegensinn der Urworte" (antithetical meaning of primordial). The explanation seems to me to be the following: These—for the grownup—contrasting performances are in early stages of development not experiences of definite entities per se, but deviations of one experience toward two directions, whereby the deviation is easier to realize than the particular direction toward which it takes place. For example: Cold and warm are experienced as deviations as to temperature, tomorrow and yesterday as to not just now.   The child acquires in connection with such experiences two different words—corresponding to the two distinct objects of the grownup—and uses them promiscuously as long as the distinction is not definite.   He does not "confound" the words; both belong to the same experience.   The more the child learns to differentiate the objects (simultaneously with development of abstraction) the more he uses the different words correctly.

There are further factors by which the development of language is determined, which become understandable if one considers them from the viewpoint of organismic development in general.   Development proceeds *from less differentiated to more differentiated phenomena*, with other words, from more simple figure-ground configurations to more complicated ones. Movements continued to the extreme possibility which the organization of the muscles, etc., allows are simpler than those which must be stopped at a certain point.   They do not demand as much precision.   Hence, it becomes understandable that the sounds produced by extreme movements occur first.   For the same reason voiceless sounds appear first, and the vowels get earlier voice than consonants.

Those performances occur earlier which are determined by perceptions. Perceptions in general are of great influence on development.   Without incitement from outer world stimuli the child would scarcely develop, and such is the case also with language.   This does not mean that the first activities are imitation of perceptions.   Imitation presupposes a certain development of motor performances (see p. 73).   The first speech activities correspond to the use of the inborn capacities of the organism, e.g., of the possibilities in which the muscles can be innervated.   Those activities are repeated and preserved which furnish the organism with experiences which help it come to terms with the outer world.   Because they are not suited for this purpose, the sound complexes of the babble tongue are lost (see p. 35), and only those sounds are preserved which serve this purpose. The first influence from the outer world seems, as far as language is concerned, to be derived from *visual* stimulation.   There is an earlier fixing of those sounds which can be controlled visually, i.e., those produced by lip movements (the *lips* of others can be easily observed, as can one's own with —and, to a certain extent, without—the use of a mirror).   Later the control by kinesthetic and acoustic experiences sets in.   Learning by imitation of heard sounds and words, etc., does not belong to the first state of development, even though acoustic perceptions are significant for the final development of language. The relation to the outer world stimuli diminishes increasingly with development. Speaking occurs, then, without control by sensory experiences (see p. 83); it is incited by a certain attitude and performed on the basis of acquired pattern (the instrumentalities, see p. 25). It is important to note that the development of *some sounds precedes the development of others:* for instance, the acquisition of "Fricatives," that of *stop sounds*, of consonants formed farther back in the mouth presupposes the possession of those formed more to the front. Labials and dentals precede velar sounds. The infant in the beginning produces stop sounds instead of "Fricatives," says, instead of "f," "p," of "s," "t."

The later appearing sounds may be substituted by the earlier ones. The infant has only one posterior nasal consonant, while he may have several anterior consonants. For the posterior "k" he may substitute the dental "t." As Jakobson has pointed out, in some languages the anterior stop sound system is better developed than the posterior one; in no language are the plosives missing. There are, however, languages which do not possess "Fricatives" (see 157, p. 37).

Considering the fact that the later developing sounds represent more difficult performances, it will be understandable that even after the child is able to produce a later appearing sound, he will stick to an earlier appearing one if he can fulfill his task in this way to a sufficient degree. Thus (cf. 157, p. 35), one observes a dominance of the sound "a" even after other vowels have been developed, and a preference of occlusive sounds to the Fricatives. Even after "y" has been developed and may be used under certain conditions, it may be avoided; the child may say "esh" instead of "yes." It is important to know that under other conditions the sound so avoided may appear in words where another sound would be correct, as, for example, the child may say "yook" instead of "look." We understand these facts from an analysis of the condition in which the one or the other performance occurs. We observe the same phenomena in aphasic patients.

The explanation of these phenomena may be that movements which can be controlled visually are easier to perform than those where such is not the case—which can be controlled only by muscle-sense perceptions. Thus, the anteriorly produced sound is easier than the posteriorly produced one. Precision is better guaranteed there, which is an important factor for phonematologic purposes.

It is something of a mystery why some languages do not build up certain sounds. Do they not need them for expression of experiences?

It is further significant to note that there is not only a definite succession in development, but that the later appearing sounds do not develop if the earlier ones are not developed: *the first presuppose the latter*. Our retraining has to take this fact into consideration, if failure is to be avoided.

In the beginning, meaning, phonemic value, is related to one sound, later to two or more sounds. But combining sounds to a new phoneme is not a simple step. The German child may be able to say "e" (English pronunciation of long "a") and "i" (English long "e") and may be able to pronounce them together but as separate entities as "e-i" (English "a-e"), but may have the greatest difficulty in combining them to form "ai" (English long "i"). The diphthong combination "ai" and differentiation from "e" and "i" which is necessary in writing is a step which is not easily taken. A German child may be able to say "bi" (English "be") and "te" (English "ta"), but not be able to combine them to "bitte" (pronounced "betta").

New sound complexes are built in two ways: by adding two sounds together in (as it is called) syntagmatic way (e.g., if b and l are combined to form bl), or by substitution of one sound by another in a paradigmatic way (e.g., sing, sang). The syntagmatic formation occurs, according to Jakobson (157), prior to the paradigmatic one. This corresponds to the biologic rule that successive performances are "easier" than simultaneous ones (see p. 121). In brain damage, the successive performances are better preserved than the simultaneous ones.

In a certain state of development, one sound is usually the carrier of phonologic value, usually a consonant, while the vowel may not yet be important. We find similar phenomena in patients; patients confound words which for us, because of differences of phonologic characteristics, are definitely distinguished.

In the same way as Jakobson mentions a child may be able to use in one word two different consonants or two different vowels but not both differences in one word, with other words the number of differences between vowels and the consonants is restricted. If, for instance, the first vowel in the word is palatal (or velar) then all other vowels of the word have the same quality; a word consists either of voiced consonants or voiceless, but not of both types. The same is frequently observed in aphasics.

All these aforementioned phenomena are examples of the general biologic rule that several processes of the *same* kind are easier to execute than a *change;* similar performances correspond to simpler figure-ground formations. In pathology, only these latter are preserved.

This is also the reason why aphasics often speak vowels and consonants without voice. The consonants lose their voice (Ombredane, 220a, p. 407) and the voiceless consonants are better recognized than the voiced ones. An attempt has been made to explain this defect by the fact that voiced pronunciation needs more energy. I think it is not so much the effect of diminution of energy in the patient as it is impairment of voluntary attitude. Voiced pronunciation needs more voluntary attitude than voiceless, which would explain why this loss of voiced characteristics is to be observed particularly in patients with impairment of abstract attitude (central motor aphasia) (see p. 208).

Very early there may be observed a discrepancy between production of sounds in "intended" speech and speech not intended, i.e., instigated by outer world stimuli, or particularly as expression of inner events (expressive sounds, "Lautgebaerden"). The child utters sounds or sound combinations unintentionally in this way which he is unable to produce intentionally. Thus, for instance, as Jakobson mentions, the child who does not yet have velar phenomena in his speech may produce them as expression of well-feeling in "go-ga," etc., or in onomatopoeic utterances, as, for example, in imitation of the croaking of the raven in "kro-kro." The liquida "r" may still be missing in language, but may appear in imitation of the voice of a bird. Children who do not produce "e" may be able to imitate chirping birds in "bebe," "pepe," etc.

A similar difference between intentional language and more involuntary utterances of sounds and also in voluntary repetitions is often to be observed in patients with aphasia, too (see p. 208). The patients are occasionally able to produce sound combinations which they are not able to produce on demand and intentionally (e.g., voluntarily to repeat involuntarily repeated words immediately afterwards), I think, for the same reason as the child—namely, the intentional production or voluntary repetition presupposes an attitude which the child has not yet developed, and in which the patient is impaired (see p. 215).

When we consider the sequence of the appearance of sounds in the development from all the aspects mentioned before, the *law of Schultze* appears valid. It has then, indeed, a different meaning, insofar as the evaluation of the effort to produce a sound presupposes the consideration of the performance in relation to the total organism, and hence brings the *question back to the analysis of the performances involved in each sound in relation to the special purpose of the organism.*

The foregoing description of the development of language in children should be considered only as illustration of some principles by which the facts can become understandable if one applies the organismic point of view. Completeness is not and cannot be intended. The material is presented with the end in view of inducing a definite procedure in our consideration of the rules of dedifferentiation of language in patients. Some of the phenomena mentioned can be compared directly with findings in aphasic patients, but our discussion of the latter should be considered merely as a basis for further detailed studies.

(5) *Some Similarities between the Development of Language and Defects in Aphasics*

Some facts which show the similarity between the phonemetic structure of the sounds and their development in children on the one hand, and defects in aphasics on the other, may be summed up in the following:

1. One of the most frequent and earliest losses in aphasics is the ability to distinguish the liquidae, l and r (Froeschels, Head, Pick, Jakobson, personal experience). This is the case also with patients who are able to speak an uvular r. The sounds preserved the longest are a and m. The sounds built by lips are better preserved in general than the other ones.

2. The nasal vowels disappear early. (They appear in French children after the other vowels—Ombredane.)

3. The interdentals are lost early, earlier than the sibilants (according to Head the patients speak zis for this). The consonants are often pronounced voiceless.

4. The consonants of the anterior part of the mouth are longer preserved than the palatals. The velar occlusives become dentals. The posterior occlusives, l, e.g., becomes t, d (Gutzmann, Head, Pick).

5. The affricates are lost first, then the Fricatives (Ombredane, p. 948). Instead of the aspirants, explosive sounds appear, but the opposite confusion never occurs. (Bouman and Grünbaum, p. 328.) Bogorodicky reports the same from Russian, Ombredane from French patients (f becomes p, s becomes t).

6. In the same way as the development of some sounds presupposes the development of others, the later developed sounds are lost earlier in aphasics and cannot be retrained unless preceded by the reacquisition of others (Jakobson, 157, p. 45).

7. Aphasics may be able to speak or read or repeat different sounds, but not combinations of these. On the other hand, production of isolated sounds is frequently more disturbed than the production of the same sound in words, production of isolated words more than of the same words in sentences or in series Speaking in series can, in some cases, be more disturbed than speaking individual words. This seemingly contrasting behavior of patients points to the differences of damage in aphasics.

8. Confounding of sounds performed by contrasting movements, of words with contrasting meaning is a frequent phenomenon in aphasics.

9. Voluntary language is early disturbed. The intended production of sounds, words, etc., is lost earlier than production incited by sensory stimulation. In some cases, repetition of words heard are preserved longer than spontaneous production (see p. 292). In some cases (of motor aphasia), imitation of seen sounds is easier than of heard ones. In other

cases, repetition is particularly disturbed, voluntary speech better preserved (see p. 229).

All the phenomena discussed should be considered for an understanding of the phenomena presented by a patient with motor aphasia, whom we usually meet in a state when the defect is partially restituted (see p. 81).

E. THE ORGANISMIC APPROACH TO THE PROBLEM OF LOCALIZATION OF LANGUAGE AND LANGUAGE DISTURBANCES

The problem of localization in the cerebral cortex stood, for a long time, much in the foreground of the discussion of aphasia. This was only too natural, considering how much this problem was connected from the beginning with research in aphasia. The discoveries of Broca, Wernicke and others determined not only the interpretation of the symptoms but became the basis for the doctrine of circumscribed centers in the brain to which definite circumscribed mental functions were supposed to be related. This assumed relation found expression in the "brain maps." Its results in the field of aphasia were the various diagrams. If one considers the immense amount of research concerning this problem, the result appears very poor. As a matter of fact, only very gross localizatory distinctions are possible.

Particularly after the criticism of von Monakow, based on his enormous knowledge, and my own discussion of this problem with a more detailed analysis of the clinical pictures, it hardly seemed possible to maintain the classic theory of localization. The question of the relationship between the symptom complex and a definitely localized lesion again became a problem, no longer, however, in the form: where is a definite function or symptom localized? but: *how does a definite lesion modify the function of the brain so that a definite symptom comes to the fore?* This problem can be attacked only from a discussion of the function of the brain matter in principle, which, in turn, depends upon a concept not only of the function of the nervous system, but the total organism also.

From this organismic point of view, I have tried to consider the problem of localization in general and that of aphasic symptom complexes in particular. Because to my opinion the findings in an individual case can be judged correctly only if one considers the points von Monakow and I have stressed, I think it may be useful to give here at least a short discussion of the concerned problem.

First, I must (particularly in respect to the brain maps) refer to an argument which has a general bearing: We are by no means justified in inferring directly from a correlation between a localized defect and a defect in performance a relationship between the concerned area and a definite performance corresponding to the defect. The facts allow only *localization of defects*, but not a localization of performances. The latter remains a theoretic interpretation which can be tried only after a careful analysis of the functions corresponding to the performance, and of the defects. Such an analysis induces a concept about brain function and its relation to performance which, unsatisfactory as it may have been until now, differs in principle from the concept of circumscribed localization (see later, p. 50). When I use the term *localization* in the following, I mean always *localization of defects*. Even this, however, meets with enormous difficulties.

We are confronted with two realms of facts which we try to bring into relation: *anatomic findings* and *observation of disturbed performances*. Investigation in the two realms in a normal condition reveals very little material for such an endeavor. The microscopic studies leave no doubt as to the cerebral cortex containing tissues of highly diversified structure; furthermore, that these differences of structure hold a special significance for different functions. The differential complexity of that structure in vertebrates, the differential structure in the various areas of the cerebral cortex, the indubitable relationship of certain characteristically stratified fields (like the sensory and motor regions), to certain performance fields, these, and many other facts point emphatically to differences in function.

If we survey the material, we can assume with a fair degree of certainty that there are areas which are designed to receive stimuli from the outer world, and others to mediate motor performances. We find a one-to-one correspondence between certain sectors of the periphery and certain areas in the cortex, i.e., an *"anatomic localization."* But it remains unsettled how these cortical areas, which I called the *periphery of the cortex*, do function. Analysis of the defects in lesions of this part does not at all allow us to bring a circumscribed defect into relation to a circumscribed lesion, still less to localize a definite performance in a definite group of cells, etc.*

Besides this periphery of the cortex, we have large sectors which, judging by their structure as well as by their relatively loose connection with the projection system, point to a significance of their own, relatively independent of the peripheral cortex. They represent, so to speak, domains of a higher order. I called them the *central part of the cortex*. This comprises the parietal lobes, the insula Reili, and particularly the frontal lobes, which we find especially well developed in the higher mammals, and particularly in man.

Besides this differentiation as to central and peripheral parts, there seems to be within the stratified structure of each area a differentiation insofar as the different strata apparently have a different functional signifi-

---

* See especially, concerning this problem, the new research of I. P. Murphy and E. Gellhorn "Multiplicity of representation versus punctate localisation in the motor cortex." Am. J. Physiol. *146*: 376, 1946.

cance. This is expressed in the differences of fiber relationships of the various strata of an area to other parts of the brain. Van Valkenburg has expressed the opinion that the cortex consists of six organs, corresponding to the layers. Whether this is correct or not, the assumption of different functions for the different layers is most probably justified. Ramon y Cajal could show that the first layer consists of association fibers within the cortex, layers II and IIIa are in connection with the corpus callosum, IIIb is a perceptive layer, layers III, V and VI have effective function. Kappers, on the basis of comparative studies, brought the fourth layer into relation to perception, layers V and VI to motor function. Thus we had to assume in each area a perceptive and a motor layer related to the periphery, belonging to the "periphery," and a more "central" part. We distinguish the so-called motor and sensory areas from the other ones by the fact that here particularly the "peripheral" functions are represented, on the other hand, in the "central parts"—the "higher" mental processes. This "laminal physiology" of the cortex (Walshe) does not receive enough attention.

Besides these very general results we can deduce very little from the anatomic differences as to the dependence of the performances on the various areas of the brain. Even these results do not permit the assumption that separate parts of the cortex are related to separate functions, but only that the different parts contribute differently to the functions of the brain (see p. 50).

The concept of circumscribed localization is based (more than upon the anatomy) upon the results of the effect of experiments of stimulation and destruction of circumscribed areas and upon observation of patients with circumscribed brain lesions. As I have stressed on another occasion, the results of the stimulation experiments, no matter how important they may be for some practical purpose, are, from the theoretic point of view of localization, highly unphysiologic and very ambiguous and not at all understandable as to effects of the stimulation of circumscribed areas alone.

The so-called classic theory of localization is based mainly on the material gained from postmortems. It should be observed that the objections against the theory stem first from a more careful consideration of the *pathologic-anatomic* data. There are the so-called negative cases: on the one hand, absence of symptoms in a lesion affecting an area which was considered characteristic of this locality; on the other hand, appearance of symptoms without the presence of a correspondingly localized lesion. A critical consideration of these numerous cases shows that they are inexplicable if one considers the symptoms as simply depending upon *locality*, *extension of the lesion*, but only if one considers them from a more qualitative viewpoint. A lesion of a special locality in different cases may differ very much regarding the degree to which the substratum in general is affected, and particularly its different strata. Such a selective character of the process may be of paramount significance for the development of symptoms. It is very difficult, indeed, to evaluate the degree of damage; it is not only dependent on the direct destruction of the nerve cells but also on the condition of the glia, blood vessels, etc. Further, we have no idea of the relationship between a definite anatomic condition and a specific performance. We are far from being able to decide *whether the preserved tissue is still functioning sufficiently to allow for a certain performance or not.* We have no definite criteria for this decision. We are facing here a methodologic difficulty which seems scarcely surmountable.

Whether certain symptoms will appear or not on account of a local injury certainly depends on many factors other than locality: i.e., on the nature of the disease process, on the damage of all or only some structures of the cortex, on the condition of the rest of the brain, on individual differences in cooperation of both hemispheres (see later, p. 51), on the state of circulation in general, on the functional reactions of the organism to the defect (see p. 10), on the psycho-physical constitution of the personality, etc.

The objections to the classic theory of localization are even greater when we take into consideration the *clinical symptomatology* on which it is based.

There is first the question: Are all symptoms which we observe in direct relation to the locality of the lesion? We have seen before (see p. 8) that this is the case only for one part of the symptoms. Another part is due to the effect the lesion has on the function of the remaining undamaged central nervous system which now functions differently because of the influence of isolation, and to the effect of the reaction of the organism to the defect (see p. 10). The distinction between symptoms which are directly related to the defect and those which are not has a definite bearing on the problem of localization.

Mention should be made of a further phenomenon which is suited to complicate the problem. The organism may react to the functional defect under certain conditions in such a way that the symptoms due to the localized defect may be easily *hidden.* One example among many is the appearance of the total visual field in hemianopsia and the organization of the pseudofovia in such cases observed in ordinary vision of the individual and under certain experimental conditions (see 105, p. 47). The defect may be easily overlooked, which would certainly be disastrous for any attempt to localize. We are faced here with a very difficult problem since we know so little about the structure of the individual performances and the reaction of the organism to cover up a defect. (See also what we have said about the possibility of covering the impairment in word-finding, p. 63.) Much work must be done here.

The above should indicate the frequent difficulty in enucleating from the multitude of symptoms those which are related to the locality of the lesion, i.e., those which we are justified in using for our attempt to localize. In any event, we shall be able to do this only if we analyze each symptom carefully according to the different possibilities of origin mentioned before. Unfortunately, such an analysis is very often neglected. Thus, a great number of cases published may be considered as incomplete and of little value for our task.

In the evaluation of the symptoms and selection of those which were brought into connection with the locality, there was frequently a theoretic bias. Otherwise, the localization of so-called images in definite centers could not have appeared justified, and the theory could not have become plausible that the various forms of aphasia, etc., are due to a destruction of definite circumscribed areas (see p. 26).

Already, Jackson had objected to the whole procedure and to the theory of images (see before, p. 26). Unfortunately, not enough attention was paid to his criticism. This criticism had to be taken up again later; Head, Pierre Marie, and I all tried to demonstrate the untenability of the theory. The effect of the criticism was great scepticism regarding localization in general. From the very beginning I was dissatisfied with such a negativistic attitude (see 105, p. 260). I tried to show that the considerations on which the objections are based have not only freed us from a theoretic strait jacket by which research in this field was hampered for a long time, but brought to the fore new facts which were overlooked or neglected by the adherents of the old theory, and which seem to be highly suited for building *a new concept of localization.*

I have discussed this problem in detail on another occasion (see 97, p. 656) with respect to analysis of individual cases. Here I can only refer to this discussion and repeat some results at which I arrived.

The symptoms which are related to a localized lesion cannot be understood from the destruction of so-called residuals of previous performances; they cannot be understood simply as due to memory defects; they are consequences of a *diminution of function of the brain matter, which finds its expression in a dedifferentiation of performance.* The more cases were analyzed, the more this old concept of Jackson found confirmation. Careful analysis of the phenomena in dedifferentiation of performances has led us to note the characteristic modifications of performances corresponding to the various degrees of damage of the brain matter. We have learned to understand them as effect of changes of function of the brain matter on performances and to understand from this point of view the modifications of performances as effect of dedifferentiation to a lower level (see before, p. 4).

We learned further that the *kind of modification of performance is in principle the same in all performance fields.* It may concern different material, motility, sensation, speech, etc. (see before, p. 5).

A lack of a special performance in one field does not appear any more as due to a special localization of a lesion but due to a particular degree of dedifferentiation of the function of the involved area. The more complicated performances suffer first, i.e., those which demand the better function of the brain matter.

For this standpoint, *each performance is due to the function of the total organism in which the brain plays a particular role.* In each performance, the whole cortex is in activity, but the excitation in the cortex is not the same throughout. There is a definite configuration in which one part of the cortex is in that particular excitation which corresponds to the "figure," while the rest is in that excitation which corresponds to the "background" (see p. 5). Distribution in this configuration varies depending on whether motor activity or perception or a mental attitude is requested. A *particular locality* in the brain matter is characterized by the *influence which the structure of this locality exercises on the total process,* by the contribution of the excitation of this locality to this process—as effect of its particular structure. Thus, for instance, the area striata contributes to this process something which is necessary for the experience of vision, the frontal lobes, something which is the presupposition for the mental phenomenon we call abstract attitude, etc., but, to reiterate, we may not localize corresponding functions in these parts of the brain.

To different localizations of lesions correspond different symptom complexes because the different performance fields are affected in a different way by the process of dedifferentiation.

Our discussion will have shown that as much as the rejection of the old concept of circumscribed localization is justified, such a rejection is *not in contradiction to an assumption that to each performance corresponds an excitation of definite structure in the cortex,* indeed, not in a circumscribed area but *widespread over the whole cortex,* differently in each performance. *This is what we should term localization.* Now, it will further become evident that we are able to localize definite symptom complexes in definite areas, but with that reservation which consideration of the mentioned anatomic and symptomatologic complexity demands.

As much as our concept of localization differs from the assumption of a simple relation between a symptom and a lesion in a circumscribed area, it leaves *unaltered* the usual procedure of localization of symptoms or symptom complexes for *practical purposes.* The gross localization, as far as aphasic symptoms are concerned, is sufficient for the localization of a brain tumor, etc. A motor speech defect will mostly be correctly localized in the expanded Broca's region of the left hemisphere (in right-handed individuals). But we should not be surprised if sometimes we err, because we have not or could not take into consideration all the factors which modify the relation between the aphasic picture and the lesion (cf. p. 45). On the other hand, symptom complexes with outstanding sensory speech disturbances will mostly be correctly localized in the temporal lobes, etc. (see the anatomic remarks to the description of different clinical pictures, p. 219).

Our discussion has not yet taken into consideration a factor which has often confused the issue of localization, namely the *role which the "other" hemisphere plays* for the development or nondevelopment of symptoms and for "restitution" of performances disturbed in the beginning.

Since the discoveries of Broca, Wernicke, et al., particularly of H. Liepmann, there is no doubt that defects of the higher mental performances, and hence particularly of language, occur in lesions in one—the "leading" —hemisphere. Thus, we are almost always correct if we localize the lesion of a right-handed aphasic patient in the left hemisphere, and vice versa. That we are sometimes mistaken, e.g., that the lesion in a right-handed aphasic is found in the right hemisphere, can have various causes. It may be the effect of a lack of conclusiveness of the methods to determine the "handedness" and the prevalence of the hemisphere.

But this is not the only factor which may confuse the issue of localization. The evaluation of the significance of an area for a definite performance will be different as the opinion is different concerning the significance of the other hemisphere for the loss and particularly for the restitution of a defect. If postmortems showed a damage of an area which one considered significant for a performance, and the latter was restituted, then often the assumption was made that the *other hemisphere had taken over the function. It is evident that the question whether or how much this assumption is justified is of great significance for a decision in localization.*

The problem is somewhat complicated. Frequently, restitution of a lost performance is wrongly assumed. Only a careful analysis will make it possible to decide whether we are not confronted in recurring performances with the effect of roundabout ways which might erroneously be considered as restitution (see p. 2). The role which the other hemisphere plays in recurrence of lost performances is not at all easy to determine. Whether such a performance must be attributed to the function of the other hemisphere or not, depends upon whether we consider a lesion suited to destroy a specific area in the one hemisphere totally; this again depends upon which extension we ascribe to the area and how we judge the lesion from the anatomic point of view (see p. 48). A definite decision that a present performance is the effect of function of the other hemisphere is justified only if one hemisphere or at least the specific area is *totally destroyed.* This is usually not the case.

We are further not at all certain whether a returning performance is not due to the fact that that part in the other hemisphere which is important for the performance has always functioned together with the corresponding part in the other hemisphere; in other words, that the concerned apparatus has comprised corresponding areas in both hemispheres. As we have explained before (see p. 9), under this condition a lesion in the dominant hemisphere may, in the beginning, set the total apparatus out of function, but after a certain time (or elimination of scars, etc.), the other side, released from the shock, may begin to function again. For instance, in a case like that of Zollinger, where after extirpation of the dominant hemisphere the patient was able to utter a few everyday phrases a few days after operation, it seems very doubtful whether we are justified in speaking of taking over of function by the other hemisphere. It is more probable to assume that these utterances were always guaranteed by the other hemisphere. Improvement would be due to recovery from a temporarily inhibited function. We have scarcely definite means to decide whether in an individual case this has occurred or not. This deliberation makes it also doubtful whether we are dealing with a real taking over of function when, after recovery from aphasia due to an insult in the dominant hemisphere, the symptoms disappear again after a second insult in the other hemisphere. Such cases are not rare. Nielsen has published a very instructive one (213, p. 146) and drawn the conclusion that the minor speech area took over the function after the lesion in the dominant one had occurred. From our foregoing discussion, another explanation appears to me at least possible. The lesion in the left hemisphere, according to the autopsy, was of such kind that the preserved brain would have been well suited to guarantee motor speech, as Nielsen points out (p. 150). Thus it is not necessary to assume that the recovery was the effect of a "taking over." The appearance of the aphasia after the lesion in the other hemisphere occurred could be explained by setting the apparatus combining both hemispheres out of function; this appears even more plausible as the left-sided part certainly was not normal. We are also not even sure whether this damage would not have had also a temporary effect. The patient lived only two days after the second insult. Possibly he would have recovered as to language if death had not occurred so rapidly. I mention this case particularly to show how difficult it is in a special instance to come to a certain judgment about "taking over."

We could assume a real taking over of a speech function, a new learning by the other hemisphere only under the following conditions:

1. If the patient had a definite premorbid prevalence of one hemisphere (that allows us, within definite limits, to assume that the other hemisphere did not act together with the "leading" one);

2. If we can assume a total destruction of the leading hemisphere, or at least of that part which we bring into relation to a certain performance;

3. If the symptomatologic defect was of a longer duration and recurrence of the performance took place slowly, possibly under the influence of definite training.

If we would find in such condition that the recurring performances show certain characteristics, we could use these as criteria for the assumption that in other cases, where a decision concerning these conditions is not possible, the recurring performances are the effect of a function by the other hemisphree. Till now, we have known very little about such characteristic performances, but experiences indicate that further studies may be successful in this respect. It seems that under this condition, as effect of relearning, a primitive form of repetition with motor difficulties in pronunciation can return (see p. 296).

The assumption that a number of performances could be taken over by the other hemisphere was emphasized particularly by Niessl von Mayendorf and in recent times by Nielsen. I agree with Nielsen that the minor cerebral hemisphere assumes the function of the major in language with great facility in some instances, with difficulty in others, and not at all in some persons. But this statement does not help very much; its generality does not permit the making of a decision in a particular case. And only if we can find the means for making such decisions can we avoid the often arbitrary assumptions which produce such confusion in the literature. The cases published, particularly those of Niessl von Mayendorf, do not allow definite decisions. Hence, a detailed discussion of them is out of place here. I think it will be better to say "we do not know," than to produce the erroneous impression that we have a right to assume such a taking over for some function in general. Our uncertainty in this respect is regrettable. A greater certainty would not only be significant for the problem of localization but for our procedure in retraining. We need a different procedure if new learning is to take place or if we are to expect recurrence of functions only temporarily hampered by shock. In the latter instance, elimination of shock would be more important than retraining.

In this state of affairs it may be useful for further research to consider at least the theoretic possibilities. We believe it is justifiable to assume that directly after birth and till to the end of the first years both hemispheres act together in all performances, or, more correctly, that the whole brain cortex represents a unitary apparatus in which functional differentiation between the two hemispheres does not exist. This is suggested by the fact that at this age, stimulation of the motor area of each hemisphere is followed by twitching movements in both sides of the body; that in spontaneous and reflectory activities of one side, usually concomitant movements also appear in the other side, that both hands are used in about the same way, etc. As far as pathology is concerned, this assumption is confirmed, for example, by the observation that in lesion of either side, aphasic symptoms occur; on the other hand, restitution takes place quickly and often totally.

Apparently in this early stage, stimulation of the sense organs is transmitted to both hemispheres, although the effect in the one, the crossed hemisphere, because of constitutional prevalence, may be stronger than in the other one and may leave a stronger after-effect. Motor activities in both sides of the body are related to both hemispheres. In addition, areas important for the higher mental functions may comprise both hemispheres, and the motor and sensory areas of both sides may be connected with both.

It seems that the development of dominance of one hemisphere parallels the development of the higher mental functions. The differentiation in use of the hands begins at the time when the child develops in this respect; it is retarded, or does not take place at all, in mental retardation or lack of mental development. Such a relation between dominance and higher mental function is suggested also by the fact that "handedness" is a characteristic property of man.

Pathology reveals now a definite difference between the hemispheres, particularly in respect to the higher mental functions. They appear particularly in lesions of the dominant hemisphere. Simple motor and peripheral disturbances concern only one side in lesion of one hemisphere.

If one hemisphere has attained an increasing significance for the higher mental functions, the other is more or less set out of function. However, this never takes place totally. The dimension of function of the "minor" hemisphere differs in *degree*, particularly as to the different performances. The sensory stimuli of both sides of the body are significant for the higher mental functions; therefore, we are justified in assuming that the stimuli from the sensory areas in both hemispheres are transmitted to the area important for the higher mental function in the major hemisphere, after the predominance has developed. In the same way, this area must remain in relation to the motor areas in both hemispheres. We can activate both motor areas from the dominant hemisphere. The relations between the motor and sensory areas to the area important for mental function in the "minor" hemisphere gradually lose their significance. We can assume that after one hemisphere has gained dominance, all new performances are related particularly to the latter, and thus the difference between the two hemispheres becomes increasingly more outspoken.

Because both sensory apparatuses, e.g., both calcarina, always operate together, and the calcarina of one side is sufficient to guarantee vision (see 105, p. 47), it is understandable that as long as the connection of one calcarina with the area for higher functions in the dominant hemisphere is guaranteed the process of visual recognition may not be disturbed; visual agnosia does not occur in lesion of the "minor" hemisphere and occurs in lesions of the calcarina in the dominant one only if the corpus callosum fibers are severed, too. The same holds true for the occurrence of sensory aphasia in lesions of one or the other hemisphere (see p. 217). The situation is different regarding the voluntary motor activities. Here stimulation of the area important for higher mental functions causes a prevalence of the dominant hemisphere for the more complex motor functions. The func tioning of the major hemisphere seems to be necessary for the cooperation of the motor apparatus in both hemispheres as basis of performances which concern both sides of the body in a unitary activity. This holds true particularly for language. It finds its expression in the prevalence of the aphasia area in one hemisphere. Persistent motor aphasia in a lesion restricted to the dominant hemisphere leads to the assumption that the corresponding area of the "minor" hemisphere cannot be directly stimulated by the "mental area" of the dominant hemisphere. The synchronous function of both apparatuses of both sides in motor speech seems to be guaranteed by a connection of the dominant hemisphere with the motor center of both sides in the medulla oblongata (see p. 201).

Interruption of the fibers of the corpus callosum may leave the higher mental performances untouched. Indeed, the use of the stimuli from the "minor" hemisphere may be disturbed. This may result in a tactile agnosia in the "minor" hand (see 79, p. 729). Further, particularly the synchronous activities suffer, and the activities of the "minor" hand which are directed by the dominant hemisphere.

Speech may not be disturbed at all in lesions of the "minor" hemisphere. Defects of the acoustic area in the dominant hemisphere are without effect as long as the stimuli from the other side reach the "central speech area" located in the predominant hemisphere. Destruction of the "motor speech area" in the dominant hemisphere sometimes disturbs motor speech only temporarily, if the areas in both hemispheres represent a unit. If the "central speech area" is destroyed in the dominant hemisphere, sensory speech performances do not seem to return. Indeed, in all the mentioned points, there is little unity among the authors. While, for example, Nissl von Meyendorf considers recurrence of repetition of heard language as an effect of the function of the "minor" hemisphere, Liepmann and Pappenheim have assumed the opposite. Other authors, e.g., Mendel and Long, considered that the two hemispheres have a different significance for different functions: the one more for the motor part of speech; the other more for understanding, writing, internal speech. The great discrepancy in the assumptions is due to lack of consideration of all the factors which we have mentioned before. Further research, taking these factors in their entirety into consideration, will be necessary before deciding whether a defect or restitution is related to the function of one or the other hemisphere.

CHAPTER IV

Survey of the Various Forms of Disturbance of Language in Pathology

B EFORE considering the different clinical pictures in which modifications of language due to brain damage present themselves, I should like to present a survey of the various forms of change of language in patients in general. This will help us toward a better understanding of the phenomena in individual cases which often show very complex features.

From our point of view all these modifications correspond to states of dedifferentiation of language. We shall consider separately the symptoms which appear as results of dedifferentiation of abstract attitude and of the instrumentalities.

A. DISTURBANCES OF LANGUAGE BY IMPAIRMENT OF ABSTRACT ATTITUDE

This defect finds expression in a great number of symptoms. In principle, the effect of impairment of abstraction on language is always revealed in the same way. The symptoms differ because in the individual case the capacity of abstraction is damaged to a different degree and so the patient may fail in some performances and not so much in those others which presuppose less abstraction. Differences as to the symptoms may occur, further, because the various speech performances need more or less abstract attitude, and the defect can be covered in different performances in different ways by concrete procedure, although this may not be readily apparent to the observer (see, in general, p. 12). Here the amount of individual premorbid "knowledge of speech" plays a leading role (see p. 25). The most characteristic appearance of damage of abstract attitude is impairment of meaning of words. The patients may be able to utter words but they are unable to use them as symbols. Therefore, these patients are impaired in the naming of objects (see p. 61). Instead of the names, they utter circumlocutions which describe the objects in a concrete way, or use "pseudonames". The same word cannot be used in different situations because the nature of double meaning cannot be grasped. In the same way, the metaphorical use of words is lost. Particularly impaired is spontaneous speech. The patient may not be much disturbed in conversation but fails highly in starting to speak; for instance, difficulty in starting, on command, a series which he will recite fluently after the first one or two members of the series are presented to him.

The more a speech utterance is determined by outer world stimuli the better it will be performed.   This does not mean that repetition is always the best preserved performance.   The complexity of repetition about which we shall speak later (p. 70) creates here a particular condition.   Emotional language is usually better than propositional (cf. p. 59).

Understanding is more or less disturbed, too.   Not enough attention has been paid to these defects.   Whether the patient fails or not in understanding can be understood only with a careful analysis of how much abstract attitude is necessary for understanding a special speech utterance.   For this reason, frequently some sentences are better understood than single words.   Particularly difficult is the grasping of a conversation in which shifting of the attitude is necessary.   Words belonging to objects are usually identified, but they are not taken as names, etc.

The concrete language is not at all normal.   It shows a more compulsive character.   The patients find it difficult to stop voluntarily, e.g., at a certain point in a series.   The patient may not be able to find some very well known words, sentences or series which usually are elicited under a certain attitude when he has to utter them under other conditions.   In time, he may even lose "speech knowledge" if the abstract attitude is impaired. A particularly characteristic example is the loss of the multiplication table in patients who have lost the value of the number.   The reason for the loss of learned material is that the patient, because of his impairment of abstract attitude, cannot control the correctness of the automatisms.   Therefore, the latter disappear (see p. 8).   The relation of the automatisms to definite attitudes is particularly important for relearning the lost automatisms.   The patient has the greatest difficulty in learning them by simple memorization.   It is easier for him when their concreteness is guaranteed otherwise, for example, through the teacher in whom he has confidence; this means by the abstract attitude of somebody else.

If in this way the instrumentalities suffer, the picture may become somewhat similar to that in dedifferentiation of the instrumentalities themselves. Additionally, spontaneous speech may be impaired here, particularly because it represents the most complicated performance in the field of instrumentalities (see p. 81).   A distinction between the two forms of defects of the instrumentalities is not always simple, particularly if in cases of disturbance of abstraction the automatisms are also damaged primarily, as in some forms of motor aphasia (see p. 85).   Because retraining must be totally different, depending upon whether one or the other defect is the cause of the patient's incapacitation as to the instrumentalities, this distinction is of great practical value.

B. Rational and Emotional Language in Pathology

The dependence upon the attitude finds an expression in the phenomenon that patients who are scarcely able to speak any word voluntarily may utter correct words and even sentences in connection with emotions. Jackson was the first who pointed to this phenomenon and saw in it an expression of disintegration in brain damage from a "higher" form of language, the "rational" language, to a "lower" form, the "emotional" language. One is inclined to help such patients regain rational language by using the words uttered in emotions. Such attempts have not proved very successful. The reasons for these failures, then, must intrigue our scientific curiosity. Jackson was very correct in his distinction between two forms of language of different complexity, but the difference between both forms of utterances is more complicated than he assumed. The difference is *not well characterized as greater complexity of the performance in rational language, but is due to the difference of the attitude* in which both conditions of speech take place. We are not dealing with different languages, but with different conditions of the total personality.

It is a widespread idea that outcries of emotions represent the basis of all language. From the time when the Greek philosopher Democritus proclaimed this idea it found many followers until the present. The primitive outcries were supposed to be used later as "language". The development from emotional to rational speech is a process of gradual objectivation, writes Laguna. Such theories were accepted particularly because they allowed human language to be considered as essentially the same phenomenon as "animal language" (Gardiner), only, however, as a development of it. We have mentioned before that Herder, who had emphasized the origin of language from emotional outcries, has denied the possibility of a simple development from the cries to language, and considered another higher mental function necessary for its origin.

Cassirer has stressed the impossibility of considering human language and what is called animal language from the same point of view, and pointed to the fact that even authors who advocate the origin of language from emotional utterances could not help admitting that the difference between interjections and language (i.e., rational, human language) is much greater and much more conspicuous than their supposed identity (35a, p. 117). The similarity lies in the use of a similar material, the difference in the attitude in which human language takes place, an attitude which is totally alien to the nature of animals. It is scarcely perceivable that an event belonging to emotional experience could become "representative" of something. Emotional experience occurs in a totally different condition of the total organism, in a totally different attitude than representational speech; a direct transition from one attitude to the other is not possible. We may be able to use the same word in emotions and in rational language. But if we do this, the word has another character, even though it may appear the same by face value. Pathology has taught us that words can undergo such change, can lose the ability to be used as symbols (see p. 61).   Patients may have words in "concrete" language, but may not be able to use them in conditions where meaning is involved.

Emotional speech belongs to concrete behavior.   Therefore, it shows similarity in its occurrence with that of concrete behavior in general.   However, there are some differences.   Emotional speech has this in common with the other speech automatisms: after it is started it runs as a whole; if interrupted, it cannot be simply continued.   However, it does not depend upon the abstract attitude in the same way as does concrete language, and it is much closer related to the total personality.   Therefore, impairment of abstract attitude does not disturb emotional utterances as much as the other automatisms. The difference between emotional and other language in patients may appear particularly great because we naturally compare emotional language with voluntary language, and the latter is severely disturbed.   Thus, it may appear as if a particular form of language is preserved, another form disturbed.   From this, it would seem more correct to speak of *disturbance of language belonging to the abstract attitude and of language belonging to concrete behavior*, than of rational and emotional language, and to consider emotional language a particular form of concrete language.

Though making a sharp distinction between "emotional" language and "rational" language, I would not deny the possibility that words uttered in emotional language may be used in other forms of language taking place in normal language, and that the patient, in spite of damage of volitional language, may be capable to a certain degree of such utilization to improve his motor defects by means of utterances in emotional situations.   Our procedure in retraining makes use of this possibility (see p. 325).   Indeed, this is particularly successful if the patient is not impaired in abstract attitude, if he is merely suffering from a motor defect; it is less successful if he is impaired in the foregoing capacity.

C. DISTURBANCES IN FINDING OF WORDS

Disturbance in finding words is a frequent symptom, and very different origins can be ascribed to this defect.

We must distinguish between the *facile summoning up of words* in fluent language when many of them are uttered without our being aware of any special activity, and *voluntary searching for words*.   But if, in the "automatically" occurring flow of words, we stop for any reason, we must always search for words to some degree, for single words or word sequences, etc., and among the words which may come to our mind in this search we have to choose those which fit best.   Word-finding is different in emotional expression, in intentional speech, in speaking of motor series, of phrases in familiar connection of words, in looking for words belonging to concrete objects or abstractions (naming), in repetition, etc.

Our behavior in respect to word-finding differs as to *different categories of words,* e.g., some words occur with particular ease in fluent language, the so-called small words, prepositions, pronouns, articles, grammatical forms, etc., while we meet in this condition greater difficulties with other word categories, as, for instance, names, proper names, etc. This difference between the word categories is not the same in the different situations of word finding. Some words, which occur easily in fluent speech, offer particular difficulty in voluntary word-finding, as, for example, the mentioned little words (see p. 68). Their correct use usually represents a difficult problem for those who learn a foreign language, etc. In the various forms of voluntary speech, as in conversation, description of facts, naming objects, etc., the subject matter is different. Hence, the problem of finding words is a very complex phenomenon. It depends on different underlying processes: on the readiness of speech automatisms, mental attitudes, organization of the processes in thinking which precede word-finding, emotional condition. Each item in our discussion of the evolution from non-language mental processes to speech plays a role here.

Accordingly, disturbances of word-finding can be due to different pathologic changes and *one cannot speak in general of disturbances of word-finding* but must distinguish different forms. Some failures depend on defects of special instrumentalities (see p. 65). But in other cases the disturbance in word-finding occurs without such defects, or if the patient shows such disturbances, the defect in word-finding is independent of them. In every case, the origin of the defect in word-finding must be revealed if one is to avoid an erroneous interpretation of the symptom and, hence, a misconception of its relation to an anatomic lesion and a wrong procedure in relearning.

A review of the ways in which word-finding may be disturbed in patients allows for the distinction of the following forms.

There are cases where words (those for concrete objects, sometimes even more those for abstractions) are almost totally lacking. The defect becomes apparent especially in the *task of naming objects,* not so much in conversational speech. Here, there are no other speech defects, particularly no motor defects, no paraphasia. The words presented to the patient can be repeated and brought into relation to the corresponding object, but he cannot produce them in naming, even shortly after correct repetition, etc.

This form of defect in word-finding is, as Gelb and I could show, not explainable as an effect of impairment of speech instrumentalities, of so-called word residuals. It is not a primary memory defect; it is one expression of impairment of abstract attitude. The patient cannot find the words because he cannot assume the attitude in which they normally appear. Even then, if he is able to find the word which belongs to an object, these words are not normal, they have lost "meaning" as analysis has revealed (see p. 62).

One may be surprised that naming demands an abstract attitude, but according to the findings in our patients there can be no doubt that such is the case. The nature of naming is often misinterpreted because one does not differentiate between *naming* and simple association of a word with an object (*pseudonaming*). It is, on the surface, very difficult to say whether an uttered word is a name or such an association. Analysis of patients with difficulty in finding words has revealed that there is an essential difference as to the attitude of the individual—corresponding to the differentiation we make. When the patient truly "names" an object, he has the experience of a word which "means" this object, considers the object as representing a category. Otherwise, he experiences the word as a sound complex belonging to an object. He frequently pronounces the word in the way we pronounce a word of a foreign language, the sound of which we know but which has no definite meaning for us (see p. 258). This difference becomes particularly evident in patients whose speech is not exceptionally impoverished, who have a fairly ample vocabulary and verbal knowledge. Such a patient may be able to bring out many words in relation to objects as reaction to the question, "What is this or this?" and is also able to describe his intention in uttering the word. As much as it may seem in such cases as if the patient names the object, his description shows clearly that actually he does not (see p. 62).

A patient of mine* correctly named familiar objects as well as colors, but the latter only when they were quite "pure." Only then would she designate them as red, blue, etc. She declined to extend the same name to the several shades of the given color on the ground that it would not be correct "to call these red, blue, etc." In short, she had not used the word as a name for an idea, as it might have appeared at first, but only as a sound pertaining to one particular object.

That the words used by the patient in a seemingly normal way are yet always of a totally concrete character may be further illustrated by the following examples. Asked to mention the names of some animals, the same patient was at first unable to do so. Not until we had given her such examples as dog, cat, mouse, did she reply to our question. Then suddenly she said: "A polar bear, a brown bear, a lion, a tiger." Asked why she named just these animals, she said: "If we enter the Zoological

* Published by E. Rothmann.

Gardens we come, at first, to the polar bear and then the other animals." Apparently she had called up from memory the names of the animals as they were situated in the Zoological Gardens, and used the words only as they belonged to the concrete situation. In this regard, it was very characteristic, that she did not say: "bears," a word which expresses the category of all different kinds of bears, and which we would call when asked to name animals—but that she called the words "polar bear, brown bear."

We found the same thing when the patient was asked to call different female first names. She said: "Grete, Paula, Clara, Martha," and, asked why she called just these names, answered, "Those are all G's" (G was her family name), and went on, "One sister died with a heart neurosis." This example demonstrates very clearly that the patient did not think of names but only words which belong to the particular situation, not used words of generic character, but "individual" words which fit only a definite object.

How very concretely such words are taken may be demonstrated by another example. When to such a patient a knife was offered, together with a pencil, she called the knife a "pencil sharpener"; when the knife was offered together with an apple, it was to her an "apple parer"; in company with a piece of bread, it became a "bread knife" and together with a fork it was "knife and fork." The word knife alone she never uttered spontaneously and when she was asked, "Could we not always call it simply knife?", she replied promptly, "No."

Another insight into the change of the character of the words comes from the use of words which have several meanings. For example, there is in German the word "Anhaenger" meaning a lavalier which hangs on a chain around a girl's neck, or a follower of a personage, or the second car which is attached to the first streetcar, as is usual in Germany. My patient was unable to use the word for all these objects. When she had understood the word in one sense, for example, "Anhaenger" as follower, she could not understand that we might also use it as meaning lavalier or second car.

Observation of such patients shows strikingly that the words which a patient may utter may not be words of categorical meaning but may belong exclusively to individual things. As we have said, the patients with this form of disturbance of word-finding have not lost the words but are unable to use them in a categorical sense, because they cannot assume the abstract attitude. It might be argued: it may be true that words as such have not been lost but that they have lost meaning, and that the disturbance of the abstract attitude is merely the result of the change of the words. There are sound reasons against such an assumption. We find side by side the change in the use of words and the disturbance of abstract behavior in general, and also in non-language performances (see p. 258). Because the change in words is basically of the same kind as the change of the behavior in general, it seems to be more reasonable to consider both changes as expressions of the same basic disturbance, neither primary nor secondary. To have sounds *in an abstract meaning as symbols for ideas means the same concerning language as to have the possibility of approaching the world in general in abstract attitude.*

If one compares the behavior of patients with this defect, there is one outstanding phenomenon which needs special consideration: the inconsistency so characteristically a symptom of these patients, their sometimes being able to name a thing, sometimes not, being able to name one thing, and not another thing, and the still more perplexing phenomenon that some patients will be practically unable to name any object, whereas other patients find relatively numerous words for objects. Do these differences not point to different degrees of memory defects as causes, and are they understandable from our point of view? The patient's possession of some words becomes understandable from our theoretic aspect when it is noted that the words he uses have the unmistakable character of connection with individual things, i.e., words like "strawberry red," "sky Blue," "to write," etc. These can be easily recognized as "individual words." But investigation shows that even when patients use words which are normally employed in a categorical sense, in their speech they have a quite concrete meaning. That is certain, for example, when they use the word "thing." This does not mean, as it may mean for us, a category detached from individual objects, but rather the word with which the patient points to one particular object if he misses the right word. He behaves as children do, who have learned this word from grownups and do not know its correct usage. This may also occur with grownups under the same condition.

Inequalities among different patients in the difficulty of finding words, are explained further by another factor, i.e., by *the different capacity of the patients to cover up* their defect. This variable capacity is conditioned by the patient's premorbid linguistic knowledge. The better this has previously been, the more the patient will be able to cover up the defect by this externalized use of words as simple associations. On the other hand, the greater the disturbance of the patient is as to instrumentalities also, the more obvious the difficulty in word-finding will be by the concomitant impairment of language memory itself, which may make awakening of words difficult (see p. 65).

From both a theoretic and practical standpoint the discussed phenomena deserve careful attention. Nondiscrimination between these two forms of disturbances in finding words has given rise to the contention that word-finding is not related to abstract attitude in the way we assume, but is an effect of loss of memory. This opposition is based on the fact that patients with amnesic aphasia may not show impairment of abstract attitude. One would think that as we are dealing with facts such controversies should not be possible. The difficulty is that whether we get facts of this or that kind depends on how carefully we analyze the reactions of the patients. The analysis usually is lacking in two respects—in respect to language and to the behavior in general.

We have just discussed the language of the patients and the different reasons why we may be deceived as to the character of their utterances.

Now, concerning the general behavior, there is particular discrepancy regarding the phenomena we observe in the sorting tests (see p. 170).

The first objection states that the concrete approach to the solution of the sorting tests is not sufficient to permit us to assume that the person is able to use solely a concrete type of behavior. Also, some normal persons, to whom we cannot really deny the possession of this ability, may, on occasion, behave in the same concrete way as do the patients. We do not deny this fact. Indeed, a pupil of mine, Dr. Weigl (311) (see also 101 and 115) has experimentally demonstrated that this sort of behavior is found quite frequently in very intelligent persons. But (and of great importance) all these normal persons, when they see that the task cannot be fulfilled by this procedure, or when asked to sort the test material abstractly and to change from one way of sorting to another, are able to do so. The amnesic aphasics were never able to bring themselves to such an abstract attitude, or to meet a situation demanding a change in their attitude. Hence, it seems that the criticism which was raised particularly by Kuenburg and Isserlin concerning the possibility of a concrete attitude in normals does not touch upon our conception as to the nature of the disturbance in the amnesic patient.

More serious is the objection which asserts that our explanations do not correspond to the facts in so far as patients, suffering from a difficulty or lack in finding words, may behave very well abstractly. This criticism has been advanced particularly by Kuenburg from examinations of her patients. Weigl and I have studied very carefully the protocols published by Kuenburg and are convinced that these protocols fail to confirm her conclusions. It is not necessary to repeat here the explanatory proof of this statement which Weigl (311) has given. However, a brief report of the critical conclusions may be useful.

(a) It could be demonstrated that it is very doubtful as to whether the patients in whom Kuenburg reports this abstract attitude *are really amnesic aphasics*. The protocols are insufficient to permit a definite opinion as to whether these patients were cases of amnesic aphasia, or whether they were suffering from some other form of disability in finding words which had nothing to do with amnesic aphasia. If the patients are not amnesic aphasics and do not behave concretely, their abstract behavior cannot be used as contradiction to our theory.

(b) But taken for granted that some were amnesic aphasics, it cannot be assumed with certainty from the protocols that the patients behaved in an abstract way. We are confronted here with a problem of general and great methodologic significance. Only a careful analysis of each reaction can determine whether the patient, in his sorting, proceeds abstractly or concretely. I pointed out many years ago that a likely source of error lies in judging the disability solely on the basis of the verbal answers of patients (see also Goldstein and Scheerer). Weigl demonstrated through a very careful analysis of single cases that the verbal answer can in no way be considered proof that the patient was really behaving in an abstract fashion. There are several obvious possibilities of error which are often overlooked. There is the error based on false judgments of the words which the patients use. As we pointed out above, the same word may be used both in a concrete and abstract sense (see p. 61), and we may be decieved as to how the patient really used it. Only a very accurate examination can give us a definite and clear result, as for example, in the case which E. Rothmann has published (see later, p. 259). The protocols published by Dr. Kuenburg give no evidence of such critical analysis, and many details reported make it improbable that those patients who were really amnesic aphasics used the words in an abstract sense. Another frequent source of error comes from a false interpretation of the results of the sorting test. Sometimes the patients put objects together in a way that may at first suggest an abstract attitude, a sorting according to concepts, but upon closer analysis proves to be an expression of a very concrete procedure (cf. Goldstein and Scheerer). Weigl has demonstrated in great detail that this is true in certain of the reports of Kuenburg, although Kuenburg uses this argument as proof of abstract character in the behavior of her patients.

From my study of the material presented by those who have objected to our conception of amnesic aphasia, I must say that in all the presentations of patients' behavior the errors which we have just stressed have not been avoided. A very critical reconsideration of more recent cases, with due attention to all these objections, has in no way forced me to modify my original concept; on the contrary, it has strengthened my belief in its verity.

Because all misunderstanding arises from an unsatisfactory analysis of the facts, in the future a much more thorough analysis of each individual response of the patient must be sought before a judgment of the basic disability of the patient may be given with assurance.

When later (see p. 246) we shall discuss the symptom complex of amnesic aphasia we shall say more about the anomalies of patients' language and the general personality changes accompanying the form of defect in word-finding which is related to impairment of abstract attitude.

In contrast to the described form of disturbance in word-finding are those forms where abstract attitude is primarily intact and *the difficulty is due to damage of instrumentalities of speech*. In these cases there is in the foreground—besides a greater or less difficulty in finding words—a distortion of the words (literal paraphasia) or a substitution of another word for the correct word (verbal paraphasia). The patient may be able to produce the first sound or other characteristics of the word, a characteristic vowel or consonant; he may be able to say whether the word is long, short, etc. His defect is due to the distortion the instrumentalities have suffered (see p. 25). His defect is not particularly and exclusively revealed in naming, or in difficulty in finding nouns, verbs, etc. Additionally, the small words, conjunctions, article, etc., are impaired too. The patient will not be able to repeat a presented word correctly, though presentation may improve the performance. He shows the same difficulty in series. But, however distorted the words may be, they have preserved meaning.

The deviation of the uttered word from the demanded one can be understood from the underlying defect of the instrumentalities and the effect of the latter on the process of thinking (see p. 101). Lotmar has studied these "derailments" particularly in a case which he erroneously termed amnesic aphasia, but which belonged to the form of disturbance of finding words we have just been discussing. His patient showed a prolongation of the time which passed till he found the word for an object, or a word which belonged to a certain sentence. Lotmar could unveil the relation of the uttered word to the demanded one by determining the ideas which arose in the patient during the prolonged interval. Some of the derailments were due to the fact that words came to the fore which were similar as to their motor or sensory structure and were easier to pronounce, or by any reason easier to evoke. Some—and these are particularly interesting—were the effect of emerging images, ideas, of "spheres" to which the correct word belonged. These images, ideas, may arise as "between-experiences" in normal individuals also, but in so transitory a manner as not to influence the finding of the correct word. However, they come to the fore abnormally if the correct speech performance is hampered. Then the individuals utter these words, or are delayed in uttering the right one which they may finally produce. These anomalies are to be observed particularly concerning words which belong to objects which cannot be visualized ("unanschaulich"), abstract concepts, objects like "correctness," "courage," "love," "law," etc., apparently because these "objects" are much more closely connected with words than are concrete objects. In concrete objects, language does not play such a definite role as in abstractions (see p. 257). It is apparent that in these patients the thought processes may be disturbed secondarily (see p. 101). This coming to the fore of words belonging to the sphere, instead of the right one emerging, is particularly striking if it takes place in the task to repeat heard words (see later, p. 313). As important as these studies of Lotmar are for understanding disturbances in word-finding (particularly verbal paraphasia) in some patients, they do not affect the correctness of our theory of disturbance of word-finding in amnesic aphasia.

There is to be mentioned another type of disturbance in word-finding which superficially shows a resemblance to that found in amnesic aphasia, insofar as the patients here also show no other anomalies of language other than the difficulty in word-finding. But there are characteristic differences: while the patients with "amnesic aphasia" are disturbed in naming of most common things, these patients usually find these words and show the defect only or particularly in respect to more rare words, or (as old people with this anomaly) to words they have acquired in the last years. The essential difference is that the words the patients utter have *not lost meaning* and that the abstract attitude proves to be normal. It may be difficult for the patient to assume this attitude in situations where there is normally a close connection with the words, but in other situations where language is not involved the patient behaves normally, as, for example, in the performance tests for examining abstract attitude. This picture is to be observed particularly in acute brain injury, in abscesses secondary to ear diseases, in abnormal fatigue, in old people. It can be considered as due to a memory damage concerning particularly the speech instrumentalities.

It may be useful to look for some definite criteria which allow a distinction between the type of word-finding in the form of amnesic aphasia and other types. In this respect, I would say: The difficulty in finding words itself is not manifested in the same way in the two forms. Whereas it is characteristic of amnesic aphasia that periphrases occur in place of words not found, periphrases are much rarer in the second type. The characteristic phenomena are mutilations in the line of verbal or literal paraphasia. Patients suffering from the latter disorder are often helped by being given the initial letter or some key-letter of a word they cannot find. No such prompting is of help to a true amnesic aphasic. Finally, the second type also exhibits these differences: speech difficulties other than in finding words, motor impediments in pronunciation, disturbances in repetition, writing and comprehension of a kind which cannot be understood as effect of the defect underlying the amnesic-aphasic type of disturbance of word-finding.

The mentioned non-amnesic anomalies in word-finding occur in motor, sensory and central aphasia. They show characteristics of these forms.

In motor aphasia, motor difficulty and disturbances in words more difficult to pronounce are to be found. The picture may be similar in central aphasia, but here the motor difficulty is not so much in the foreground. Verbal paraphasia is to be noted particularly. The patient, in addition, often has great difficulty not only in finding the word spontaneously but in repeating it. Under the first condition, e.g., in naming, he may even behave better. The words substituted for the demanded ones may belong to the same sphere (see p. 101). Frequently in these cases, typical amnesic defects occur beside the mentioned ones.

In so-called sensory aphasia, there exists no difficulty in word-finding if we are dealing with pure word deafness. The other form, which is closer to the central aphasia and distinguished from the latter only by a greater defect in understanding, shows similar disturbances of word-finding as central aphasia. One difference is that the words which are found are uttered more quickly—however much paraphasia, literal and verbal, they may show. The patients are often not aware of the defect, in contrast to the cases where disturbances of word-finding are due to motor defect.

Still other forms of disturbance of word-finding are secondary to disturbances of the thinking process and of the process of transformation of thinking into language (see p. 309). Under this condition, those words are lacking which correspond to the failure in the process of thinking and the transformation into language.

Disturbances in Finding of the "Small" Words

We mentioned before (see p. 60) that some patients may have a special difficulty with the so-called small words, prepositions, articles, pronouns, grammatical forms, etc.

Saloz, in his autobiographic "mémoires d'un médecin aphasique," reports that the speaking of short words has caused him great difficulties, especially if several such words follow in a sentence (with these short words he particularly meant the mentioned small words). I have stressed several times that some patients are not able to speak, to read and to write these words, some cannot even repeat them, and that the behavior of patients differs in respect to these words according to the different underlying defects.

Froeschels has reported that patients with motor aphasia could neither write nor speak such words as "ich," "du," "er," "sie," "es." Isserlin has often observed the difficulty accompanying the use of these and other small words in patients with difficulties in the motor act of speech; when suffering from "peripheral motor aphasia," these words are missing apparently because—as Isserlin has stressed—the motor difficulty induces a definite attitude which concentrates on those words which are sufficient for being understood. This means certainly also a change of the process in thinking, in which this lack of definite words has to be taken into consideration. From the origin of the defect in these patients, it is understandable that the lack of these words shows particularly in spontaneous speech and not so much in reptition, reading or writing. But it can occur also in these performances. A patient of Minkowski (to whom we shall refer later in more detail; see p. 144) with motor aphasia, who was best in reading, had great difficulty in reading these words and frequently left them out.

In central motor aphasia, the patient has great difficulty when he must speak or write these words, particularly when they are demanded in isolation, and this is because he is impaired in his abstract attitude. To understand, to use these words isolatedly (which are usually used only in a definite connection with other words), presupposes the abstract attitude. From this origin of the defect in these patients it becomes understandable that a patient may be able to produce them, understand them, etc., in the concrete condition in which they usually appear, in definite combinations with other words. Thus, a patient of ours who showed the defect in speaking, repetition, reading and writing, could produce words like "an" (on), "der" (the), "in" (in), "das" (the), if they appeared in the address of a letter, and under similar conditions. That we are not dealing here with a primary motor defect, but with an effect of a missing attitude, becomes further apparent in a case where such words as "four," "one" could be produced in isolation, but such similar words as "for" or "an" could not be produced. Another observation is particularly elucidating in this respect: After I had explained to the patient time and again the character of these words, had demonstrated their "belongingness" to some situations, had induced him to copy, to repeat them in isolation, I dictated again some of the words. Now he seemed able to write the words; but he did not write down that word alone which I had dictated, the word "in," for example, —but wrote instead a number of words which belonged to this group "in, aber, auf, unter" (German). He apparently produced all words which he remembered as used in the several examinations. That his production was not based on having the words individually at his disposal became evident by the fact, that also afterwards he was not able to write them isolated on dictation. The individual words were as strange to him as before. This observation is a good example of how easily we can be deceived in respect to a capacity of a patient if we consider only the result of a task, not the way in which the result was reached (see p. 2).

Bouman and Grünbaum have reported the difficulty in producing these words isolated in a case where the motor speech defect was not due to a primary motor disturbance, but was due to an impairment of the function of the brain in general (see p. 76). The patient, in reading aloud, had difficulty with all short words and particularly with the "small words." He could speak these words together with others with which they built an articulatory unit, but not outside of such a unit. Bouman and Grünbaum have explained the defect in a similar way as I, by the difficulty of the attitude towards those words which, isolatedly presented, are "senseless".

Another factor plays a role, according to Bouman and Grünbaum, in the difficulty to pronounce such short words which are not senseless. Words with several syllables are easier to *speak* because the articulatory units are more "prägnant" (precise) than those consisting of one syllable. The long words "roll down" better ("rollen besser ab") than the short ones (if there is a primary motor defect). This greater fluency facilitates the pronunciation of the elements of which the word consists and which have to be produced in articulation. This factor may be valid particularly in cases of the type of the patient of Bouman and Grünbaum. Whether this factor plays a role in cases of other causation is doubtful. In ordinary motor aphasia the patients show greater difficulty with the long words; also in central aphasia repetition of long words is not performed as well as that of short words.

In respect to the small words, there is a difference between the cases where the instrumentalities are impaired in their function (primary or secondary, as in the case of Bouman and Grünbaum) and the cases where the defect is due to impairment of the non-language mental function—as transcortical aphasias or amnesic aphasia. Here the small words often represent a great deal of the spontaneous speech of the patients. They come to the fore even in an abnormal way, because they represent the only means of overcoming the distress due to the defect in speaking in an ordered way (see p. 12).

Our knowledge of the behavior of aphasic patients in respect to these small words is limited. Further studies would be of great interest.

D. Disturbances of Repetition of Heard Language

Repetition of heard language is more or less disturbed in many patients. To understand this we have to consider the many factors upon which repetition depends. It is not at all a simple phenomenon as often has been assumed.

For correct evaluation of the functional defect underlying any failure in repetition, we must first define what we expect an individual to do when we ask him to repeat a sound or a word, etc. We can demand a strict repetition of the acoustic percept, a performance which would be better called *imitation*. Or we can demand that he perceive the acoustic phenomenon, recognize it as language, understand it, and repeat the presented words. In this case, we usually do not pay attention to whether the repeated product corresponds exactly to the acoustic presentation or not. That is, for example, the usual form of repetition we expect in the so-called repetition tests.

The correct performance in both phenomena is dependent upon a number of factors. As to the differences of the disturbance of one of them or of several concomitantly, the deviation of repetition from the norm varies greatly in patients.

The factors involved are sensory perception, motor speech capacity, inner speech, the relation of the material to be repeated to "understanding," the 'attitude' of the individual, the educational level of the individual, the situation in which repetition occurs.

Both—repetition as well as imitation—presuppose perception, but imitation to a higher degree than repetition. We can imitate only what we have perceived well, but correct perception is not necessary for repetition. We are able to repeat the words presented even though we have not perceived them completely and correctly. If the acoustic perception gives only a hint we are often able to utter the right words, although not to imitate the heard ones exactly.

Even if perception and motility are normal, we do not always repeat exactly. Our repetition shows more or less the characteristics of our own pronunciation. Correct imitation occurs only when we pay special attention to the acoustic and motor phenomena. Hence, there results a difference in repetition between educated and uneducated (less literate) individuals. The first, more accustomed in general to pay attention to what they are doing, and especially to speech, are more correct in imitative repetition, if it is demanded, than uneducated people. These latter have much more difficulty in simply imitating what they hear; they are much more inclined first to ponder what the word means, and then to repeat it. It takes longer for them to repeat, and they do not repeat the heard sounds exactly but utter the word in their own way of pronunciation, for instance in their dialect. Children behave similarly. The normal individual is so accustomed to consider language from the aspect of understanding that he must abstract himself from this point of view when he wants to concentrate on the sound and motor activities which is presupposition of exact imitative repetition. Uneducated individuals find the performance of this abstraction particularly difficult. This shows that somehow the reaction in imitative repetition is not at all the simplest performance. It presupposes a higher mental attitude. In this respect, it is very different from pathologic echolalia (see p. 303).

Under pathologic conditions, in impairment of abstraction, the patient may be able to repeat only those words whose meaning he understands, even when perception and motor activities are undisturbed—or at least not so much disturbed as to make repetition impossible. If he is able also to repeat senseless material, he "imitates" it with difficulty and effort (see p. 70). His repetition has some echolalic character but does not show the compulsive-passive form of typical echolalia (see p. 303).

There is another factor to be considered which may produce differences in repetition.   People who are easily capable of abstraction may repeat easily. Those who have difficulty in this respect, who are not so accustomed to abstract, may refuse to repeat at all, if they cannot repeat correctly, because they are afraid to do something which appears to be incorrect.   This often occurs also in educated people; they may try to imitate, but experiencing inability to carry through the performance, they hesitate or refuse to repeat at all.   This occurs especially in patients who, as we said before (see p. 12) try particularly to avoid all unclear situations.

The more difficulty one has in perceiving the presented word correctly, i.e., in a way which is recognizable as a known sound complex, the more one tends to try to understand it first, believing that understanding may facilitate perception and repetition.   This is demonstrated particularly in patients.   Here the defect of perception may not awake a definite word with a definite meaning, but instead the "sphere" to which the word belongs according to its meaning.   The patient repeats, then, not the presented word but one which belongs to the "sphere" and which for any reason comes to the fore (see p. 101).

There is a difference between voluntary repetition in examination and involuntary repetition in conversation or in everday life.   The uneducated individual may repeat words unknown to him—senseless sound combinations—even better than the educated one in the latter condition.   Thus, he may learn words of a foreign language easier from hearing than the educated one (only a certain kind of language, indeed—the concrete language, see p. 25), and pronounce the words better than his educated fellow.   He is, in his use of language, not as disturbed by all the implications which the word contains for the educated man.   The same thing happens in patients. They may be able to repeat some words or even sentences involuntarily, but not if demanded to do so.

In general, there is a greater difficulty in repeating unknown words than familiar ones.   But if we are able to concentrate on the sound (disregarding whether we understand the presented sound complex or not) we may imitate totally unfamiliar words, if they are not too difficult to perceive and to pronounce, even better and more correctly than familiar ones.

Whether a word is, for an individual, more or less familiar as to perception, pronunciation, or attitude toward it in general, depends upon the general level of education, but also upon an accidental acquaintance with the word and—it seems—upon an inborn greater or lesser gift for language.

There are words very familiar to us which are not often pronounced, e.g., the technical words which we read and to which we react in a definite way but which we never or seldom speak.   In spite of the fact that we understand their meaning, it is frequently difficult to repeat them.   For less literate persons, the names of the letters belong more or less to this group.

A patient may have particular difficulties in repeating words which usually occur in a definite connection, if they are presented isolated. In cases showing difficulty in repetition, sentences may not be repeated as well as words, but sometimes sentences may be repeated better than *isolated* words.

Repetition in both forms presupposes adequate motor capacity; particularly high development of motor capacities is necessary for imitation. Usually we do not imitate but speak by using our "automatisms," the "simpler" motor phenomena.

When a normal individual imitates a sound complex, abstracting from the content and thus from his own personality, and tries as much as possible simply to repeat the acoustic presentation parrot-like, the relation between the production and the producing personality never gets completely lost. The automatic activity is always under some control of the abstract attitude (see p. 8), and is possible only within this frame.

There are conditions of very strong impressive stimulation when even normals come into a repeating behavior which develops compulsively and almost passively. This occurs when people, without being aware of it, repeat words or music. It may particularly be observed as repetition of actions induced by seen actions, for instance, if the individual is exposed to the sight of very impressive movements. Here there occurs some kind of "isolation" of the reaction from the personality, which then shows the characteristics of performances of isolation. But these are exceptional situations in normals. Such isolation of the reaction from the personality is produced by pathology in some patients: these patients are not able to "repeat," but imitate parrot-like, passively, in a compulsive way. The presupposition seems to be not only a lack of understanding of the contents of the presented material but also a lack of any voluntary reaction (see p. 301).

Imitation will be correct only if the instrumentalities are intact. But even if this is not totally the case, some defective speech will be produced in the form of echolalic imitation (see p. 303).

The ability to imitate must not be wrongly interpreted as an expression of good recollection, e.g., if a patient can repeat a normal number of digits in the repetition test. This repetition can be a passive phenomenon which must not have any thing to do with attention, memory, etc. It is then an expression of abnormal stimulus boundness (see p. 4). This may become immediately evident when the patient is asked to repeat the numbers with pauses between them, or to repeat them in reverse. In both cases, he fails, because these tasks can no longer be solved by senseless imitiation, but presuppose some mental activity on the order of abstraction.

One remark may be added: Not all imitation must be meaningless and passive as that of the mentioned patients. Imitation of normals may even presuppose a particularly high mental attitude.

E. Disturbances of the Expressive Side of Language

The expressive side of language may be damaged in the following ways:
1. By paresis of the muscles used in speaking;
2. By damage of the motor speech instrumentalities;
   a. by *damage to the after-effects* of previously built performances (motor speech "Gestalten") or decrease of their excitability;
   b. by damage of the *specific function* of building motor speech performances;
3. By *isolation of the motor instrumentalities* from the other speech instrumentalities or by *damage of them;*
4. By *damage of those mental processes other than speech*, or isolation of the instrumentalities from them.

The symptom complexes corresponding to the effect of the first kind of damage are those which are usually called *dysarthria,* those due to the second kind of damage, *motor aphasia,* those corresponding to the effect of the third represent the *disturbances of motor speech in defects of inner speech* and *sensory aphasia.* Those corresponding to the fourth kind of damage represent the so-called *transcortical motor aphasia.*

(1) *Dysarthria*

The motor speech performances are executed by the activity of muscles which are used not only for this but for other purposes also. It is evident that any paresis of these muscles must produce speech disturbances. These disturbances show in defects of those sounds whose production is dependent upon normal activity of the muscles which have become paretic. The effects of the paresis of the concerned muscles on non-language performances may be combined with dysarthria. However, some preserved functions of the muscles may be sufficient for the other performances but not for production of the more complicated sounds. Thus, we may meet a somewhat isolated dysarthria. This difference, indeed, may be partially due to the fact that it is easier to recognize defects of speech than of the other performances. However, there are cases where dysarthria occurs apparently without definite disturbance of the use of the muscles for other purposes.

In these cases, the speech defect shows particularly in production of isolated sounds. The words may become so distorted that communication by means of expressive language may be severely disturbed, while otherwise the patient may be completely normal and able to communicate by other means in a normal way. The patient may not be able to produce some sounds at all, or the sounds may appear clumsy, sluggishly blurred, the voice hoarse, weak. The tempo and rhythm of speech is modified. Frequently there are difficulties in breathing (regarding the problem of dysarthria and its treatment, see particularly Froeschels).

Our knowledge in this field is not very satisfactory. We shall be able to understand the clinical pictures better with an increased insight as to which muscles and which sounds are defective in cortical lesion of the concerned motor sphere. This is not simply a matter of chance. We are dealing here also with a dedifferentiation of function so that the more complicated performances are more disturbed than the less difficult ones. But there are still other factors involved. The machinery underlying the production of sounds and sound combinations in language is very complicated. It consists of a number of parts in addition to the special muscle activity which produces the sound: the configuration of the place where the sound is performed (place of articulation, lips, nasal-pharyngeal cavity, etc.), the strength of expiration, etc. We know very little about the influence of cortical lesions in all these respects.

A particular problem is the ease or difficulty with which individual sounds can be produced in the *sequence* of a word. This is not guaranteed by the ability to produce individual sounds. The relation between the sounds plays a role here, the greater or lesser similarity of the sounds occurring in a particular word; the degree to which definite sounds can be produced in a sequence within a word seems to be governed by the rule which we have mentioned before, namely, that the production of the *same* and *very different* performances in a sequence is easier than the production of *similar* performances, i.e., the latter is more difficult because it needs a more precise differentiation of the sounds. A functional damage which may impair the capacity to differentiate may make it impossible to produce "similar" sounds in a word, but leaves undisturbed the production of the easier sequences. Thus, the same sound may be pronounced correctly in one word, while in another it is omitted or "assimilated" in one simpler to pronounce. This phenomenon is demonstrated in a patient of Bouman and Grünbaum, whom the authors investigated particularly in respect to this problem. I think it will be valuable to give a little more detailed report of this case, particularly because there is scarcely another so careful examination of such a case in the literature.

It is true that in this case the motor speech instrumentalities are not damaged themselves. The disturbances in speaking are the effect of a damage of the brain function in general. But this is not important for our discussion here.   This general damage of the brain function has on a special field, in principle, the same effect as a direct damage of this field (see p. 48).   I think we are justified in drawing from this observation also some conclusion as to the behavior of sound production in word sequences in cases where the motor sphere is damaged directly.   Whether this is entirely accurate or not, the case is valuable because it should stimulate further studies.

The patient, 27 years old, an accountant, suddenly acquired paresthesia in the right hand and could not recognize objects by touch.   He had attacks of fainting and sensations of the world turning around before his eyes.   Difficulty in uttering a complex sentence and in thinking developed.

At admission, he had a right-side paresis and astereagnosis on the right side. Clinical diagnosis was a localized process in the middle third of the left Gyrus post-centralis, expanding probably posteriorly and to the precentral region.   A suspected tumor was not found by exploration, but a lesion in the 'center' for the left hand; an extirpated piece was microscopically diagnosed as encephalitis.   The *day after operation* the patient understood, but *could speak only "yes," "no."   Speech improved greatly, repetition coming first.*   Examination some time later revealed the following symptoms: the patient spoke spontaneously very little and apparently with great difficulty.   His speech was slow, the procedure of pronunciation seemingly demanding a great effort.   After he said some few words he stopped talking and continued after a pause.   His speech appeared disjointed, as if cut into pieces.   He spoke more and better when he was asked to tell definite things—to communicate something—and particularly in reading.   Therefore, the *special examination* concerning the motor speech was performed particularly *in reading.*

Visual perception, acuity, visual field, visual recognition was normal in every respect.   The patient understood the words of a printed text when he looked it over with his eyes *with no attempt to articulate the individual letters* (as could be tested by questions).   *The word was apparently visually grasped as a whole* also if the words were presented crossed by lines.   He recognized senseless words, visually presented, as seen before when later they were presented again.   He distinguished wrongly written words from correctly written ones, but only after a long time could he discover what was wrong.   The same was true as to sentences with wrong words.   He had *greatest difficulty in reading aloud.*   Under this condition, he spoke the words by combining the letters, or by forming the letters with his lips without producing sounds before he spoke aloud.   Unknown words or senseless combinations of syllables produced particular difficulty.   He read parts, stopped and showed motor paraphasia (see p. 83) if he was forced to continue.

He was not *able to produce a word—which he could produce as a whole—by pronouncing each letter separately.*   If letters were omitted in a word, he produced what he saw but one could observe that silently he spoke the ommitted letters, too.   Reading a word divided in syllables was well performed.   *Long words were better produced than short ones,* words consisting of one syllable were more difficult to read than those consisting of more than one.   Speaking of words which are usually used only in combinations with others necessitated considerable effort; he might even be unable to read them at all, as, for instance, naam, het, op, in, mech, toen, hen, heb, de (Dutch).

The speaking of *isolated letters* was *more difficult* than that of *words* containing the same letters. Isolated vowels were well read, *not so isolated consonants*, while he read consonants in words without difficulty. He could speak the consonants in repetition.

Repetition, as a matter of fact, was his best performance, but somewhat different in different presentations. Known, senseful, long words were always correctly repeated, short senseful words only if they were presented several times. Senseless words produced great difficulty.

Usually the patient did *not* show *much paraphasia* but it became apparent when he was forced to utter a word which was difficult to speak. Sometimes he was successful after trying in different ways. He recognized his failures by hearing, and tried until he spoke more correctly.

Besides his difficulty in speaking, the patient presented *anomalies in the non-language mental performances*. He had no defect in immediate recognition and recollection. He was able to reproduce 5, 6 digits after half a minute correctly and quickly. He understood sentences which can be understood if one grasps one paramount content, but in more complex sentences *containing different contents which have to be grasped and computed, he failed;* he might understand the general meaning in a vague way, but not the true meaning of the whole. He had difficulty in reacting to *two things and in grasping their relations to each other*.

In the Abelson test, where a triangle, square and circle are presented in such a way as to have some parts in common, the patient could show a place which was located in the triangle, square, etc., but had difficulty in showing a point which was common to two or three of the figures. He explained that he understood the name triangle, etc. If there were two or three objects with which to be dealt, he had difficulty, he must ponder in order to distinguish the names and, therefore, was not able to fulfill the task. He did not forget even long sentences "for himself," but he had difficulty to understand them.

The patient had no difficulty in distinguishing left and right, but in tasks where he had to make a differentiation between left and right he found it quite difficult. He said, "Left and right are very much related to each other." The same idea showed in other spatial distinctions. Thus he could demonstrate up, down, etc., but had difficulty in showing "below in the middle" (of a place) or "right, down," etc. The disturbance was not in right-left, or up-down, etc. orientation but rather in *recognition and distinction of two types of spatial determination*.

His attention was sometimes good, sometimes bad. He was determined by the total aspect of the stimulus situation and had difficulty in dealing with *parts* of a whole, hence, likewise in directing his attention to the parts. All performances were more difficult which demanded operations with parts within a total situation. As a special effect of this defect it should be mentioned that in the Bourdon test where the subject has the task of crossing out definite letters in a text, he behaved better when the text was senseless than when it was senseful. In the senseful text, his attention was directed to the words as wholes and their meaning; this hindered his attention toward the letters. In the senseless text an opposite situation prevailed, and therefore he behaved much better.

In thinking processes he might fail because he stopped when he had grasped the structure of the whole and was not able to consider the part elements.

In *arithmetic* he was about normal when he did *not* have to think about the procedure. He failed when he was forced to abstract the elements of the problem and keep them in mind during the arithmetical operation. It was hard for him to find his way when he was confronted with a greater number of digits which had to be considered in the operation, or when two different operations were needed. He understood immediately the following problem: If one adds to a number another and subtracts the second again, then one gets the first one. But he had the greatest difficulty in understanding that division is the reversed operation of multiplication; e.g., he answered immediately, "5 × 7 are 35," but asked how much is 35 : 5, he said: "I cannot do that so quickly." He fulfilled immediately the same problem when presented in written form.

The authors have investigated the causes why the words are sometimes produced incorrectly in experiments; their remarks deserve special attention.

They worked from the assumption that individual sounds are more or less similar in respect to the energy of the stream of expiration, the strength, localization and duration of the resistance which this stream finds at the place of articulation and the kind of resonance in the speech organs. Words or wordlike combinations of sounds which are presented differ in kind and degree as to phonetic relations. Definite difficulties, disturbances of pronunciation, may occur when the articulatory mechanisms are damaged. These mechanisms may be sufficient to build words in which the sounds belong to one sphere and to produce definitely different sound combinations, but not to build similar sound combinations, particularly if they have to be uttered quickly one after the other. This corresponds to the general rule we have mentioned before (see p. 39). Referring the reader to some of the interesting protocols, I would like to give here some of the important results which confirm the assumption of the authors, and also the general rule.

The patient, who said without difficulty "mamma," "papa," had great difficulty in pronouncing such combinations of syllables as paba, bapa, mana, nama; a particularly great effort was necessary before he could even produce the second consonant.

If the combinations consisted of consonants of different places of articulation—as in pata, pada, laka—then the patient read the words without effort.

A labial consonant took the place of another labial, or a cerebral of another cerebral.

Syllables with two consonants of the same place of articulation and one vowel between them (e.g., pab, tad, kag), which are difficult for normals to speak, were produced particularly badly, the second consonant not being pronounced at all or substituted by one similar to the first one.

From these and similar experiments, which may be found in the original paper, the authors concluded that the patient's difficulties in pronunciation originated from the fact that he had *the articulatoric total Gestalt but was impeded in producing finer differentiations in the latter* (p. 528). These studies are particularly important for understanding paraphasic distortions in motor aphasia.

The authors consider the disturbances in the field of speech as the same as in all other performance fields, namely as a result of a change of the form of function of the damaged brain matter. They characterize this basic formal change as "Stehenbleiben des psychischen Prozesses auf einer fruheren Phase seiner normalen Entwicklung und zwar in der Richtung von einem amorphen Gesamteindruck zu differenzierten und prägnanten Ausgestaltungen derselben" (a stoppage of the process in any performance before the end is reached which would correspond to the normal performance, and in direction going from an "amorphous" general reaction to more differentiated and precise ones).

From this it results that performances which can be executed in this "amorphous," general sphere may be well performed, but not those where a differentiation of particular parts within this whole is presupposition for correct performance.

From this viewpoint, the authors make particularly understandable the failures which become apparent in that form of paraphasia we call motor paraphasia. The causes for some forms of dysarthria are to be seen here, also.

They point out the similarity of the change in their patient to the change which Goldstein and Gelb have considered as the basis of the defects in their case of "visual agnosia" and of the change in the cases of Woerkom. They confirm the idea of Goldstein that in brain lesion it is not individual performances which are damaged, but functions, and that the individual performances in all fields are disturbed to the degree that their normal execution is dependent on the disturbed function (see p. 5).

Usually, one distinguishes strictly dysarthric disturbances from the *aphasic* disturbances by the definition that the aphasic patient has no paresis but has lost the capacity to use his muscles especially for the production of language; as the French authors say: "L'aphasique ne sait plus parler, l'anarthrique ne peut plus parler."

This *difference between dysarthria and motor aphasia* is not at all as clear as it is often stated, and does not do full justice to the complexity of the phenomena observed in patients.

Some patients cannot use the concerned muscles voluntarily in a definite way, either in language or in non-language performances; only the reflex movements are preserved. Such a patient may not be able to bring a piece of bread voluntarily by mouth and tongue movements to the pharynx, but in the moment it accidentally touches the latter or he brings it there by means of his hand, the reflex process of swallowing takes place normally. He may not be able to produce swallowing voluntarily. Likewise, he may not be able to produce any sound, but makes noises by pushing air through the vocal cords, etc.

Other patients are unable voluntarily to produce non-language movements, e.g., screwing up the mouth, closing the lips (as in pronouncing the letter m), moving the tongue voluntarily, puckering, etc., while they *can* produce these movements as *language* performances.

In a third group again, non-language actions can be performed but not language actions.

These different pictures can be understood if we consider that sometimes we are dealing with paresis, sometimes with apraxia or a combination of both. Both factors may have a different effect on language and non-language performances.

Paresis may show particularly in the motorically complicated language performances, and not so much in the other ones: apraxia—in the form of difficulty voluntarily to produce isolated movements—in defect of isolated non-language performances which we usually ask the patient to perform in our tests and which are difficult because we are not accustomed to produce them voluntarily. We have, on the other hand, learned to produce isolated sounds, and hence they may be easier to utter. Because it is easier to produce sounds in words, the patient may be able to produce the sounds thus, but not isolated. If paresis and apraxia exist combined, it may be very difficult to decide which defect is due to paresis, which to apraxia (see such cases from my hospital as described by W. Riese).

(2) *Motor Aphasia*

Now what do we call *motor aphasia*? I think we should reserve this term for that difficulty in uttering sounds and words which is due to a *defect of the learned specialized motor speech performances*, i.e., due to a *defect of definite motor "Gestalten,"* or of the function by which these motor complexes are built. By this we distinguish motor aphasia from apraxia of the speech muscles. There may be cases where the difficulty in speaking is due to apraxia. But this is not the usual clinical type of motor aphasia; both types should be disinguished separately. In the commoner type, the symptoms are the expression of dedifferentiation of motor speech performances. Only with this assumption do the symptoms become understandable and hence the success of treatment by training the motor performances (see p. 328). Such treatment is much less useful (or not at all) in cases where the defect is due to apraxia. This concept of motor aphasia does justice also to the anatomic findings which have been discussed so frequently and with which we shall deal later (see p. 199).

We can distinguish *two types of motor aphasia:* those cases where the previously acquired motor speech "Gestalten" is dedifferentiated, and those where building of new ones, i.e., the function of building them, is damaged. Usually we find a combination of both defects, but there are cases where particularly the process of building is damaged (see, regarding the relation of both forms of damage, p. 114).

In the first type, the patient in the beginning often shows a total lack of spontaneous speech as well as in repetition, reading aloud, etc. Some few words, even short sentences, uttered in emotional situations as "My God," "Mother," "Yes," "No," etc., some swear words (the recurring and occasional utterances noted by Jackson) may be preserved, but the patient is unable to utter even these intentionally.

With time, the sounds reappear more or less, usually in a definite sequence (see p. 000). (For understanding the sequence and other peculiarities of the speech of these patients, see the previous explanation, p. 000, concerning the structure of motor speech, its development in children, the phonologic character of the individual utterances which should be taken into consideration, etc.) The uttering of words gradually increases, but for a long time there remains difficulty in pronouncing the sounds correctly; this difficulty is often more notable with isolated sounds than in words or sentences. Even if the patient has regained a great number of words, he will omit in spontaneous speech definite word categories (which in repetition he may be able to speak), particularly if the omission does not hinder communication. In his speech we miss particularly the "small" words, prepositions, articles, etc., while names and verbs predominate. The patient speaks in *telegram style* (see p. 194). It is hard for him to find the grammatical forms; he prefers the simplest ones, for instance, infinitives (motor agrammatism). There are no disturbances of the syntactical structure. At this time the patient may be able to repeat most of the words, although more or less distorted by motor defects. The same situation may be observed in the speaking of series, which often is particularly disturbed.

The picture in the state of recovery is usually very complex, and each performance or defect is understandable only if one always takes into account the total situation in which it takes place, particularly the influence which the attitude of the patient has on the motor efficiency. The final result in cases with the best improvement may show that the patient is almost normal in the different aspects of speech, but his talking necessitates voluntary effort—it lacks, to some degree, the mechanical effortless character of the normal; the patient has to think too much in speaking (see the case reported on p. 195 ff).

Sometimes patients may *stutter*. This symptom is to be considered as an expression of the emotional distress into which the patient comes when he is aware of his defect. This condition is the same as most of the cases of stuttering in nonorganic conditions of psychologic origin. It is important to realize this because it must be considered in our procedure of retraining.

Reading ability is intact as far as understanding is concerned. *Reading aloud* shows similar defects as speaking, but is often better; it reveals motor defects, however. Although in some cases understanding is better when the patient reads aloud, at times the opposite may be true (see p. 82).

Writing is individually disturbed in different ways (see p. 131). The patient may be able to write some words correctly ("writing automatisms"), others not, or with the same mistakes as in speaking. Writing on dictation is often better than spontaneously. Copying is intact.

The degree of improvement depends upon a number of factors: extension and character of the lesion (traumatic lesions in general have a better prognosis than vascular ones), degree of cooperation of the other hemisphere, presence of more or less learned automatisms, the general psychologic and physiologic condition, retraining (see p. 325).

The use of instrumentalities can be impaired by *heightening of the threshold of excitability.* This is demonstrated *particularly in difficulties in voluntary speaking,* but less if speech is stimulated from the outside. It was Bastian who introduced (1898) the functional factor into the theory of aphasia for explanation of the different preservation of different performances in a defect of a "center." Although we do not agree with him in the concept of "center," he is correct in assuming that in the severest damage the brain matter does not react to any stimuli; in less severe damage, it reacts to direct sensible stimulation (not to voluntary or "associative" stimulation); in still lesser damage, to all stimulation except voluntary. Hence, even a gross lesion can damage the different functions in a different way. This corresponds with what we see in a recovering case of motor aphasia, namely, that the patient is able to repeat words or sounds which he is not able to speak spontaneously. This picture is usually called *transcortical motor aphasia.* As we will see later, this is only one way in which the picture of transcortical motor aphasia originates (see p. 293).

Concerning the *third group of symptoms,* in the expressive side of language, we should discuss first the modifications of motor speech due to sensory speech defects, a phenomenon which has often been discussed in the literature. According to a theory accepted by most authors, from the "classic" period of the study of aphasia until recently, motor speech depends upon acoustic experiences or residuals (see p. 83), and a defect of *the latter* is the *cause* of paraphasia.

(3) *The Origin of Paraphasia*

Wernicke considered the function of the motor speech area to depend upon the sensory speech area, our speaking to be controlled by the acoustic speech images.   Kussmaul, Freud, et al. assumed that speaking always follows in the path of these images; as Granich recently said, to formulate most words, we must have recourse to a "quiet" projection of the word as an auditory pattern—'re-auditorize' the word (p. 11).   I explained years ago (see 83) that this theory is theoretically untenable and not supported by clinical facts

There is no doubt that acoustic experiences play an important role in the development and normal use of speech, but not, however, in the starting or control of speaking; their function lies in the finer elaboration of pronunciation of sounds, rhythms of speech, etc.   Speaking is based on motor performances which are learned by motor activities.   The beginnings of speech in infants are active phenomena, are active motor performances, not imitations of heard sounds (see p. 35).   Later, for perfection of speech, the hearing of others' and one's own speech is important.   But lack of hearing does not disturb the structure of the word, the right position of the letters in the word, disturbances so characteristic for paraphasia.   In fluent speech, we do not experience acoustic speech images.   If, however, there occurs any difficulty, then we may refer to images and try to use them as a basis for speaking (see p. 26), and in this respect, intentional "re-auditorization" may be helpful for relearning.   But this does not justify the assumption that such re-auditorization plays an essential role in normal speaking.   The lack of images does not play any role as long as the motor activities are undisturbed.   Further, the assumed control would not, as I have explained previously, be useful because it would always come too late.   It could be effective only if there were an interval between the intention to utter a word and the actual utterance.   In everyday fluent speech, this is certainly not the case.   It is even disturbing if it occurs. If we want to say something and begin to think about the words, then our speaking is impeded; the words we utter may even become strange to us.

Experiences with patients give no evidence for the mentioned theory of paraphasia.   Generally speaking, observations of patients with sensory aphasia have been used as basis for this theory (see p. 87).

Before we discuss these observations, it is necessary to consider the phenomenon of paraphasia more carefully.   We shall then see that there are different forms with which to be dealt.

(a) In one form, the patient has difficulty in pronouncing even sounds and letters correctly; in attempting to speak motorically in a fluent manner, he hesitates, distorts letters, leaves one out because he is not able to pronounce it correctly, perseverates on others which he can speak, misplaces letters, etc.   This form of aphasia is due to motor difficulties.   It should be called *motor paraphasia*.   This form was carefully studied by Bouman and Grünbaum.   Because he is easily distressed due to his motor difficulty, the patient may stop speaking entirely, or try to find aids to

better speech.   One such helpful mechanism is the omission of some words
which the normal person would speak in a definite sentence.   To utter
all words would demand more energy then he could summon and he would
not be sure whether he could produce the words correctly enough to be
understood.   Therefore, some words are omitted.   These are not at all,
as one might think, the motorically most difficult ones, but rather those
which are not absolutely necessary for communication.   Thus, he is able to
concentrate on words which are important in this respect and to produce
them better.   This is one cause of motor agrammatism, the telegram style
(see p. 81), to which Isserlin has drawn attention.

There is another possibility utilized by the patient for improving his
speech: the use of speech images.   This may be a further cause of paraphasia.   Normals refer to images when they have difficulty in speaking a
word, i.e., to acoustic, visual and motor images.   The patient is often inclined to do likewise because his motor difficulties are constant.   This
becomes evident by the similarity of his paraphasic mistakes with the
deficiencies of the images of normals.   It is apparent particularly in writing
words on dictation, when a patient—who is accustomed to speak silently
before he writes—because of his defect in motor speech is not able to proceed in this way and copies his visual images of the words which he wants
to write.   Many paraphasic distortions can be explained in this way.

(b) One other *cause of paraphasic distortions is impairment of inner
speech.*   This will have to be discussed in more detail when we discuss dedifferentiation of this part of language.   Here I wish to mention only some
characteristics of this distortion of motor speech which differ from distortions due to the motor defect and its substitutes.   First, there are no real
motor distortions of the letters.   The characteristic hesitation of speech is
absent, the paraphasia does not occur so much in production of the learned
motor automatisms, series, etc.   On the other hand, there is more a lack of
letters or misplacing of the letters within the word in the foreground, the
rhythm and accentuation of the word is wrong.   The distortion and dis-
placement do not follow so much the laws we have seen effective in defect
of the *minor* hemisphere, but rather correspond to the dedifferentiation of
the "concepts" of words.   Usually, a verbal paraphasia exists beside the
literal paraphasia, i.e., wrong words are uttered which are, however, somehow related to the right ones.   This relation is not only that of similarity
as to motor or sensory structure but also as to meaning (see p. 23).

This form of paraphasia is the most frequent one.   It occurs in patients
with motor or sensory aphasia, if the lesion does not affect the motor or
sensory part of the speech area alone, but also the area important for inner
speech (see p. 249).

(4) *Central Motor Aphasia*

In this group of motor disturbances of speech, the patient's speech does not present severe motor speech defects; he may show some motor paraphasia (see p. 83), but pronounces many words correctly, even series.   In spite of this he is in general much more hindered in the use of language than the patients belonging to the other groups.   Particularly *spontaneous speech* is severely hindered, frequently almost *totally lacking*.   The spontaneity in general may be reduced, too, and the patient also shows mental defects other than language which reveal impairment of the abstract attitude (see p. 56).   While the patient may be able to speak if his speech occurs in the concrete attitude he may fail totally if he has to utter something in the abstract attitude.

I have called this form of aphasia *central motor aphasia* in contrast to the *peripheral motor aphasia* which corresponds to the usual type, the *pure motor aphasia*.   One could doubt whether it is justifiable to call these cases *motor* aphasia at all, because an essential cause of the difficulty in speaking is a defect in the non-speech mental processes.   However, the terminology seems to me justified (see p. 198), not only because the defect in speaking is in the foreground of the clinical picture but also because among the patients described as motor aphasia cases in the literature there is a considerable number who belong in this group.

This form of aphasia is similar to some cases where the defect of non-language mental performances is in the foreground.   The concerned patients are severely changed in all voluntary actions, and the defect of speaking is only the expression of this more general defect; the patients with the central form of motor aphasia are not so much damaged in general as these; the motor speech disturbances, on the other hand, are more in the foreground.   By the latter defect they gain similarity with the peripheral forms of motor aphasia, but differ from them by some peculiarities of the motor speech disturbances (see p. 208), and particularly by the lack of any non-speech mental defects.   The central motor aphasia, further, is similar to the before-mentioned form of "transcortical motor aphasia" (see p. 82) insofar as in both forms spontaneous speech is impaired, but the latter type is different because of the lack of general mental damage.

Table 1 presents a short review of the main symptoms in the various forms of motor aphasia which allow clinical differentiation.   This differentiation is important because the underlying anatomic processes and the prospects for spontaneous improvement and retraining are different.

The mentioned form of transcortical motor aphasia is very often of traumatic origin, or due to tumor abscess and similar processes pressing on the brain.   Sponanteous improvement takes place, if the cause is elimi-

TABLE 1.—*The Main Symptoms in Various Forms of Motor Aphasia which Permit Clinical Differentiation*

	I. PERIPHERAL MOTOR APHASIA	II. DAMAGE OF MOTOR SPEECH AREA WITH TRANSCORTICAL MOTOR SYMPTOMATOLOGY	III. CENTRAL MOTOR APHASIA
Spontaneous speech	Severely diminished, but intention to speak great. The patient *tries to speak*, even though the words he utters are motorically defective. Sounds and words show severe motor defects.	*Severely diminished:* what the patient speaks does not show severe motor defect.	*Severely reduced, often totally lacking.* Motor defects present, but not so outspoken as in I.
Conversational speech	Not essentially better than spontaneous speech.	Better than spontaneous speech.	Much better than spontaneous speech.
Voluntary effort	Improves speech. No involuntary movements of the lips in the attempt to speak. Voluntary movements show 'trial and error.'	Does not improve speech.	Does not improve speech. Correct involuntary movements of the lips in the attempt to speak. No possibility to repeat words voluntarily.
Motor series	Particularly defective. Presentation of the first members does not improve performance.	Presentation of the first members improves performance but there remain difficulties.	Impossible to begin, but, when the first members are presented, often continuation with normal rhythm and few motor defects.
Repetition	Sometimes better than spontaneous speech, but *in principle the same defect.*	*Much better than spontaneous speech.*	Much better than spontaneous speech.
Grammar	Telegram style. Grammatical forms damaged.	—	Telegram style, but motor grammatical forms not severely defective.
Non-language mental performances	Intact.	Intact.	Defective, particularly impairment of abstract attitude.

nated.   The central motor aphasia can have various causes, the region
between frontal lobe and motor speech area being affected; prognosis depends on the character of the underlying process, but is in general poor,
and great improvement by training is not to be expected.   The usual motor
aphasia is commonly due to a vascular lesion, and prognosis varies widely
(see p. 199).   Improvement by retraining is often very successful.

(5) *Severe Motor Aphasia Due to Lesions in the Temporal Lobes*

Mingazzini has described (1908) three cases of bilateral lesion of the
temporal lobe which showed, beside word-deafness, a severe motor aphasia.
The patients were able only to utter a few syllables in an explosive way.
Similar observations were published by Liepmann, Niessl von Meyendorf,
Agosta, Ugolotti and others.   Mingazzini considered the motor defect as
a consequence of bilateral destruction of the "acoustic word center,"
which, indeed, he considered localized not only in the posterior two-fifths
of the first and second temporal convolutions but for which he claimed
Heschl's convolutions also, and possibly the posterior half of the Isle of
Reil.   Broca's convolution can, deprived of all acoustic impulses, in his
opinion guarantee only very primitive performances, which are to be
considered similar to the first sounds of the infant.   Niessl von Meyendorf,
who considers "paraphasia" as a product of the right acoustic word center,
assumes that not paraphasia but word-muteness occurs under the mentioned condition.

If the defect in the acoustic sphere were really the cause of paraphasia and
word-muteness, one could expect that the motor speech would become more
outspoken if the acoustic sphere were more severely damaged.   As Bonvicini (21) has stressed, this is not the case.   He mentions correctly that
even bilateral lesions of the posterior parts of T I and T II or diffuse processes of both temporal lobes must not be accompanied by paraphasia or
other changes of motor speech.   That, on the other hand, some patients
with temporal lesions show paraphasia or so-called jargonaphasia there is
no doubt.   It seems that in those cases where more muteness than paraphasia was present the lesion was more extended and affected both Heschl's
convolutions and the inferior parietal lobe (cases of Berger, Bischoff, Mills,
Mott, Liepmann, Bonvicini).   Liepmann held the opinion that this was
explained by the fact that in these cases the motor speech area was deprived
of all sensory stimuli and therefore did not function.   I believe that the
severe motor aphasia was due to the fact that in the extended lesions also
the central speech area was set out of function.   We know that in central
aphasia, motor speech is particularly affected.   This may be especially
true if both areas are damaged, as we can assume in these cases.

The cases of severe motor aphasia in bilateral temporal lesions are certainly not explained sufficiently. Further studies of such cases are very desirable.

F. DISTURBANCES OF THE RECEPTIVE SIDE OF LANGUAGE

Understanding of heard language is based on perception of sounds and sound complexes. Sensory aphasia exists if sound and sound complexes are perceived in a normal way but are not *recognized as language*, or, if this is the case, are not comprehended in their *meaning*. Three forms of sensory aphasia have been distinguished: *pure word deafness*, where sounds are not recognized as language; *sensory aphasia proper* ("cortical" sensory aphasia, Wernicke's sensory aphasia), a complex picture where perception of sounds as language is somewhat preserved, but not so well that the patient would be able adequately to recognize the heard language—he cannot perceive the heard words in order to recognize what they mean. This sensory defect is accompanied by other speech defects, particularly paraphasia. In a third form, the so-called *transcortical sensory aphasia*, perception of language is perfect, but the words do not evoke the right meaning.

This distinction is somewhat theoretic, although there is no doubt that in different cases the defect of one or another of the above mentioned performances may be in the foreground.

It cannot be said definitely how much hearing is necessary to guarantee appreciation of speech sounds, i.e., to recognize them as known speech. Word deafness should not be assumed if it is not proved that the patient hears enough to perceive the sound complexes underlying speech.

It is widely assumed that for recognizing sound complexes as language the normal perception of at least b^1–g^2 (the so-called "sixth" of speech) is presupposition (Bezold). Probably one octave higher or lower has to be heard. But not only the correct distinction of tones is necessary, but also a definite intensity and duration of perception of the tones. Sensory aphasia can be assumed only when perception in this respect has proved normal. Indeed, much work will be necessary before we shall be sure about this relation of hearing tones and perceiving language sounds as such.

These speech sound complexes represent phenomena of the type of "Gestalt." How the system of acoustic "Gestalten" is dedifferentiated in pathology is not yet well known. Here again further studies are necessary. The expression of this dedifferentiation is *pure word deafness*. The presence to some degree of other speech disturbances in a case does not speak against the assumption of word deafness. These disturbances may be secondary to this defect (as lack of writing to dictation, lack of repetition), or the effect of other concomitantly existing defects. Each observed speech defect present in a case has to be evaluated in respect to the primary disturbance of speech-sound-Gestalten, whether or not it has anything at all to do with the latter.

This, indeed, is often not easy to decide. It may be considered as a criterion of distinction that deaf patients try to repeat the distorted perceived sound complexes, while patients with sensory aphasia do not make this attempt, or, when urged, do it very hesitatingly (see p. 217). It speaks further against primary defect in hearing when the patient perceives some words—and always the same words—correctly and others never, and when this phenomenon is not related to defect of definite tones. Particularly if the patient perceives some words but not acoustically very similar ones, we are dealing with an aphasic patient. One of my German patients, for instance, always understood the word "hund" (dog) and never the similar one "hut" (hat).

There is a relation of acoustic speech-Gestalten to other acoustic Gestalten, as noises or music. The different acoustic phenomena are certainly not isolated from each other; they are different expressions of the activity of the *acoustic perceptual sphere*. Whether all acoustic Gestalten are disturbed or only some depends upon the degree of dedifferentiation of the sphere. Usually in word-deafness, appreciation of other noises is preserved, although not always in full degree. When both forms of noise appreciation are affected, usually speech sound Gestalten are more disturbed than the other noise Gestalten. But even this is not always true, inasmuch as sometimes certain speech sounds may be recognized, certain noise Gestalten not. Here again, further studies are necessary in respect to the greater or smaller complexity of each preserved or disturbed phenomenon. Such studies should consider the different, even individually varying familiarities with the concerned phenomena, etc.

Thus, already, the correct appreciation of the effect of dedifferentiation in the perceptive acoustic sphere faces us with a very complex problem. The difficulty increases if we include the problem of *understanding of the meaning of the word*. Meaningful understanding is not at all in direct relation to the correct hearing of the word, for even defectly perceived words may transmit meaning. On the other hand, meaning can be disturbed by damage of factors which have nothing to do with the appreciation of the heard word (see p. 23).

In the unitary process of understanding heard language, we distinguish somewhat abstractively phenomena like speech perception and speech understanding which normally never exist separately as such. Only under special conditions are we normally aware of the acoustic phenomena, i.e., if we are especially interested in them, or if the process of understanding is not running normally as when we hear a foreign language. Meaning is usually in the foreground if we hear somebody speak.

In pathology, this unitary process can be dedifferentiated in different ways. The different symptom complexes correspond to different states of dedifferentiation whereby the general rule is valid that the more complicated phenomena suffers. But whether a performance is disturbed or not in a special degree of dedifferentiation depends not only on the dedifferentiation in the acoustic speech realm but also on the relation of each performance to other performance fields, but in conjunction with the activity of the total organism and with the condition in which speech occurs. A word may be purely perceived and cannot be repeated, but it may be effective enough in the sphere of meaning, so that as reaction to the heard word, another word may be uttered which belongs to the same sphere (see p. 226). This is only one example which points to the significance of the total situation—inside and outside of the individual—for understanding, this must be considered carefully to understand a concerned symptom.

We owe to A. Pick's careful investigations the distinction of different steps of defects in appreciation of heard language which a patient may show in relation to different degrees of damage of the acoustic speech sphere. The complex process of understanding speech may be stopped at various steps and patients may, accordingly, present different pictures. The following brief survey concerns these different possibilities by which the process may be disturbed, and confirms, in the main, Pick's investigations.

In severest damage the patient may not react to speech sounds at all; he may show a lack of attention to them especially. Under such circumstances, he may perceive speech sounds as noises, as unknown alien noises, or he may differentiate them from other noises without recognizing them as speech. Sometimes he has the impression that he is confronted with a foreign language. Polyglot aphasic patients may recognize their mother tongue as language, other known languages as unknown sounds or words. Even if the patient recognizes sounds as language, he may not understand the words, or is unable to repeat them. He may grasp some sounds but not the words, or he perceives the words if they are not spoken too quickly. He may recognize them only if they are spoken in a pronunciation known to him, e.g., if they are spoken by somebody belonging to his part of the country, but not if spoken in another regional dialect, and still less by a foreigner.

The words may be grasped as known but not understood. A patient may repeat words which he understands, not those he does not understand. If he is forced to repeat them he shows defects in repetition. The patient may not realize that a word presented some time before is the same when presented a short time later.

He may be able to repeat automatically sounds or words in an echolalic way without understanding them. Repetition may occur more voluntarily, and the words may be understood after repetition. In this state, the word may be understood only under certain conditions, for instance if the word belongs to an object he sees, or if he is confronted with it among other words, or if it belongs to the situation in which the patient is and in which he has understood certain other words.   Sometimes understanding of the word may improve the acoustic perception of the words secondarily.   The patient may not yet be able to perceive the word so well that he is able to understand it or to repeat it, but sufficiently enough so that the sphere of meaning to which it belongs is elicited, and the patient may summon up another word belonging to this sphere.

The different word categories are not all understood in the same way. In a state where a patient may understand a great number of words, he may not understand the "small" words.   He may not be able to repeat them, even to differentiate between different words which are presented to him (see p. 68).   The same words may be repeated if presented in a sentence which the patient understands.

The relations between defects in understanding of words and of sentences cannot be characterized in a general way.   Words are often better comprehended than sentences, but the opposite may be the case, too.   In this case, the word is not understood if presented separately, but only in connection with others in a meaningful sentence, particularly if the sentence is related to the situation.   If a sentence contains a number of words which present difficulty for understanding and these words represent the essential parts of the sentence, the patient may understand some of the words better if individually presented than within the sentence.   If some words within the sentence—particularly in a definite situation—suggest the meaning of the whole sentence, these words are better grasped in the sentence than presented separately.

Our knowledge of the behavior of patients in dedifferentiation of the perceptive side of language undergoing increasing damage is certainly incomplete.   Nevertheless, observation along these lines will show that the occurrence of a special defect is not at all dependent only upon the degree of damage but rather upon a number of other factors which all must be taken into consideration for the understanding of any individual performance of a patient.

It would be very useful if in cases with increasing or decreasing damage of the substrate, exact and continuous protocols about the behavior of the patient would be taken.

Disturbances of understanding can occur even if the instrumentalities are not damaged.   They then are due to a "loss of meaning" as in amnesic aphasia (see p. 246) and to a damage of the processes of thinking—so-called transcortical sensory aphasia (see p. 293).

G. Disturbances of Inner Speech

The term "inner speech" is often used ambiguously in the literature. The reason for this is, on the one hand, the fact that the term originated in research of two different disciplines, in philosophy of speech and in psychology, particularly psycho-pathology of speech; on the other hand, because the complexity of the underlying processes gives rise to considerable misunderstanding.

The interest of philosophers and psychologists in the problem of the inner processes which precede speaking differed, and led them to place different phenomena into the foreground.   To avoid misunderstanding, it is of paramount importance to make clear what one has in mind.   Unfortunately, different phenomena were often named with the same word.   One should distinguish between the phenomena meant in philosophy of speech and term them "inner speechform," according to W. v. Humboldt who has created this term ("innere Sprachform"), and inner speech" with which term are designated the psychologic phenomena which we experience and which are disturbed in some aphasic patients.

W. v. Humboldt considered as "innere Sprachform" the structure of language which, according to his investigations, reflects the special way in which people who speak a language look at the world, grasp the world and are accustomed to communicate their own feelings, thinking, etc., to their fellowmen.   It corresponds to the specific "world perspective" of a people in language.   This is expressed in a special organization of the forms, by which general communication with other people by language takes place (the special way how tenses, flexions, articles, are used, time and space are expressed, combinations of words to new words are used, the preference which is given to words of general character or words for concrete experience, the difference in rhythm, sentence formation, etc.).

When we speak here of "inner speechform," we do not mean the inner experiences of the individual who speaks or understands language, but his system of forms.   It differs not only as to different languages but—at least to a certain degree—also as to different groups which speak the same language, even as to individuals.   The special attitude with which the group or the individual looks at the facts of life, the special interest and communicative behavior in general, finds expression in peculiarities in the structure of their means of communication, in their language.

Our knowledge of the inner speechform may become more valuable for our problems if the phenomena observed in a patient are compared with the peculiarities of the variation of inner speechform in different languages. Until now, this has found little consideration in research of aphasia.

Inner speech belongs to the experiences which precede speaking, and is elicited by the hearing of speech.   According to the differences of opinion concerning the structure of these phenomena, inner speech has been considered differently.   For those authors for whom the central phenomenon of speech is images, inner speech was silent speech, silent experiencing of images.   Thus, Dejerine wrote: "Notre langage intérieur s'effectue à l'aide des images auditives et motrices, et c'est l'union intime de ces deux espèces d'images qui constitue ce que l'on appelle la notion de mot."   According to Charcot, we have to distinguish different types of individuals as to the paramount role which acoustic or visual or motor images play in their mental life.   Following this concept, it was assumed that in some individuals inner speech consists especially of images of one or the other kind.   Most of the authors, as, for instance, Bastian, Kussmaul, considered acoustic images as the most important constituents of inner speech (see p. 83), a theory which, up to the present, has had many adherents.

Wernicke—dissatisfied with this concept—tried, on the basis of new experiences with aphasic patients, to define inner speech as a special association complex composed of motor and sensory images.   He distinguished this complex from the motor and sensory processes in language and termed it "Wortbegriff" (concept of the word).   Since that time, the problem of inner speech has usually been discussed in the form of "concept of the word."   For normal speaking and understanding, the "Wortbegriff" must be intact.   Characteristic symptoms of a defect of the "Wortbegriff" were for Wernicke paraphasia, disturbance of reading and writing.   Later (1906) he brought additionally the disturbances in understanding in motor aphasia (to which Dejerine had pointed) into connection with a defect of inner speech.   This explanation did not find general acceptance.   Wernicke himself later abandoned this theory.   Kleist at first followed Wernicke.   The two components of which the "Wortbegriff" consists were to him even more closely, inextricably linked together.   But Kleist, too, later relinquished this idea. In a very interesting paper which did not find as much attention as it deserved, S. Freud spoke of a unitary phenomenon as the center of language, in which associations take place "in a complex way which we can no longer understand."   Around this unitary phenomenon, the sensory and motor language phenomena are grouped.

In contradiction to all these concepts, another concept of inner speech was emphasized by Storch (288) and myself (83).   This concept denied that the "Wortbegriff" is composed of images; it denied the significance of any such association-phenomena and considered the *Wortbegriff as an experience in principle different from sensory and motor phenomena.*   Storch worte: "My inner experience knows only of concepts of words which sometimes are awakened by acoustic stimuli, sometimes precede phonetic innervations and come to the fore in discharge of motor phenomena."*   I myself characterized this central phenomenon of language in a similar way. It was scarcely possible at that state of our knowledge to describe it in

*Translated by this author.

very positive terms.   More important was its usefulness in describing some clinical symptom complexes in a clearer way than before.   It was particularly the occurrence of the so-called plus-symptoms in sensory and motor aphasia (see 87 and 96) which could not be explained as secondary to defects in acoustic and motor speech processes, and which found a new interpretation as expressions of a defect of a special psycho-physical phenomenon which I saw in the "Wortbegriff."   That we are dealing with a symptom complex which is not secondary to motor or sensory aphasia is evident from the fact that it can persist after the motor or sensory disturbances have disappeared and that it can occur without such disturbances at all.   The symptom complex of so-called "Leitungsaphasia" (conduction aphasia) now found a new and plausible interpretation by the assumption that we are dealing with the effect of damaged inner speech.   I called the symptom complex *central aphasia* because inner speech seems to me to be the *central phenomenon of instrumentalities of speech.   Inner speech is the totality of processes and experiences which occur when we are going to express our thoughts, etc., in external speech and when we perceive heard sounds as language*.   Inner speech is, on the one hand, in relation to the "non-language mental processes" (see p. 104), on the other hand, to the external instrumentalities (external speech).   The first relation finds its expression in the organization of inner speech according to the "inner speechform," in the selection of definite word categories by a special language, in its syntactical forms and in its grammatical structure, in the adaptation of the particular speech to the general and special situation in which it takes place, its dependence upon the environment, the listener, etc.   It has a definite character when we speak to somebody whom we can expect to have in general the same attitude towards the things we are talking about, who grasps the present situation and the means of communication in the same way as we do.   Correspondingly, we omit words, we stress others, we form the sentences in a special way, etc.   Inner speech differs in a definite way when we speak to ourselves, when we read or write, when in writing we want to communicate with somebody we do not know, and even when we expect to have an individual reader of whom we cannot be sure whether he is in a condition to understand only hinted contexts.   The words written may have a different meaning for writer and reader; therefore, we have to express ourselves in another way than in speaking, if we want to be understood.

All these characteristics of inner speech are determined also by its relation to the structure of the non-language mental processes.   Therefore, the correct formation of inner speech will occur only if the processes of thinking are correct.   The speaker must have an adequate insight into the whole situation, the relation between speaker and listener and insight regarding the development of speech of himself and the hearer.   In abnormalities of these non-language mental processes of the speaker, definite speech disturbances occur (see p. 292).

The relation to the external instrumentalities produces other characteristics of inner speech. The phenomena of inner speech are not at all mirrored by the motor and sensory instrumentalities. The latter have their own systematic structure, as we have explained before (see p. 74).

Inner speech and instrumentalities are not always developed equally. Special development of one or the other modifies speech. If motor speech is particularly developed, then it gains a certain independence, and speech may be determined by motor automatisms, stimulated by thinking but not following the finer organization of inner speech. The speaker may cover a lack of development of inner speech by excessive and rapid speaking. Thus, some phenomena observed in patients with damage of inner speech find an explanation (see p. 208). Poor development of motor speech, on the other hand, may hinder the expression of the processes in inner speech and may hence secondarily impair the process of thinking, etc.

The complexity of the problem of inner speech makes it understandable that we must look for further information concerning its structure. Such we may find in observation of language in infancy.

There is general agreement that the words of the infant are closely related to individual objects. A particular word is a kind of property of a certain object, just as the object has other properties, and the word accompanies activities performed with the object. Such words can scarcely be separated from the object; they do not "represent" objects, they are not "names" (see p. 61), have no meaning in the sense of the words of grownups.

Correspondingly, it is to be assumed that the inner experience of the child in using or hearing language will differ from that of the grown-up.

Already the development of the first sounds shows that they belong closely to the immediate relationship between the child and the environment (see p. 38). They are "social" phenomena, indeed of a very primitive type. The child and the world around him are not separated; the child's activities are embedded in a unitary totality of himself and the environment. This concerns language, too. If the child is aware of his speech at all, this may be experience of motor and sensory phenomena belonging to a state of satisfaction in his trend to come to terms with the environment.

This interpretation of the language of the child in the first state of development of speech is not in accord with the interpretation of such an excellent expert of child psychology as Piaget. He calls this first speech "egocentric" speech and considers it an event which is not determined by a relation between child and environment. The child thinks and speaks for himself. It is for this reason that his language is so incomprehensible for the adult. His "speech," as it were, has no function of its own and decreases gradually with the development of social contacts of the child. It changes at about school age. Language becomes more and more socialized and thus understandable. From the organismic point of view, it is not very probable that, in a state of life which is so important for the child's development in general, it should have a language which has no special function in this development. This seems to make Piaget's concept somewhat implausible. This concept has been criticized particularly by Vigotsky on the basis of observations and experiments with children and, as I think, in a convincing way.

Vigotsky points to the difference in the development of the semantic aspect of speech and the external, the vocal aspect. The child first speaks in words which it combines later into sentences. It proceeds thus from less complex to more complex phenomena as far as the external performance in concerned. Concerning the development of meaning of these words, the development takes an opposite direction. The words have the meaning of sentences, which idea was particularly stressed by W. Stern. Only later does the child perceive the meaning of individual words, learns to "direct his formerly undifferentiated thoughts into a series of separate verbal meanings." These facts show the discrepancy between the development of semantic speech and external speech. "Egocentric" speech of children is related, according to Vigotsky, to inner speech, it "does not merely accompany the child's activity but serves the purpose of mental orientation of conscious understanding, of overcoming of difficulties and obstacles" (p. 38.). It is from the beginning a social phenomenon. "It increases when in the course of an activity difficulties arise which demand consciousness and reflection." Between the third and seventh years, the general "egocentric" attitude of the child gradually disappears, language— if it were egocentric in the sense of Piaget—should diminish and the child's language should become more understandable. This is what Piaget has asserted. Vigotsky has tried to study the phenomena under conditions which weaken and strengthen the social situation, and has shown that in the first case "egocentric" speech diminishes, in the latter it increases. The "illusion of understanding" is functionally connected with egocentric speech, and is important for its appearance. If the child *cannot experience that his speaking is understood, speaking diminishes* and vice versa. Vigotsky has given evidence that Piaget's assertions are not in accord with observations. The speech of the child of seven is less intelligible than that of the child of three. "Egocentric" speech diminishes, but "behind the symptom of dissolution (decrease of egocentric speech) lies a progressive development, lies the formation of a new speech. . . . It is a speech which abstracts from the sound, which imagines words instead of pronouncing them" (see

304, p. 40). Speech is now, one could say, more and more a phenomenon of inner life, which can be transformed into external speech according to the demands of the situation, but which the individual is no longer forced to externalize, as the child did before. With increasing individualization, i.e., distinction of the ego and the world, speech (transformation of thoughts into language) becomes more and more an internal phenomenon, it detaches itself more and more from the external instrumentalities.

The inner speech in the first state of development is much more closely related to these instrumentalities. They are very necessary for the attempt to come into, and remain in contact with the environment. This contact is of paramount importance for this state of development. Therefore, the instrumentalities develop enormously during this time, even those which currently have no meaning for the child but which it can use like other objects in a practical way. It is a known phenomenon, particularly stressed by Piaget, that the child possesses a number of words long before he understands their meaning, e.g., "because," "in spite of," and others. We observe a similar discrepancy when we learn a foreign language as adults. We use a number of words or sentences correctly, i.e., fitting a definite situation, without completely understanding their meaning. We have experienced their usefulness as a means of coming to terms with the situation, but did not understand the "meaning of the situation." We may, therefore, make severe mistakes when the situation appears the same to us but possibly means something totally different and therefore demands another interpretation by language. Our inner speech in such occasions is similar to that of the child.

According to the concept of Vigotsky, Piaget's "egocentric" speech is the predecessor of the later speech and is transformed into the inner speech of the adult. I would prefer to say that the inner speech of the child (which corresponds to the behavior of the child in general) is from the beginning a social phenomenon, and is transformed into the inner speech of the grownup (corresponding to the behavior of the grown-up in general), particularly in regard to his different social relations.

We note what is going on in inner speech in an individual, if we cannot get direct information from the speaker, by observing the special form of external speech. This information is impossible to obtain in children and not very reliable in grownups. At any rate, there has not been much research in this respect, and thus we must depend on the external speech. The language of the child corresponds to the primitive way in which he is able to understand the total situation and the way he reacts to this situation in which his speaking takes place. The language of the grownup is determined by his totally different insight into the situation and changes according to the differences of the latter (see p. 196). Inner and external speech always changes in such a way that the apparent speech allows for best self realization in the given situation.

With the development of the child, i.e., increasingly better adjustment to the total situation, the inner speech frees itself more or less from the dependence upon external speech. The speech of the grownup shows—in spite of the fact that it increasingly acquires external instrumentalities—more or less restrictions in this respect. Here the correspondence is to the structure of inner speech which does not at all contain in detail everything which one wishes to say. Contrariwise, there is a selection by an adaptation to meaningful interpretation of the total situation. Vigotsky has pointed in this respect to the specific tendency toward abbreviation, for instance, by preserving the predicate and omitting the subject and words connected with it, which does not disturb understanding, but rather alleviates it because it takes the situation of the listener, his expectations, into consideration.

I agree with the concept of inner speech developed by Vigotsky not only because it is supported by good evidence but also because it is in conformity with the ideas about human behavior in general and language in particular which seem to me most accurately to represent the facts. It also seems pertinent to me to understand, at least to a certain degree, some symptom complexes which we are inclined to consider as expression of dedifferentiation of inner speech and to give hints as to how they should be studied further.

There is much evidence that the speech of patients has the character more of communication with others than of "speaking to oneself"; it has lost its adequacy to the total situation (a characteristic of normal inner speech); it is abnormally determined by the acquired and preserved instrumentalities; the modification which our speaking goes through by the organization of inner speech is more or less lost. The syntactical organization, for instance, is determined more by the motor automatisms to the patient's proposal than by the structure developed in the normal inner speech. The "fundamental syntactical form of inner speech" (Vigotsky) is disturbed, the patient's speech may contain even more words than normal speech under the same conditions—if he has the corresponding automatisms and is determined more by them. The reduction which inner speech makes possible is impaired. The defect then is compensated, if that is possible, by an increase of speaking.

In pathology, there is often a great discrepancy between inner speech and external speech. The external instrumentalities can be defective (as in motor aphasia, see p. 190), though inner speech may not be altered; inner speech can be disturbed (as in central aphasia) without motor speech being correspondingly disturbed; the motor automatisms then gain an abnormal independence (see p. 229).

All the phenomena we have mentioned represent modifications of the *function* of inner speech in normal speech. Besides these functions we have to consider that inner speech consists also of *material fixed more or less by previous functioning of the "apparatus," by experience.* The concepts of letters, words, phrases, are more or less fixed wholes, patterns which we are aware of *in the framework of an inner speech attitude* and used as wholes to start the speaking activity. These patterns are developed to a different degree in different individuals. They can be impaired to a greater or less degree in dedifferentiation of inner speech. In this field, dedifferentiation follows also the laws of impairment of figure and ground configuration valid for pathology in general (see p. 5).

The word is normally experienced as a phenomenon of a characteristic structure in which the sounds follow in a definite sequence; it is not composed of parts, it is experienced as a simultaneous whole of a definite structure. This applies for speaking, not writing or reading.

In pathology, the character of simultaneousness is lost (simultaneousness suffers early in damage of the brain, see p. 118), and the word is dissolved into different parts, into letters or syllables; or, again, one part experienced before as background may gain the character of figure and gain abnormal importance. The first part of the word may still be well structured, the other part partly or totally lost or destroyed, etc. The individual must proceed in a successive fashion—the legato is lost and he has to proceed in staccato, as Rieger has put it. The result of the different ways in which the word is destroyed is a great variety of abnormalities of the word.

The word may possess the previous length, rhythm, some characteristic outstanding sounds, but the inner structure is loosened or even broken up. The parts of which the word consists do not occur immediately in the right sequence. The first part of the word may be produced correctly but then disorder takes place. Some letters may fall out totally, others come to the fore abnormally and at the wrong place. This destruction of words produces certain characteristic phenomena of literal paraphasia: omission of letters, misplacing of correct letters, occurrence of incorrect letters due to increased "assimilation" as an expression of dedifferentiation, premature end of the word, etc. But this is not the whole story. The patient will try to perform as well as possible. If he experiences failure in proceeding in the customary way, i.e., speaking according to his previous "simultaneous" capacities, he will try to compensate by proceeding in the successive way. He will attempt to use the different means whichare at his disposal: images of different kinds, visual, motor, etc. (see p. 28). This may help him to a certain degree but it will also produce some new characteristic failures which correspond to the *deficiency* of *normal* images. One part of the paraphasic defects is due to this procedure (see p. 84).

When we speak about fixed patterns, we should not forget that the maintenance of the pattern is guaranteed by the ability to control them, as is the case for all patterns (see p. 8). If this control by impairment of the function of inner speech is missing, the pattern will suffer. The control is diminished because of the impairment of the analyzing and combining function, which is a characteristic defect in brain damage. This function is particularly important for reading and writing. The spoken or heard word must be broken down into components when we learn to read and write; and when later we want to read and write unknown words, these components must again be combined to words. In fluent reading, we are not aware of all parts, we recognize the words more or less as characteristic wholes. But if there is any hindrance for this whole-recognition, e.g., if we are confronted with "unfamiliar" words, we have to analyze and synthesize. If the normal procedure is impaired in patients, the symptom of *paralexia* results. The defect becomes still more apparent in writing. Writing is an active motor procedure in which the complicated synthesizing function plays a particular role. Thus we see that in damage of inner speech, *disturbances of writing* are often the first symptoms to appear.

The defects in reading and writing can be compensated to a certain degree also. The patient may be able to recognize the visual picture of a word as a known whole and thus understand its meaning and even be able to speak it; but he is not able to "read" it in the proper sense of the word (see p. 312). He proceeds as children do when they "read" words in their first reader. Sometimes he may recognize the meaning without being able to pronounce the word aloud. It is evident that some further failures in reading may occur by wrong recognition of the picture of the word.

Writing can be compensated by motor patterns which the patient has acquired before, and thus he may be able to write a word as a whole, but not in parts. This writing may then not show the paraphasia his speech presents. But this will concern usually only a few words. The patient writes them in, as it were, a circuitous, round-about way, avoiding inner speech. If this is impossible, writing will show particularly paraphasic defects even more than does speaking. How much writing is preserved or disturbed will depend on the patient's premorbid capacity to write words as wholes.

Copying will be better than spontaneous writing, particularly if the patient copies each letter. If we hinder him in this activity, copying will show paraphasia, too.

From our remarks about the reading and writing of these patients, it will appear evident that the patients will show definite *failure in tests of spelling of words and combining presented letters into words*. Here, too, some substitution is possible which in turn may produce failures by the defi-

ciency of the substitutive procedure.   The patient may spell by "sounding,"
pronouncing one sound of a word after the other quickly, i.e., using a motor
procedure (see p. 210).   Patients very much skilled in typewriting may
"spell" in this test very well.   They produce simply the motor series which
they maybe accustomed to speak before typing (see p. 272).   In both cases
one will find that the patient may be unable to repeat these sounds or letters
with intervals between them or to spell in naming the letters.   This shows
that his seemingly good performances are not real spelling.   The defect in
combining the letters into words can be substituted somewhat by visualization.   The patient may simply name the letters he visualized (see p. 145).

The damage of the concepts of words will produce *verbal* paraphasia also
(see p. 229).   The phenomenal analysis performed by Lotmar has shown
that the *inability to grasp the right word makes the patient enter the sphere of*
non-speech mental processes and summon up a word corresponding to the
sphere of the demanded word, if this new word is, for any reason, easier to
produce.

Our patients will be particularly inclined to such a digression in the
sphere of thinking, because this is a sphere which is not disturbed, the sphere
of meaning.   In this procedure, there are a number of ideas which in normal reactions (in the process of reacting to a presented word or of finding
a word) are in the background, in the "fringes"; but here these ideas come
to the fore because the procedure lacks a definite direction.   Why one or
the other idea becomes prominent, why one or the other word is uttered,
is not easy to say; however it may be, we shall not discuss it here, but in
this respect attention should be drawn again to the interesting paper of
Lotmar.

There is another phenomenon to be observed in the verbal paraphasia of
these patients, namely that the *wrong words are uttered often with less para-*
phasia than the right ones.   This is a frequent observation.   Stengl has
stressed it and given an explanation based on findings in association experiments which he has performed in his patient.   In addition, in these experiments, the patient did not show paraphasia as to the same words which he
uttered distorted in repetition.   Apparantly the defect of the patient did
not have the same influence on words which were uttered under these conditions.   Stengl has tried to explain the difference by the assumption that
thinking without direction is increased in these patients because there is a
relative increase of "Sphaerenbewusstsein" (the processes in the "sphere")
and these less directed activities (as those in verbal paraphasia and in the
association experiment) are not so much influenced by the defect of the
patient, which concerns particularly the directed behavior.   I agree in
general with this interpretation of the author and should like to describe
the phenomena in the terminology of my general point of view as follows:

In the performance where patients show paraphasia, in spontaneous speech, repetition, finding words as names they have to react in a definite way directed by a definite attitude and voluntary impulse. Concomitantly with such reaction processes, others, of a more passive, involuntary character, are going on in the background; they are represented by words, ideas, in the "fringes." If, by a defect of the directed reactions, it is the understandable trend of the patient to find a way out of his distress, he looks for substitutions; it is then that these processes in the fringes become more active and performances corresponding to them become more apparent. They are only slightly (if at all) "directed," emerge more passively and are therefore not so altered by the defect of the patient which affects particularly the directed performances. The same is true in the association experiments, in which the subject behaves in a less directed, more passive way. By this interpretation, we bring the behavior of the patient into relation with a phenomenon which we observe again and again in pathology: the disturbance of voluntary processes and the coming to the fore of more automatized phenomena (see p. 98).

The findings of Stengl are of such great significance not only because they explain why the words in verbal paraphasia show little or no literal paraphasia, but also because they present new facts for the correctness of this interpretation of pathologic phenomena in general; and finally, because they point to the close relationship between inner speech and the non-language mental processes, which we have stressed before. In the future, more association experiments should be performed in aphasic patients.

A similar interpretation may be found for the fact that sometimes in hypnosis or in slight sodium amytal narcosis, the patients speak better.

Even if the patient may finally find the right word, the time may be so prolongated that under certain conditions where retardation may bring the patient into distress, he prefers to utter the wrong word. Hence, the same word may sometimes show verbal or literal paraphasia, while under other conditions it will not.

The difficulty in finding the *right* word and the confusion which this and the destruction of the words themselves produce, will increase the disturbances of the grammatical form of speech which already is disturbed (as we have mentioned before) by the defect in the general function of inner speech (see p. 98).

From what we have said it will be understandable that the patients with this disorder always show a more or less considerable lack of *spontaneous speech*. They may, as much as possible, avoid speaking at all because they have a great difficulty to overcome and they will never be sure whether or not they are making mistakes. As much as possible they will use motor automatisms. The motor speech may be more restricted if there is a complication by motor aphasia or amnesic aphasia.

Understanding will be disturbed, too, but may be much better preserved. The destruction of the concepts of words will not injure it nearly as much as speaking, as long, that is, as the perceptual sphere of speech itself is undisturbed. Understanding will sometimes be damaged more (particularly in some phases of the disease) because the acoustic sphere—due to the locality of the lesion underlying these symptom complexes—is often damaged anatomically too (see p. 244).

There will always be a *difficulty in finding words*, not so much in the form of characteristic amnesic aphasia, but more in the difficulty of finding words which we consider characteristic as due to impairment of instrumentalities (see p. 65). The nouns which the patient utters often show a similarity to the correct words, the defect consisting mainly in paraphasia. Circumlocutions are not used frequently as is typical for amnesic aphasia.

Finally, we should mention a symptom occurring in impairment of inner speech which needs special attention because it was this phenomenon which first induced the authors to distinguish the special form of aphasia we are concerned with here: the *disturbances of repetition*. We have seen that repetition is a complex phenomenon (see p. 70) which is related to speech and non-speech mental processes. We have seen further that the correctness of the concepts of a word is very important for it. Repetition is not a simple imitation of percepts. Before we repeat—if we do not simply imitate the heard *sound*, not the word (see p. 70)—we are aware of the "concept of the word." Destruction of the apparatus "underlying the concept of words" disturbs repetition. Thus, disturbances of repetition are characteristic symptoms of central aphasia. Only seldom, indeed, does it show complete inability to repeat; usually it shows paraphasia of literal or verbal character. If the patient does not repeat at all, this may be due to an especially severe defect (see p. 284). Often it is at least partially due to a psychologic reason, the trend of the patient to avoid doing something which he recognizes as wrong or senseless.

Frequently, there is a difference reported between the severity of paraphasia in repetition and in spontaneous speech. This can be for several reasons. In repetition, the patient has to use a definite word while in spontaneous speech there is more variability possible without disturbance of the fulfillment of the task. Thus the patient may choose words which he can utter better. The words which are selected for repetition are often such words which in spontaneous speech are not uttered. In a specific case, this might be enough to explain why spontaneous speech is better than repetition. But sometimes also the opposite is true. One could consider here that spontaneous speech needs more activity than repetition and thus may appear to be disturbed more. But I think we should not overlook the phenomena which we have just discussed concerning the origin of paraphasia (see p. 82). The factors mentioned there are well suited, under certain conditions, to make spontaneous speech more difficult, under others repetition, and thus one or the other performance may appear to be more affected. Whether or not one is really more affected is scarcely to be decided with certainty from the reports, because it depends on how the patient reacts to the particular problem in a particular situation. Only a careful study which takes all these factors into consideration will allow a decision regarding the concerned problem.

H. Disturbances of "Intelligence" in Aphasic Patients

As we have seen, internal speech uses external speech—the learned mechanisms, the various possibilities they present—for the purpose of expressing what the individual wants to express in the attempt to come to terms with the environment. This makes it evident that internal speech is in closest relation to the "higher" mental processes, or better to the nonverbal mental phenomena. There was much discussion in the literature about disturbances of "intelligence" in aphasic patients, whether aphasia is an expression of a disturbance of intelligence, whether the patients are suffering from impairment of "intelligence." These problems had already been discussed in the early development of the doctrine of aphasia even before the aphasic symptom complexes themselves were clarified. Bouillaud (1825) distinguished two components in articulated speech, one being essentially intellectual, the other mechanical. Trousseau stressed particularly the intellectual side of the aphasic disturbance, characterizing it as a "trouble corélatif du language et de la pensée" due to disorder of general intellectual faculties particularly of memory and attention.

Broca distinguished between "aphemie," loss of articulated language without any disturbance of ideas, and "amnesia," loss of recognition of the associations established between ideas and words, in which cases intelligence is affected.

Bastian (6) recognized the disturbances in thinking in some forms of aphasia and explained them as due to defects in the connections between speech centers and "higher centers." Particularly did the transcortical aphasias gave rise to consideration of the impairment of higher mental functions in aphasic patients. In these cases, the speech performances themselves— perception of heard words and motor speech—could be considered essentially intact—in spite of the fact that the patients are not able to understand words and to speak spontaneously; this pointed to an origin of the speech disturbance from defects in the "higher" mental level. These

symptom complexes led Lichtheim and Wernicke to assume a center of
concepts ("Begriffszentrum") separate from the assumed speech centers and
to consider the various forms of transcortical aphasias as due to disturbances of this center or of the association fibers between it and the motor
and sensory speech centers.   A pupil of Wernicke's, Heilbronner (136), then
brought certain aphasic symptom complexes into connection with speech
disturbances observed in some psychotic patients and tried to understand
both as an expression of the mental condition.   Kleist (163) made an
extensive study from this aspect.

But this interpretation of some speech defects did not induce these
authors and their followers to consider the aphasic symptom complexes
simply disturbances of intelligence.   On the contrary, they and many
others as Liepmann, Mingazzini, Niessl von Mayendorf, etc., continually
stressed the difference between the intellectual defects in general, and the
speech defects.   It was thus that Pierre Marie found such ardent opposition when he declared aphasia a disturbance of intelligence.   Wernicke's
sensory aphasia was for him *the* aphasia.   Excluding the other forms of
speech defects from aphasia, he tried to prove that aphasia is nothing
but a special form of defect of intelligence.   It could be, and indeed, was
thought that with this exclusion of the other forms of speech defect the
theory of Pierre Marie represents only a problem of terminology.   But
this would hardly do justice to Pierre Marie's work.   For him, the difference was not at all simply a question of terminology.   The essential
point of his criticism was that there exist some speech disturbances in brain
damage which differ essentially from others, because here alone the defect
concerns that intellectual function which is essential for language.   These
symptom complexes only should be called aphasia.   Here we are dealing
with a "trouble intellectual, especially concerning speech," and in addition, troubles of "l'intelligence générale," defects in mimic, attention,
memory, association of ideas, loss of professional skills, etc.   He excluded
such forms as pure motor and sensory aphasia because here this intellectual
function is undisturbed.

Pierre Marie was correct in rejecting the attempt to understand aphasia
as loss of images (see p. 196) and in distinguishing two essentially different
forms of speech disturbances in brain damage.   Here he approached my
distinction between speech disturbances due to impairment of meaning of
words and of instrumentalities.   But, in his theory, he could not do justice
to the complexity of the phenomenon of speech and its disturbances in
patients.   He overlooked particularly the close relationship between both
groups of disturbances.   He, who stressed so much the relation of speech
disturbances to intelligence disturbance, did not clarify the issue because
what he called intelligence was too diffuse a concept.

What he calls disturbances of general intelligence are symptoms frequently observed in aphasia but they are not at all clear in their structure and their relation to the aphasic phenomena. Hence, Pierre Marie had scarcely any influence on the development of aphasia research—at least much less than he could have had if, in the attempt to reject his exaggerations, readers had not overlooked the fruitful nucleus of his discussion.

If one wants to understand the intellectual component in aphasia, a clarification of the nature of the phenomenon which we call intelligence is presupposition. This indeed could not be determined before the use of special tests was emphasized which did allow the study of mental function of the patients without interference by the speech defect, i.e., before application of performance tests.

But even this would not have been sufficient. What was needed further was *an analysis of the structure of these tests and the intellectual functions underlying accomplishment and failure.* As far as I can see, these exigencies were first fulfilled by introduction of the sorting tests by Gelb and myself in the studies concerning amnesic aphasia. Through these studies, the problem of disturbance of intelligence underlying some aphasic defects was, for the first time, based not on theory, but on facts. From here it was possible to discover how much the defects, considered as of intellectual nature by Pierre Marie, are due to disturbances of "intelligence" or secondary to defects in the "instrumentalities" of speech (see p. 23) and which structure an existing intellectual defect has.

If one spoke of intelligence in relation to speech, or of defect of intelligence in aphasia, he considered such phenomena (according to the general theory of the organization of the mind) as thoughts, ideas built up by associations between images, the products of previous experiences.

The relation between speech and thinking in general was considered in different ways. In philosophy of speech, following particularly Aristotle, identity of speech and thinking was assumed. Thus, thinking was considered either the primary phenomenon—with speech, as it were, only a reflexion of thoughts (this usually by the philosophers), or else thinking was considered as nothing else than "subvocal talking" (a theory proclaimed particularly by the psychologists of the behavioristic type).

There is another theory of language also originating in ancient Greece, namely by the sophists: the sceptical theory of language, for which mind and language are not at all identical. This theory states that if they were not different, it would be impossible to veil thoughts by language. We may have a particular idea but do not want to make it apparent. We cannot do this better, at times, than by speaking. Language is not a repetition of thinking but a particular form of expressing our thoughts.

In more recent times, the German school of "Denkspsychologie" (psychology of thinking) contributed much to the clarification of the situation by experimental research and analysis of the concepts. Experimental analysis of the thought process has given the basis for the important distinction between speechless thinking and formulated thinking in the form of sentences. In aphasia research, it was particularly A. Pick who rejected the theory of identity and made use of the results of "Denkpsychologie" for the theory of aphasia. My own research induced me to follow a similar line.

Of course also for this concept, speech and non-speech mental phenomena are closely related, but not in the simple way of association of parallel processes. Their relation is not a direct one but a secondary one, determined by their signification for the organism's coming to terms with the environment in the given situation. They represent different ways which influence each other. Therefore, investigation of the non-speech mental processes when separated from the consideration of their usability, and of their use in a given case for a given purpose, can be only of a relative value. This becomes evident if one evaluates the very careful investigations of Weisenburg and McBride who tested aphasic patients with most of the known intelligence tests, including those which do not demand language for solution. Their results give very little encouragement, particularly if one compares them with the great amount of work involved. They come to the conclusion "that aphasia is first and foremost a disorder of speech," "aphasia is a particular deterioration, not a general defect of intelligence" (p. 462), but "other types of mental functions beyond the language might be affected," too. "In clear-cut cases of aphasia there is never deterioration." The problem is: What is a clear-cut case of aphasia? If one takes into consideration only the "pure" aphasias, motor and sensory, the statement of Weisenburg and McBride may be right. I agree with them, further, that language is not only a "symbolic formulation," and aphasia not only a defect of this function. But there are other forms of aphasia than the mentioned ones where, in addition to the defect of language (of the instrumentalities), disturbances of the higher mental processes are present, and the problem is, what is their relation to the deterioration of the instrumentalities. As we have seen before (see p. 8) the "automatisms"—and the instrumentalities belong to the "automatisms"—are not independent of the "higher mental" functions.

The opinion of Weisenburg and McBride about the relation in which we are interested here does not become clearer when they say: "The extent to which intelligence may be said to be affected varies from case to case; but for aphasic patients as a group it is evident that intelligence suffers in so far as the language processes disturbed are necessary to the carrying out of intelligent behavior, and, secondary, in so far as non-verbal activities are handicapped by changes in mental functions which extend language processes and are not dependent upon them."

There are several reasons why such investigations bring so little elucidation. The cases with speech disturbances are so different particularly in respect to the non-speech disturbances that a statistical evaluation of the material cannot be of great help. Only an analysis of individual cases can bring insight into the relation of the speech defect and the other mental defects.

The application of the usual mental tests is another point, and I think the main point responsible for the failure. The construction of these tests is based on a scale of steps of ascending difficulty. The steps are meant to represent either progressive mental age levels (as in the Binet test), or performance levels of increasing complexity.

The principle of "graded difficulty" presupposes that each of the ascending steps represents quantitatively greater difficulty of performance. It presupposes at the same time that each step represents the same degree of difficulty to the average individual. Therefore, the scores which the subjects receive for their accomplishments in the different steps indicate whether or not one subject is better able to overcome the difficulties than another. The assumption that the same step represents the same degree of difficulty even for normal subjects is disputable. In the case of abnormal subjects, *such a quantitative comparison is inapplicable*. The steps of graded difficulty may represent for the patient a *qualitative* difference. A patient may fail in one subtest of a "lower grade" and succeed in a subtest of a "higher order" of difficulty, because the first task demands a mental attitude which the patient is not able to assume, owing to a qualitative change in his relation to the world due to pathology, while the step which contains greater difficulties to normals may be solved by the same patient. It may represent an easier task for him because its solution does not demand the attitude in which the patient is impaired.

The usual scoring method, based on a scale of difficulty which has been standardized on a statistical basis, offers no adequate instrument for determining the nature of the patient's impairment. One can*not* simply deduce from a test score which task represents a greater difficulty for the patient and which a lesser; a consideration of the entire procedure, the specific reasons for the difficulty the patient encounters, is imperative. Any statistical evaluation must be based upon a qualitative analysis of test results. It must first be determined what kind of difficulty a given task represents in relation to the changed performance capacity of the patient; thereupon a quantitative inference as to the degree of impairment, etc., can be made.

One could modify the usual tests in a way which would do justice to this problem. However, this would involve changing the underlying principle. Some examples may illustrate.

In the Bourdon test, the patient has the following task: In a standard text which contains a certain number of *a*'s, he is instructed to cross out all the *a*'s as quickly as possible. The number of crossings made in a certain time is recorded and used as a measurement for the degree of attention. In the test the patient may succeed perfectly, or at least may not have lower than average results. I have observed this even in severe cases, and similar observations have recently been reported by Rylander. However, this result offers little information about the mental capacities of the patient. It does not even tell us anything about the so-called attention in general, but only under an experimental condition with which the patient is able to cope.

The following change in the test shows how slight modifications of the experimental conditions may modify the results. When the subject is asked to cross out every *second a*, or every third one, little difference is noted in the behavior of normals. But it may essentially change the results of a patient. He may then behave very poorly. This modification of the test may not seem to be very important on the surface. The facts, however, show that the task must have been changed in a way which made it considerably more difficult for this type of patient. Analysis of the modified test reveals what the difficulty is. It has nothing to do with attention directly. The modification necessitates the abstract attitude which the patient is unable to assume. At first glance, it may be surprising that this attitude is needed to fulfill such a simple test, but further consideration will show it to be a necessary factor. If the test is arranged in the usual way, where this attitude does not play a role in completing the test, the patient succeeds; if the test is rearranged in the way we described, he may fail.

This simple test shows some ambiguity in another respect. With normals, one gets about the same results whether the material presented is a senseful or a senseless text, or an at random combination of letters, although the result with a senseful text may be a little better. A different situation may be observed in some patients. They may show better results with a senseless text (see case 6). If the text is senseful, they are induced to read before they look for the letters. This is difficult for them because it necessitates two simultaneous actions, a procedure impossible for these patients (see p. 6). However, this is not the case with a senseless text. Here their attention is directed only toward letters. The same ambiguity is met in another simple test, the "sentence completion test." To normals, the test presents degrees of difficulty as to different texts and different omissions in the text. But with patients, another difficulty is involved which one does not consider in testing normals: namely, whether the content of the text can be grasped in a concrete way, i.e., refers to a situation, etc., familiar to the patient, whether it concerns some personal incidents, or needs abstract attitude. Such a text may be as to the structure, omitted words, "easy" for a normal person, but possibly unsolvable for the patient (see case 6, p. 212).

Unfortunately, most physicians who adapt these and similar tests from normal psychology are unacquainted with the intricate pitfalls and do not realize that, by changing some seemingly unimportant point, a special test may represent a totally different task for the patient.

From the foregoing, it will become evident that the usual consideration of a patient's mental capacities from the result of any kind of I.Q. administration must be of doubtful value. We are facing here a problem with which we are confronted in general in investigation of the "intelligence" of patients with damage of the brain cortex. I have stressed again and again how misleading the results of the application of the usual test batteries in patients with cortical damage can be (see 108, p. 96).

The mental capacities which are needed to gain a high score are of different kind for the various subtests. If we were sure that the subject would be forced to perform each subtest in a definite, invariable way, we could form at least some sort of conclusion from the end result, and use such information for comparative studies. Unfortunately, the subject is *not* forced to proceed in a definite way. Some of the subtests can be executed in different ways without revealing the method of procedure in the result. This may not be so important for quantitative studies on normal subjects. But it makes the whole testing very ambiguous when someone who is disturbed in a particular capacity by which a certain subtest is usually performed, performs it in a roundabout way by utilizing another capacity. For instance, it may be that a subtest which is usually performed by an abstractive procedure may also be performed (although not easily) by use of memory; the time required may be somewhat longer, but no definite abnormality may be revealed. Another patient, who has poor memory, may produce poor results. In a similar way as lack of memory, the behavior may be influenced by the personality structure of the individual patient. He may not use his memory because he is unaccustomed to attack problems in this way but rather by the attitude in which he is now impaired. The I.Q. of this patient may thus appear lower than that of a patient for whom the utilization of memory was an adequate way of procedure, in spite of the fact that both have the same impairment in regard to the capacity of abstraction. The I.Q. in patients can be deceptive in either direction: it may lead one to assume too high or too low a grade of mental capacity. The results are particularly ambiguous if the reaction has to be given by language. This is in consequence of the double aspect of language (see p. 25).

The fallacy with which we are here confronted may be illustrated by the results obtained with the "proverb test." The subject is supposed to grasp and explain the meaning of a proverb, as for example: "Hunger is the best cook" "The apple falls near the tree," "A bird in the hand is worth two in the bush." This test can be valuable for disclosing lack of ability to abstract. But the results can be very ambiguous. I should like to refer to investigations of Rylander, which entirely agree with mine. If an office manager, whom Rylander observed, answers: "If anyone has a bird in his hand, it must be a tame bird," or, "If the apple is beside the tree, it has naturally fallen down from it," these answers certainly represent deviations from the normal way of thinking of an educated man and reveal a lack of abstraction. If a countryman of little education, with a concrete approach to all things, makes the same sort of reply, it would correspond to his usual way of thinking and would not necessarily indicate a defect. However, it does not follow that the second patient has no impairment of the abstract attitude. The test merely does not reveal this man's impairment.

An intelligent man, accustomed to solve problems linguistically, may give an answer which sounds approximately correct, but analysis may reveal that we are deceived by his excellent vocabulary. We may overlook the fact that he is really disturbed in his "symbolic" capacity.

We may avoid mistakes, when we begin our examination, by testing the capacity for abstraction. If we find that the patient is disturbed in this capacity, this will indicate that we should arrange the tasks for testing special functions, as, for instance, memory, motor activities, visualization (see p. 26) so that the presentation of the test allows the patient to fulfill the task in a concrete way. Thus, we may gain an insight into his capacities at least under these circumstances. We will further not bother the patient with tests he cannot fulfill if the abstract attitude is impaired.

Of course, also, careful analysis of the results gained with the usual test, e.g., some subtests of the Binet-Simon test, would reveal whether abstract attitude is impaired or not. But it is easier to determine the condition by application of the tests we have built for this special purpose. They have the advantage of containing tasks in which everyone usually proceeds in the abstract way in order to reach a correct result, or, if somebody tries it in another way, it becomes apparent in the manner of procedure. A man may be inclined by habit to proceed concretely, then, by small modifications of the tests (the subtests), which no longer allow achieving of a result in this way, it will become apparent whether he can act abstractively too, or not.

In testing any mental function, one must always remember that a similarly appearing deviation from the norm can be due to an impairment of abstract attitude (if the task needs this capacity for fulfillment) or due to a defect in "instrumentalities" in a particular field.   Two examples will illustrate: A patient may be unable to recite a series of numbers on demand because he cannot begin—due to the impairment of abstraction—or he may be unable to do it because the automatisms underlying this performance are disturbed (see p. 190).   Again: A patient may not be able to understand a word because of impairment of abstraction, if this word needs abstraction for understanding (see p. 57), or he may not understand it because his acoustic instrumentalities are damaged.

The foregoing criticism does not underestimate the value of testing special functions.   Such testing can be very significant in some cases, and the results must be considered carefully in our treatment.   However, the results obtained with the usual tests can be evaluated correctly only if the attitude in which the individual attacks the problem is taken into consideration.   It is not possible to judge the subject's capacities from the end result.

Returning to the question of the relation between aphasia and intelligence defect, I should like to stress the following points, which, for purposes of clarity, I have organized generally into six brief sections.

I. There may be present, *simultaneously, defects in speech and in mental capacities* due to concomitant lesions in different parts of the brain.   Here, neither type of defect has anything to do with the other.   In so-called pure sensory aphasia, the patient may have intelligence defects which are due to brain damage outside of the speech area and in no relation to the speech defect.   Indeed, they may secondarily influence speech and the speech defect may secondarily disturb the use of the higher mental functions.   Thus, some mental anomalies in such cases of "pure aphasia" represent the individual *reactions* of the patient to his speech defect, they are expression of the disturbance of the contact of the patient with the outer world and of avoidance of catastrophic reactions and other behavior changes secondary to the defect (see p. 10).   Frequently, these *secondary symptoms are misinterpreted* and erroneously considered as directly related to the speech defect.   One component of the picture of Wernicke's sensory aphasia is of that particular kind.   One could consider the disturbances of internal speech which belong to Wernicke's aphasia as intellectual disturbance in so far as the performances of internal speech are in principle different from those corresponding to the motor and sensory acts.   They are closer to the "mental" phenomena (see p. 94), but they are *speech* phenomena, and anomalies in this realm should be termed speech disturbances and at least distinguished from the disturbances of the non-speech mental phenomena which may be more or less present at the same time.

II. *Speech defects may be secondary to mental defects*, one expression of the mental defect. Here, not only the "intellectual" deterioration is to be considered but also the changes of emotions. Particularly, impairment of "intention"—till now a very unclear and certainly complex phenomenon—plays an important role in pathology of speech. Some forms of the complex picture of transcortical motor aphasia are expression especially of lack of intention (see p. 294).

The question of how dedifferentiation of the process of thinking does influence speech has been, until now, so difficult to explain because our knowledge of this process itself is so insufficient. The following presentation does not at all pretend to do full justice to this problem. It tries to consider it so far as the results will provide a basis for bringing some order into the various phenomena observed in patients.

The process which underlies the *origin of an image, concept, thought, etc.*, is very complex. It contains more or less of part processes which are related to each other in a definite way. Some particularly significant ones stand out, while others are in the background, supporting the first ones, and are important for the clarity and definiteness of the phenomena. All these processes build a unit of the type of the figure and ground configuration (see p. 5). This unit is based on analysis, synthesis, and order by which the "material" of thinking, the after-effects of different experiences— perceptive and motor — are organized to the *units of "higher" mental phenomena.*

Even the *perceptions* to which these units can be traced back do not at all owe their existence to simple reflections of the outer world on brain or mind. They are a product of a psycho-physical activity bound on the function of the brain matter. They do not represent the result of a simple summing up of the effects of stimulations of different senses, produced by an "object" in the outer world. They are the *result of a selection process* by which the perceived properties of the "object" are synthesized to a unit which is useful for the coming to terms of the individual with the outerworld — in the trend of self realization. They are not simple tools which we utilize in any way whatever for different purposes. They remain always related to their origin. They are dynamic phenomena which are always repeated to some degree when we need a perception experience. They may be modified if the situation demands it, i.e., if clarity, order can be achieved only by such modification.

When we want to evoke a representation ("Vorstellung"), images, ideas, etc., we usually begin with some diffuse experience which concerns particularly the "meaning" of the thing, its relatedness to other things, to other mental phenomena, other representations, feelings, activities; images of various senses may appear.   Even if we are conscious of a definite representation the mentioned phenomena may be present more or less—in the "fringes."   But their sum is not what we experience; all these experiences are grouped around a unitary nucleus of the representation.   Indeed, this dynamic process which corresponds to the evoking of a representation can be more or less substituted by a fixed phenomenon.   Representations may become more or less independent from the personality if they are used in routine-like life.   These fixed patterns of representation may produce a deviation in normal behavior if routine does not do justice to the demands of the situation.   This occurs in patients when fixation becomes abnormally manifest in pathology due to the defect in the building of representations (see p. 113).

In a similar way as we have described the building of representations, the building of *concepts* and *thoughts* is the result of a unifying activity of the personality.   We bring together various representations of objects which owe their existence to previous thinking, etc., to the unity of a concept; we combine concepts or parts of them into thoughts.   We build higher thoughts through syllogisms which we acquire by the comparison of concepts or thoughts.   As well in concepts as in thoughts, the parts from which they are formed do not disappear, they stand out more or less as to their different significance in their utility for coming to terms with the world in the present condition.

If a situation demands the evoking of a concept or thought, then the process of formation is not always repeated; *abbreviations* may take place, or even only a *fixed pattern* which corresponds to them is present.   This occurs particularly if the situation is very familiar and can be handled in routine fashion.   Concepts and thoughts once elicited follow each other in a pattern-like way.   This corresponds to the concrete behavior we have discussed before in general (see p. 6).   All characteristics of this behavior which we have described are to be observed also in the stream of thoughts; hence, particularly concrete thinking is dependent upon abstract attitude (see p. 8).

Thus also in the *non-language mental processes*, we must distinguish between *"instrumentalities"* (images, fixed concepts, thoughts, series of such in form of conclusions, etc.) *and the use of them* in abstract or concrete way. The abstract attitude may be considered a special (highest?) form of the unifying processes.   How it is related to the building of concepts and thoughts we cannot discuss here.   Such a discussion would take us too far afield and might not even be successful.   For our purpose, i.e., understanding pathologic phenomena, it seems useful to distinguish the effect of a *damage of the unifying process in general* and the effect of a *damage of abstract attitude,* as we shall see later when we discuss some observations of patients (see p. 292).

Concerning the relation of these processes to language I should like to stress the following: The more "complex" the concepts or thoughts are, i.e., the greater the number of different "objects" they comprise, the farther away they are from the concrete experience to which they owe their origin, the more often they are represented by "symbols," especially by language. *Words appear instead of concepts and thoughts particularly if we are not so much concerned with creation of new concepts but with reproduction for special purposes, thus, for instance, if we want to communicate our concepts and thoughts to others.*

Then, often, no more than the corresponding symbol is present and is uttered. *But language is not only a means to communicate thinking; it is also a means to support it, to fixate it. Defect in language may thus damage thinking (see p. 66). On the other hand, in defect of language the thought processes may come abnormally to the fore.* This shows, in turn, in definite modification of language (see p. 101).

While the concepts are represented in language mainly in *words,* thoughts are mirrored in the form of *sentences.* The formulation in sentences in language is preceded by a definite organization of the parts which are combined in the thought process (in the "syntax of thinking"). The sentence formation in the process of thinking is achieved by putting each part in a definite place in a sequence. The psychologic subject, i.e., that about which one thinks, precedes, as von der Gabelentz has explained, the psychologic object, i.e., the process which corresponds to that which is thought about the subject. Of course, the thought formation occurs only gradually. The first result may be of very general form, may be in the shape of a scheme, in which representations, images, emotions, stand out and relations between them are experienced. Then, increasingly, the scheme is filled with contents which are organized in a definite order. The sequence of the parts in ordered thought formation is then determined by the significance the thinker ascribes to the different parts in the total of the present thought, and thus may differ, to a certain degree, as to the general attitude toward the different things in the world. Thus it may differ as to the peculiarities of cultures, groups, individuals, the situation, etc. In the syntactic organization, some parts may appear in the foreground because of their objective significance, their emotional value for the speaker in the moment, etc.; others may remain in the background, in the "fringes."

III. *The order of the thought formation is not at all repeated in language.* It is *modified* by a number of factors:

1. *By the culturally and individually determined instrumentalities* at the disposal of the speaker and listener. The organization of the thought

formation is transformed by the means language offers to express the thought processes.   While in the thought processes, position in a sequence is the essential way of order, in language, besides position, use of definite words and tenses are the basis of order (syntax and grammar).   The learned mechanisms, corresponding grammar and syntax, pronunciation of sounds, rhythm, accentuation, "speech melody," are of great significance.   Defects in the instrumentalities due to pathology may thus modify the thought processes (see p. 101).   The disturbances of grammar and syntax of language produced by impairment of the instrumentalities are to be distinguished from those which are the effect of disturbances in thought formation itself (see p. 309).

2. The form of expression in language differs further *as to the attitude of the speaker toward the situation,* his relation to the listener, his intention, i.e., what he wants to achieve by his speaking; whether he wants simply to inform somebody about facts or whether he wants to induce some activities, or if he is driven by emotions, expresses his emotions, etc.   He may communicate his emotions because he cannot keep them internally, he speaks because he has to satisfy certain demands, sometimes because only by speaking he can get rid of the tension, the fear produced by the situation, etc.   Speaking differs further as the speaker uses mimic and gesture as substitute for language in different degrees according to personality, situation, etc.   An important factor in the transformation of thoughts into language is the assumption of the speaker that a number of things need not be expressed, in language because the listener is expected to complete correctly in his mind the unuttered ideas, etc. (see p. 94).   This completion is based on the known relationship between speaker and listener, on the knowledge of facts, which can be expected to come to the fore in a definite situation, etc.

A number of symptoms in aphasic patients are due to disturbances of all the factors just mentioned.   The patient may speak wrongly because he cannot grasp correctly what can be presupposed, what not, etc.   He will not understand us because we may not know how much he may be able to grasp of what we assume "can be presupposed."

3. *The transformation into language begins usually during the formation of thoughts.*   Some thoughts or parts may immediately be experienced or uttered in words.   The words which come thus to the fore may fit the isolated part but not the position of this part in the whole of the intended thought.   The emerged word may then influence the thought process in an "inadequate" way, and this change of thinking demands modification of the transformation into language.   Before the intended thought is transformed in the right way into language, a number of various wrong solutions may be experienced and more or less uttered.

If, as in pathology, there is a difficulty in eliciting words, wrong words may enter the picture and may modify or even disturb thinking and, hence, speaking. We have stressed this point when we discussed the symptom of difficulty of word-finding (see p. 59).

IV. We have mentioned the relation between *abstract attitude and thinking*. Impairment of this attitude may change thinking and language in principle in the same way (e.g., in amnesic aphasia, see p. 246). Thinking and language may not be disturbed essentially in all other respects; thus, for instance, "concrete thinking" and "concrete speech" may be nearly normal; may become even more manifest than usual (see p. 269) as substitute for the damaged abstract attitude. Abstract attitude represents the most complicated, most active function of the mind and may be disturbed first in some brain damage. In such cases the examination by the usual intelligence tests may not show any essential numerical modification from the norm, in spite of the fact that the patient has to be considered as damaged considerably in his intellectual functions. Here the ambiguity of these tests becomes particularly evident.

V. Thinking is not only expressed in language, but *language influences in turn thought formation*. Lack of words due to pathology, therefore, may become apparent secondarily in defects of thinking under conditions where thinking is induced by language (see p. 101). Under conditions where language plays no role, thinking may prove to be intact. Tests which can be performed without language are, in this respect, particularly significant (e.g., our abstraction tests). They are enlightening if we want to differentiate the cases with real lack of words due to damage of instrumentalities from difficulties in word-finding due to the impairment of abstract attitude (see p. 67).

VI. Disturbances in the realm of *emotions* influence speech. Here attention must be drawn again to what we have said about the relation of emotional life to the abstract and concrete attitudes. Under certain conditions in emotional situations, speech may be facilitated (emotional speech, see p. 57).

From this review of the main possibilities of the relations between some anomalies of speech and those of non-language mental processes, it will have become evident that it is *not possible to speak in general of any correlation between both disturbances, but that one has to reveal whether a particular defect in one field is the cause of a defect in the other field, and how.* Only a careful analytic comparison of the structure of the anomalies found in both fields will allow for any decision about relationship. *To speak of the condition of intelligence in aphasic patients in general—its maintenance or defect—is impossible.*

In the non-speech mental realm, we have to distinguish (as in language

and in all other performances) between the effect of abstract attitude and
of instrumentalities, and to consider their mutual dependence. The *instrumentalities of thinking* can be damaged concomitantly with or without
impairment of abstraction, abstract attitude without damage of the instrumentalities of thinking. Thus, different symptom complexes may occur
(see p. 92).

In our consideration of the different ways non-language mental performances and language are mutually related and how defects in the one
modify the other, we have described the phenomena in psychologic terms.
One could try to understand the phenomena on the basis of changes of the
function of the brain matter and *describe them in physiologic terms*.   We are
not yet able to do much in this respect.   I have tried to understand the
impairment of abstract attitude as reducible to a functional disturbance,
by assuming as its cause that patients are impaired in the capacity to
have "two things in mind at the same time; separated and combined in one
view, to distinguish them and to synthesize them to a new whole."   This
capacity, which I have called also "simultaneous function," represents the
highest function of the brain matter.   It is disturbed by a slowing down
of the processes, which may completely incapacitate this complicated
process.

I came to this conclusion first during the observation of a patient with
visual agnosia (see 97, p. 665), who was impaired in the capacity to do some
thing (in every performance field) which demanded "simultaneous function," while he performed well when it was possible to fulfill a task by
successive procedure. A great number of symptoms in different performance fields could be explained in this way.   "Simultaneous function"
demands a better functioning substrate than "successive function."
Therefore, it is the first to be disturbed in dedifferentiation of the brain
functions in general.

Bouman and Grünbaum have tried to explain the defects of a patient
in different performance fields, and especially in motor speech, from such
a point of view. We report the case in detail elsewhere (see p. 76).   The
symptoms of the patient in all performance fields became understandable
from the assumption that the processes come to a standstill in a more
amorphous state, and that differentiation of parts in a whole and synthesis
of these is lacking.   The patient was not able to keep elements of wholes
in mind long enough to synthesize them.   Thus, all performances were
difficult which demanded operation with individual elements within a total
whole ("Gestalt").   As long as consideration of the whole could bring
about success in a task, the patient performed well (see p. 78).   This
case is particularly valuable because it shows the fruitfulness of our point
of view for explaining the defects in the production of speech sounds, which

are not well interpreted otherwise (see p. 76).   In respect to the problem of the relationship between speech disturbances and non-language mental disturbances, it is a new proof for our assumption that both language and non-language mental processes may be disturbed in a case *without a justifiable assumption that the disturbances depend upon each other.*   They *are simply the effect of the same dedifferentiation of brain function in two performance fields* (as we could show first for amnesic aphasia, see p. 246).

I. Disturbances of Reading and Writing

(1) *Disturbances of Reading*

In *reading* a text, the words and the kind of phrasing are familiar to us; our attitude is so essentially directed toward the meaning of the language it symbolizes that ordinarily we are very little (if at all) aware of the seen letters, words, etc.   Usually, the visual impression evokes language and non-language activities.   Not all which is presented as writing or print is transposed into language; some parts, depending on their degree of significance in respect to meaning, are omitted in a similar way as not all which we want to express is transposed into language, but a definite selection takes place (see p. 94).

Some, indeed only a few, seen words or even sentences may evoke activities or ideas without any transposition into language.   A written sign, which we expect in a definite place, may produce an activity even without our being able to recognize the words—remembering of them.   Understanding of normally presented material of words, etc., is a unitary process in which we often do not experience parts.   This is different if the presented material is not understood immediately.   If the print is strange, if there are words we do not know visually, which do not evoke language or meaning immediately, then we have to proceed step by step.   We recognize the letters, combine them to words, language experiences of different types come to the fore, names of letters, sounds, sound combinations, either in form of speaking or in acoustic images, concepts of words, and finally we may get the meaning.   Even if we do not go through all this complex procedure in normal reading, the different steps must be at hand because also in normal reading difficulties may arise which can be overcome only by means of one or another part of this complex process.   Even in a familiar text, some words may be unknown and produce difficulty in immediate understanding; then they have to be spelled, etc.   This may change the total procedure of reading, and is more likely to occur the less an individual is accustomed to read.   It occurs always to some degree and in different ways in pathology when the unitary process is disturbed at one or another step.

We can say that reading can be modified in principle in three ways; by pathology in the visual material, in the instrumentalities of language and in meaning. Indeed, the symptom complexes are not simply to be understood by damage of one or another part of the unitary process. A defect of each part always also changes the function of the preserved parts which is further modified by the attempts of the individual to compensate the defect. The means used under these conditions may not correspond to normal procedures in reading. "Analysis of the way, in which an act of reading is performed under pathological conditions does not reveal the functional elements out of which it is normally composed," says Head. "The value of such analysis," he continues, "lies in the light it throws on the varieties of aphasias underlying the defect in reading." I would like to add that the analysis teaches us something about the means adopted by normals in difficult situations which cannot be handled in normal ways (see, regarding this, e.g., what we have explained before, concerning the use of images in normal speech, p. 26).

The first group of reading difficulties is due to a damage of visual recognition. This *primary alexia* (also called pure alexia or agnostic alexia) is the expression of visual agnosia in reading.

(a) *Primary Alexia*

The process of *recognition of letters* can be disturbed in different degrees. The patient may be unable to see—in spite of intact visual acuity—the simplest forms in general (so-called Gestaltblindness, see 112a, p. 753), and thus also the forms of the letters. In other cases, the "simpler" forms may be recognized, not the more complicated ones; therefore, various, in some respect, similar forms may be confused, and reading is more or less impaired. It seems that in some cases visual imagery is totally lost, in others not to such a high degree. The decision as to the degree of loss in an individual patient is difficult, due to the imperfection of our methods of investigating this capacity (see p. 27). But even if visualization is totally lost, writing may be intact (see 112a). Whether writing is disturbed or not, depends upon the individual patient, whether he is accustomed to use visual images in writing or not. But no evidence supports relating this to the question of whether the lesion is cortical or subcortical. Copying in severe cases is impossible. In cases of less severity it is possible in varying degrees. Some patients (with preserved writing) may be able to guess from imperfect perception with which letter they are confronted and produce this letter voluntarily (see the behavior of the patient of A. Adler, 1, p. 123).

In some cases, visual agnosia and also pure alexia are accompanied with other symptoms. A detailed description of the behavior of such a patient has been given elsewhere (see 112a).

However, I should like to give a short summary here of the main symptoms of this patient, beside visual agnosia and alexia: astereagnosis with good performance as to perception of touch qualities; incapacity to perceive simultaneously presented elements in the acoustic sphere; recognition of length, of height of pitch, etc., combined with good performances as to perception of qualities; loss of space experience in the proper sense, with maintenance of good reactions in accordance with the differences in space in the outer world; lack of the capacity to perceive quantities in all sensory fields and to compare them; incapacity for voluntary actions with maintenance of actions released by objects and language; loss of the value of numbers, impairment of such intellectual performances as analogies, syllogisms, with retention of many intellectual performances as long as they can be based on language or movements. Narrowing of the total personality in experiences and actions with maintenance of a fine tactful, unselfish and reasonable personality in situations with which he is able to deal with the capacities maintained.

Our analysis of the structure of the different symptoms brought the conclusion that all could be considered as the effect of a damage of the "basic function of the brain cortex," which we called the *simultaneous function, with maintenance of the "successive" function* (see 97 and 101). We could characterize the defect also as impairment of abstraction. We have tried to explain why lesions in the parieto-occipital region are suited to produce this characteristic modification of behavior in such different fields and why by this localization of the process the visual recognition is disturbed particularly. We have mentioned before the characteristic modifications in *language* which these patients show (see p. 323), and which are explained by the same damage of the brain function as the other symptoms. Whether all cases of this form of alexia show this complex symptomatology cannot be decided. Further studies are necessary.

In spite of this incapacity to recognize any letter by vision, the patient was able to "read." Analysis showed that his reading was based on the kinesthetic experiences he acquired by tracing movements. Because he did not recognize any form visually, he had to proceed with his tracing in a "planless" way, determined by the black spots which he saw with his fovea. He moved the fovea along these spots by movement of his head and from kinesthetic experiences derived from the head movements he concluded with which letter he was confronted. (See, regarding this procedure, the detailed description in the original paper, 112a).

An especially interesting aspect of the case was the patient's own ignorance of his device. Even after our discovery, we found it difficult to persuade him that his procedure was not the customary one. He showed very clearly that he considered it inevitable for people to "read" in this way.

We tried to make his procedure clear to him and to teach him to proceed more systematically.   He finally developed his tracing movements to such perfection that he not only became able to read the newspaper in this way, but also created a particular motor alphabet which made it possible for him even to read different kinds of printing and writing.   The way he proceeded in tracing was instructive.   He usually began at the left upper part of the "black spot" which represented a letter to him.   He started there because he knew from experience that many letters began in the left upper corner of the black spot.

When confronted with letters which were most conspicuous at the bottom, the patient began there, after having discovered by several trials that beginning at the upper part did not help him to recognize the letter.   After having traced the first part and recognized its shape, he pondered on what letter it might be.   If it was possible for him to guess the letter from the first part in an unmistakable way, he stopped tracing.   If the first tracing corresponded to the pattern of movement in various letters, which was not infrequently the case, he experimented by searching for some further characteristics, usually very small peculiarities, which he expected to find in certain letters.   For example, the capital letters C, G, S, E, in German, begin in print with a semicircle opening at the right side.   In the E and the C, the circle opens at the lower end of the letter.   By this characteristic, the patient separated E and C from the other letters.   If he now found that a transverse tracing movement fitted, then it would be an E; if not, it would be a C.   If the circle continued to the upper part of the left side, he judged that it was a G or an S.   He then experimented further to see whether it was possible to trace a line in the vertical direction; if that was possible, it would be a G; if not, it would be an S (see 112a, Fig. 12).

Obviously, in order to have been able to find out all these little peculiarities, he must have had an extremely good knowledge of the movements corresponding to all the various letters.   This was attained by practice. Reading was easier after he found that he could omit some letters or words, relying on the general visual appearance or on the context of a word or sentence for the meaning.   For example, he did not have to trace the second m in a word written with two m's.   He recognized the first m by tracing the three vertical strokes of the m.   He would then realize that there was a similar broad thing with an alternating white and black pattern. From this, he came to the conclusion that it was a second m.   He preceded in a similar way in words with two l's or two n's, etc.   He often omitted things which he guessed were articles or some other little words not necessary to the meaning of the sentence, or which he could guess from the context.

In teaching such a man, the best method is to start by teaching him to read words written very distinctly, preferably in a handwriting familiar to him, where tracing is easy. In time, the patient learns the motor experiences in letters of other handwriting and various kinds of printing.

Of course, this training was rendered possible by the patient's particular motor predisposition, and any success in using this method will depend upon this capacity.

The patient's way of reading became particularly evident when he was confronted with words he could "read," and the words were then crossed by some oblique lines which would not disturb reading for a normal individual. Now he could not "read" any more, because by his planless tracing he came into wrong lines, entered a senseless maze, as it were, and so could not get the right kinesthetic experiences. For the same reason, he could not "read" letters written in a form differing from what he was accustomed to, even when the different writing made no difference at all for the reading of a normal individual; for instance, he could read the familiar script k, but not K, which traced gives an unfamiliar experience.

Patients who used tracing movements to compensate difficulties in reading have been reported in the literature by Westphal, Nielsen and Gibbon, and recently by A. Adler. The purpose of tracing varies in the different cases with the kind of defect in visual recognition, and is correspondingly performed in a different way. As we said, our patient who did not see any form had to trace planlessly. Other patients who see some form, though defective (as the patient of Adler), proceed on the basis of what they see of the form; tracing is only a help—it facilitates recognition of forms which are not seen with normal precision. The patient will in this way recognize details which he may otherwise overlook because of the defect of perception and which he must grasp for correct recognition of letters. Tracing aids further, as A. Adler says, "by successive addition of parts" if the simultaneous perception of the parts in the whole is impaired. A. Adler's patient often perceived only parts and had to complete them by guessing. In copying, she did not copy what she saw, but wrote in her own handwriting what she had guessed. Therefore, she could guess and write down the correct letter only if it were presented in a normal position, and would guess another if the same letter were presented in a different position. She guessed, for example, e, "because it has a space on this side," pointing to the right. If the same e were presented to her upside down, she said, "That is a small a because the space is on the other side," pointing to the left. Both guesses were based on visual experiences. Our patient could never do this. He guessed, too, but from kinesthetic experiences; if these did not correspond to his experience of a definite letter, e.g., when he was induced to trace in an unfamiliar way, then he did not recognize the letter at all and came to a wrong result when this tracing produced a kinesthetic experience belonging to another letter or another form known to him (see 112a, p. 27).

In other cases of alexia, the difficulty or incapacity to read is not based on defects in the visual sphere. Here the defect consists of a failure to relate the visual experiences to the intact speech performances.

These patients recognize the presented letters as such, they distinguish them from other forms, they may be able to match letters of different types (written, printed, capitals and small letters, etc.), but they are unable to find the corresponding sound or name. There are cases where this defect does not improve. Here retraining is often helpful (see p. 333).

There are patients who are able to read letters but are not able to combine them into words. Here we are not dealing with a defect in the visual sphere but with a defect in language. If the motor speech performances are intact, then the patient is suffering from an impairment of inner speech, with a defect in spelling and combining letters into words. The patient may be able to read some words as wholes, but when he has to proceed by spelling, he shows defects, paralexia (see p. 312).

The opposite phenomenon—better reading of words than of letters— may have various causes. In one group of cases, the cause is not a reading defect; the patient recognizes the letters and can utter corresponding sounds. The failure is due to impairment in word-finding. This picture is a part of amnesic aphasia (see p. 246).

In other cases, the patient may have a visual alexia and not be able to recognize the letters but some words familiar as visual pictures may reproduce definite speech performance. This "pseudoreading" is mostly restricted to a few words, as the patient's own name, the name of some acquaintance, etc. That in these cases we are not dealing with reading becomes evident when the patient "reads" his first name as his family name and vice versa.

Even if the patient recognizes the seen letters, he may read words better than letters. This is the case with patients who are impaired in their capacity of abstraction. The letters have become so strange to them outside of words that they cannot read them. They do not awaken language activities. The case is different with words which are familiar, concrete to them. That this interpretation is correct becomes evident by the fact that the patients may be able to read only such words which produce a concrete experience, and not those which do not. Thus, patients may not be able to read the "small" words (see p. 68). How many words a patient will be able to read depends on his visual capacity as to written or printed material. The patient we mentioned on p. 312 was able to read many words because of his excellent capacity in this respect. But even here we are not dealing with real reading.

(b) *Secondary Alexia*

In the various forms of disturbances of the instrumentalities of language, reading will be disturbed in different ways. However, besides the effect the special speech defect has on reading, an individual factor is to be considered: the greater or lesser dependence of reading upon the speech performances.

In peripheral motor aphasia, reading aloud is disturbed, but the patient may understand all he reads. But there are individuals who are so accustomed to speak aloud or silently when reading that the motor speech defect makes understanding of written material more or less impossible.

In central motor aphasia (see p. 208), reading aloud may be better if the motor capacity is not severely disturbed; the patient may even read aloud better than he speaks. But in these cases, the more concrete words may be read better than the more "abstract" words, e.g., the "small" words may not be read at all or only as parts within a senseful sentence (see p. 69). In these cases, it may be observed further that if the patient is induced to read aloud, he may not understand what he reads, while he understands better if he is allowed to read silently. The energy may be sufficient to produce one performance but not both (see p. 4).

In transcortical motor aphasia due to reduction of the function of the motor speech area (see p. 293), reading is usually better than spontaneous speech. It corresponds approximately to the capacity to repeat.

In peripheral sensory aphasia, reading is intact in every respect.

In central sensory aphasia, the change of reading is like that in central aphasia. It is the direct effect of the defect in speech—thus, it shows paralexia both literal and verbal—and the different effects which the difficulty of spelling and combining letters to words exerts on the various words.

There are patients who recognize the letters as known forms, the letters of different alphabets as belonging together and who have no speech defect but are unable to relate the seen forms and language. They may be able to read a few words by recognizing the form of the whole word and its belongingness to a certain spoken word, but they cannot read a word or even a letter. This defect, the theoretic interpretation of which is not quite clear, is of practical importance because training in a definite way is successful (see p. 333).

The disturbances of reading in other speech disturbances is dealt with in the description of the special cases.

(2) *Disturbances of Writing*

Cases of more or less isolated disturbances of writing were published in the last century first by French authors. Particularly Charcot's and Pitres' cases became well known in the literature. Then came the publications of Wernicke, Binswanger, Gordinier, Oppenheim, et al. Already during this time the problem arose whether the disturbance concerns only one hand or both. The cases differed in this respect. In some cases, only one hand was affected; in others, both (see p. 128). Even the character of the defect could differ in both hands, as in the case of Heilbronner, where the patient had, in the right hand, a total agraphia, while with the left hand he could not write spontaneously nor on dictation but could copy. All the problems involved found a better clarification only after the structure of voluntary performances in general and the structure of the writing mechanism in particular became better known. Liepmann's publications on apraxia were of the greatest significance here. Only now was it possible to discuss the different clinical pictures on the basis of the lesion of the dominant hemisphere and of the different parts in it.

Writing is a complex performance. As motor phenomenon, it has in principle the same structure as any other motor activity. It consists of voluntary and automatized processes bound together to units. An impulse is necessary to bring it into action, which impulse originates from the desire to communicate by language in the written form. The forms themselves are executed by innervation of various muscles in a complex and very precise combination. This combination is determined by the "ideas" of the forms of the letters.

These "ideas" of form can be executed by any movable part of the body, we can write with either hand, with the legs, with movements of the head, etc. It was Wernicke who first pointed to this fact. However, one part of the body, in righthanded individuals the right hand, is particularly trained for writing. Motor automatisms of the right hand make writing so fluent and the individual acts in producing letters somewhat independent of the "ideas of forms." They are set in process without our having to innervate them voluntarily. Words, even sentences, are innervated more and more as wholes and gain increasingly a stereotyped character. Indeed, the dependence of some voluntary influence never gets totally lost. This is demonstrated in the differences of handwriting in varying conditions of the individual and in disturbances if, in pathology, this influence is damaged. The relation between the voluntary and the automatized part varies as to the different conditions under which writing is performed. In the usual writing of an individual very much accustomed to write, the automatic part is very much in the foreground when the person performs writing for everyday communication. Writing of isolated words on dictation is less automatized, still less that of isolated letters. If we are asked to write a definite letter, our attitude is much more voluntary than when we write the same letter within a word. Even the form of the letter differs. This concerns words too. The same words may be produced much more fluently in sentences than when isolated. This is demonstrated particularly in pathology which makes the writing of some isolated words impossible, while the same words in definite (familiar) combinations may be well written. This difference is related to the fact that the motor performance is not the goal in itself in writing, not even its effect—the written letters, words, etc. All this is only the means to communicate something by awakening meaningful language. Those words which are meaningful even in isolation are easier to write than those the meaning of which is not so immediate (see p. 69). This occurs particularly if abstract attitude is impaired, which defect deprives definite words of any sense if they appear in isolation, i.e., outside of a concrete situation (see p. 56).

The correctness of written words and sentences is, thus, partially dependent upon the perfection of motor automatisms. But there are, in all writing, parts for which such automatisms do not exist; new combinations of letters in words and of words in sentences are necessary. In this respect, writing remains dependent upon language and reflects activities of the latter in the form of spelling, combining letters to words, and the influence of synthetical and grammatical structure. With modification of these language processes, new automatisms may originate.

It is evident that such a complex structure as writing can easily be disturbed and will be disturbed in different ways if the one or another of the "parts" of this unitary process is damaged. This, indeed, does not simply away with this part but modifies the whole process of writing, particularly the various kinds of writing, spontaneous writing, writing on dictation, copying, writing with block letters, etc., differently. Accordingly we meet different forms of agraphia.

We distinguish two main groups of *agraphia*, one in which the motor act of writing is *primarily* damaged, another in which the disturbances of writing are *secondary* to such of language.

(a) *Primary Agraphia Due to Impairment of the Complex Motor Act of Writing*

The symptoms differ as to which part of the motor act is damaged by pathology.

The *lack of "impulse"* ("Antrieb") (see Goldstein, 97, p. 822) in some forms of transcortical disturbances (see p. 294) may find expression in a somewhat isolated defect of writing, because writing needs more intentional impulse than the other voluntary acts. Particularly, beginning to write is hampered; the impulse may further be sufficient only to produce one part of the word, not the whole. The patient may stop in the middle of the word or of a sentence. If he is in the process of writing and very much automatized words, etc., must be produced, he may write more fluently. If he is able to produce letters, their form may not be changed. Writing on dictation, particularly copying, will be better than spontaneous writing, because it does not need so much spontaneity.

In impairment of abstract attitude, the defect may objectively be similar insofar as the patient may often have difficulty in starting. But this is not such a general phenomenon here as in the form mentioned just previously. It occurs particularly (possibly only) if the patient has to write words which have lost meaning because of his impairment of abstract attitude, e.g., the small words in isolation (see p. 68). He may write "concrete" words much more easily. Because the letters may have become strange to him, he may not be able to produce them in isolation but may write them well within a word. Dictation and copying may be about normal.

In *ideatoric apraxia*, the idea of the form of letters is disturbed. The patient shows defects in the production of letters, he makes wrong hooks, arcs, etc. This form is usually combined with ideatoric apraxia. Sometimes the defects may show more in writing than in other activities. It may not be so apparent if the patient has to write words for which he possesses very good motor automatisms. Dictation is not better than spontaneous writing. This defect in writing always concerns both hands equally, and shows also in attempts to write with another movable part of the body (see p. 226). Copying is disturbed too, but less than spontaneous writing. In this condition, the patient mostly has difficulty in recognizing letters; he has some alexia. He is not able to distinguish letters similar in some parts, does not see the failures in wrongly written letters. But these disturbances are less developed than the defect in writing.

There are cases where the patients have difficulty in producing a letter, while, after a certain time, they may gain the ability to produce it. It seems that they cannot recollect the form of the letter; they seem to ponder about the form before they can produce it. Sometimes they produce a wrong letter but this in a correct form. They never produce a wrong form. They recognize immediately the letters and distinguish promptly a wrongly written from a correct one. I tried to explain this type as due to a difficulty in awakening the intact ideas of the form of the letters. I called this type *amnesic-apractic agraphia*. These patients have a similar difficulty in the voluntary production of other forms of objects, while they are able to recognize them. We are dealing here with a slight form of apraxia, which should not be confused with amnesic-aphasic disturbances of writing (see p. 252).

The observation that the patients with ideatoric apractic agraphia show the same defect in both hands in a lesion of the dominant hemisphere is explained by the dominance of this hemisphere in the process of ideation for performances on both sides. As we have mentioned before (see p. 126), there are patients observed who could not write with the other ("minor") hand spontaneously or on dictation, but could copy. It seems that it depends upon the severity of isolation of the other (minor) hemisphere from the dominant one whether this function is also damaged. Copying may be guaranteed by the function of the minor hemisphere but can be set in action only if the impulse is not damaged too. Such may be the case if particularly the relation to the frontal lobe of the dominant hemisphere is severed. This becomes evident in the differences between Heilbronner's patient and my patient with total interruption of the corpus callosum who could not write at all. Incidentally, in my case ideation itself was intact as was evident by the intactness of writing with the right hand, but the influence of ideation on the function of the other hemisphere was totally impossible.

All the mentioned forms of apraxia concern the preparatory state of writing, while the innervatory phenomena may be completely intact. The patient may be even able to compensate the defect partially by use of the motor automatisms. In other cases, damage of these automatisms is the cause of the agraphia. The patient can innervate the muscles by which writing is performed for other purposes but not for production of letters. This is the form which usually is called *pure* or *motor agraphia*. It is the effect of damage of complicated motor mechanisms and corresponds thus to the peripheral motor aphasia (see p. 190).

The lesion in this form is localized in the part of Frontalis II which is located anteriorly to the motor area of the hand in the anterior central convolution. It is a particular part of this area.

This localization was first postulated by Exner (1881). There are a number of cases published with this localization of the lesion. Particularly the collection of cases by Henschen (139) leaves no doubt about the significance of this localization for the development of this particular form of agraphia.

The defect concerns (in right-handed people) the right hand, sometimes also the left.

The patient of Pitres (1884) could write with the left hand. Pick's case, published in 1897, could not. There seems to be a great irregularity concerning the affection of the other hand. There are a number of factors to be considered if we want to understand this irregularity. The localization of the lesion may be different, and, correspondingly, we are not at all dealing with the same functional defect in all the cases. The cases with defect of ideation, e.g., should be excluded. We have seen before that, in principle here, both hands are affected.

When we restrict ourselves to the cases of motor agraphia, there are patients who can write easily and fluently with the other hand but produce mirror writing. There are other patients who write normally but slowly, with difficulty and with defects in the form of letters and with omissions. One has the impression that the individual letters are produced by them with great effort. In the first cases, we can assume that the other hand, in learning to write, was trained concomitantly with the major hand. The effect of the same movements in the other hand is mirror writing. We can observe among normals a group of persons who, induced to write with the left hand, produce mirror writing without being aware of it, while others write in the normal way. If an individual of the first type is suffering from motor agraphia, he will instigate the learned movements of the other hand, and mirror writing will appear. This reveals an automatic character of "normal writing"; the individual is not deliberating about the forms of the letters and writing is rather fluent, particularly if one considers the unfamiliarity of writing with the other hand. If one asks this person to write with the other hand in the normal way, he may not be able to do so, if he is of the motor type. He will write like the other type with effort if he can use his visual images.

In all these respects, the writing with the left hand of the other types of patients differs. It is a deliberate production of performances. It seems, as far as we know it, based on imitation of visual images. This explains the fact that it is not mirror writing, that it is slow, that mistakes occur due to the imperfectness of the images and the lack of training of the motor acts. If such patients do not have good images, they are not able to write with the other hand at all.

Thus, the questions of why a patient is able to write with the other hand (or why not), and how he writes, will be understood only by careful analysis of the total personality of the patient.

Particularly interesting are the cases where *agraphia concerns the minor hand only*. Such cases have been published by Liepmann, Maass, Sittig and myself. My case leaves no doubt that the anatomic cause of this picture is a destruction of the corpus callosum, as Liepmann first showed. This case is further significant because the right hand was free from any paralysis and any difficulty in writing. The total agraphia of the left hand was accompanied by apraxia of the left side of the body, or, to put it otherwise, was one expression of this defect. The agraphia of the patient was of the same type as his apraxia (see original publication). The patient was able to hold the pencil correctly in her left hand (effect of a preserved motor automatism), but was unable to produce any correct form of a letter; she produced rings, lines in various directions (horizontal, vertical or oblique). Presented with such forms, she was able to "imitate" them (though in an imperfect way), but not to copy them. The forms she produced in the task showed not the faintest similarity to presented letters or numbers. She wrote in "abduction"; i.e., writing from right to left, she thus belonged apparently to the motor type (see p. 130). Ideation was intact in this patient, as is proved by the normal behavior of the major side of the body. The agraphia as well as the apraxia was due to the destruction of the relations of the left hemisphere to the right motor system.

The autopsy revealed a total destruction of the corpus callosum and of the adjacent parts of the right hemisphere, particularly in the frontal lobe, by an embolism of the right arteria cerebri anterior. The extension of the softening was similar to that in the Ochs case of Liepmann and Maass; in their case it was located in the left, in our case in the right hemisphere.

In contrast to other cases of left-sided agraphia, where writing was somewhat preserved, particularly in copying, the defect here was total. The difference can be explained by the assumption that in the former cases, some relations to the major hemisphere were preserved.

There are a few published cases where apraxia and agraphia of the right side was observed in left-handed individuals with lesion of the right hemisphere (cases of M. Rothmann, Gans).

There has been some doubt as to whether it is justifiable to consider the left side agraphia as an expression of apraxia. Poetzl has stressed that, in general, agraphia does not develop parallel to apraxia. Considering the left-handed agraphia, this does not seem to be correct. The cases of Liepmann and Maas (case Ochs), Maass, Rose, Touchard, Sittig and my own case show both disturbances. It seems that agraphia can appear earlier than general apraxia, as in a case of Sittig (K.R.); this is understandable from the particular complex character of writing. If such a patient is seen at a time when the general apractic symptoms are not outspoken, the idea may seem to gain support that agraphia is independent from apraxia.

When apraxia without agraphia occurs in a case, one has to consider carefully the character of the apraxia. If it concerns only the right side in the form of defects of expressive movements and of showing how to use objects—as in the case of Vix—it is understandable that no agraphia existed. The slight defect did not affect writing, which has strong automatisms at its disposal.

(b) *Secondary Agraphia Due to Disturbances of Speech*

Disturbances of writing are frequent in aphasic patients. In all these cases the capacity for forming letters is unimpaired. The patients are disturbed in writing capacity as a consequence of defects in their language function.

There are some patients *with motor aphasia* who have defects in writing, but this is not always true. Correspondingly, an attempt has been made to distinguish two forms of motor aphasia which have been termed cortical motor aphasia with disturbances of writing, and subcortical motor aphasia without. This distinction is not at all based on facts (see p. 206). The motor speech defect in itself does not produce difficulties in writing, but there are individuals whose writing is so closely connected with speaking—whose writing is always accompanied by silent speaking—that if they acquire a motor aphasia, they are also disturbed in writing.

In individuals who normally do not accompany writing with speaking, agraphia will not necessarily accompany motor aphasia. Sometimes motor aphasia appears simultaneously with motor agraphia simply because the localization of the lesion which produces motor agraphia is so close to the area involved in motor aphasia. According to Dejerine and others, the isolated lesion of the Gyrus angularis is supposed to be followed by isolated alexia and agraphia. Niessl von Mayendorf has criticized this assumption; he explains the alexia as effect of disturbances of vision of the macula. According to von Monakow, it seemed to be necessary for appearance of alexia under this condition that the corpus callosum fibers also are severed.

There are certainly cases of alexia with intact vision of the macula (Dejerine, Schuster, the case of Gelb and myself). Alexia is, in my opinion, an *expression of general visual agnosia*, where the defect in reading is more outstanding than in recognition of other objects because of functional differences (see p. 120).

It is not quite decided which role, in this respect, lesions in the Gyrus angularis play. A new interpretation of the cases is very desirable. The cases described are, even symptomatologically, of very different types and the anatomical lesions do not at all permit the assumption that a lesion here produces isolated alexia.

Concerning the agraphia in these lesions, there is no doubt that cases are observed where visual alexia exists without disturbance of writing (see p. 120). In one group of alexia cases, the disturbances of writing are most probably of language origin, and not due to alexia. But, as we have said before (p. 120), in some individuals, defects in visualization may damage writing.

The disturbances of writing in *central aphasia* (see p. 229) mirror the speech defect. In general, writing is even more modified than speaking, but the patient may be able to write some words correctly because he possesses motor writing automatisms. In *pure sensory aphasia*, there is no writing defect at all. In so-called *cortical sensory aphasia*, the writing defect is due to the defect of inner speech. In the *transcortical aphasias*, the writing defect corresponds to the speech defect (see also p. 292). A special form of modification of writing is observed in *amnesic aphasia* (amnesic aphasic agraphia) (see p. 252).

There is a group of patients who are able to form letters, copy letters, speak sounds, but who have lost the capacity to relate language and letters. Therefore, they cannot "write" letters and words, i.e., are unable to produce them in relation to language; thus, for example, they cannot write on dictation. See the corresponding defect in reading (p. 125) and its training (p. 337).

In other cases, we are dealing with ideatory apraxia, which shows also in disturbances of writing and reading, which may even be particularly developed here (see case Bonhoeffer, 19, and p. 126). There are some differences between the symptoms in reading in visual alexia and in ideatory apraxia: in the latter cases, reading and writing is not disturbed so severely, and their failures show modifications characteristic of ideatory apraxia in general; copying is relatively good, while in visually produced cases, copying is severely disturbed.

J. DISTURBANCES OF THE CALCULATING CAPACITY

Disturbances of the calculating capacity are frequent in cases of brain damage. Calculation is a complex performance in which we can distinguish two main factors abstractively: an *intellectual* one, the ability to understand the meaning of value of the numbers, and the various methods of calculating, as addition, multiplication, etc.; and, on the other hand, *learned patterns* which play an important role in the procedures of calculation and consist of motor automatisms, sometimes writing automatisms and visual patterns. Here we find individual differences based on congenital abilities, and particular forms of learning calculations which produce different forms and extent of the disturbance in the same brain defect, all of which must be taken into consideration in retraining. Accordingly, compensation and covering of a defect also may differ and hence deceive us.

1. *Disturbances of the Intellectual Ability Underlying Calculation*

These disturbances occur in visual agnosia of the type Gelb and I have published (see 112a). Here the patients have lost the concept of the value of numbers. They may be able to deal with numbers in learned activities as, for instance, to count or to do multiplication on the basis of learned motor automatisms. But they have no idea of what numbers mean. The loss of this concept is not an isolated defect, and is also not the consequence of the visual-agnostic defect or a lack of visualization. These disturbances and the loss of the value of numbers can be attributed to the same basic modification of the brain function, the function which we call "simultaneous function" (see p. 121), psychologically considered a defect closely related to impairment of abstraction. The origin of this functional defect makes it understandable that these patients are disturbed in the understanding of the nature of groups, of the methods of calculation, etc. The patient may even not know which is the greater, 6 or 8, etc. (regarding this and other related phenomena, cf. particularly the publication of my co-worker, Benary, 8).

On another occasion (see ?, p. 753) I have tried to explain why this basic function (and with this, the defects in calculation) occur in lesion of the occipital parietal region, as I call it, the posterior part of the "central part of the brain cortex" (see p. 46).

Similar defects in calculation are observed in lesion of another region, of the frontal lobes; this is understandable because this region belongs to the central part of the brain cortex too.   I should like to refer here to cases as those of Woerkom and my own (see p. 208).

As the motor automatisms can be intact in these cases, the defect can be covered by using them.   The patient may appear to be a slow calculator because this procedure, particularly if the patient counts in a roundabout way, takes a certain amount of time.   It is characteristic that the patient does not know whether his results are correct or not.   When, for example, by counting he arrives at the result that 8 is more than 6, he assumes this to be correct because in counting, 8 appears after 6, and this is what "one calls more"; he has no idea, however, whether it is really right or not.   The following practically very important consequence sometimes results: such patients may lose, with time, the patterns of calculation because they cannot control the results and so lose confidence in their usefulness.

These patients must relearn even the simplest multiplication without insight as to its correctness, and hence learn such processes only by confidence in the teacher or by discovering their usefulness in practical situations (see p. 8).

2. *Disturbances of Calculation Due to Loss of Visual or Motor Images and Learned Patterns*

First let us consider cases which occur in occipital lesions.   To this group belong most of the published cases with disturbances of calculation (case of Lewandowski and Stadelmann, a great number of observations by Henschen and of brain-injured men observed by Poppelreuter, Goldstein, Peritz, et al.).   There are different possibilities of how, in lesion of the occipital lobe, these disturbances of calculation occur.   We have discussed those due to impairment of "simultaneous function."   All the others are in *relation to visual defects*.   The difficulty or impossibility of reading numbers certainly will make written calculation impossible; such may be the case in visual field defects and in visual agnosia.   Indeed, it is known that in visual alexia, numbers may be well recognized even if letters are not.   This is certainly not because we have different centers for letters and numbers and because the latter is preserved. The reason is the different attitude which we assume toward letters and numbers. Letters have no meaning in themselves; their significance comes from the relation of definite forms to language. Numbers, although also symbols, are more concrete objects which are in a definite relationship to the total personality. A damage in the visual sphere may therefore damage letters more than numbers. Certainly, in a severe visual alexia, the recognition of numbers also will be impossible, and thus written calculation will be disturbed; however, oral calculation may be left intact, if the meaning of the value of numbers is not disturbed and the individual was accustomed to use motor patterns in calculation. In some cases of visual alexia, the patients are deprived of the recognition of the signs for calculation, as $+$, $-$, etc. This can happen also without loss of the value of numbers and the procedures of calculations, but there must be no defect in oral calculation.

There is another possibility for the origin of defects in calculation by a lesion in the visual sphere, namely, by *disturbance of visualization;* in a slight alexia reading may be somewhat preserved, but visualization severely damaged. This may not have a definite effect in individuals who do not use visualization for calculation (for representing definite visual patterns and organization of the procedures in calculation); but those who are accustomed to work in this way may have difficulties in calculation. They may be capable of doing written calculations, but not oral ones. They present, thus, the opposite picture from the mentioned patient with disturbance of visualization. It was assumed that these observations speak for the existence of a "Zentrum für die Rechenfähigkeit" ("calculating center") in the occipital lobe (Peritz, p. 334), but this is neither necessary nor justified.

Motor speech defects can produce disturbances of calculating in two ways. People who are accustomed—and there are many such—to calculate (particularly to do multiplications) on the basis of motor speech series, will be impaired in calculation if the latter are impaired in motor aphasia. These patients may be able to fulfill written calculations because their intellectual capacities are undisturbed; but some patients are not able to calculate thus, and these are the patients who are accustomed always to accompany writing by speaking. They may be able to calculate through visualization, by use of visual patterns which they had built up before or build up now for compensation.

I should like to mention here a patient of this type.

The patient had a typical peripheral motor aphasia (see p. 190); he could speak a few words, with difficulty in the motor act. He improved in this respect, but was not able to learn motor series, particularly the grammatical series and those which one needs for calculation. His intellectual capacities were intact in all respects; he understood the methods of calculation and had the concept of value of numbers.

He could perform written calculation of all kinds, even complicated interest accounts without difficulty; the only abnormality was that he needed considerable time; his main defect was that he could not find a result in simple multiplication, addition, etc., or it took such a long time that his written procedure was disturbed.

He improved in this respect by use of a tool which he had invented himself. It consisted of small tablets on which he had imprinted numbers and their additions or subtractions. From them he acquired visual images which he visualized, and found the result in addition and subtraction with increased rapidity.

For multiplication, he used a square tablet which he divided into a hundred equal squares, ten on each side. He wrote the numbers 1–10 in the top horizontal row, and down the left-hand row. Then he filled in the multiplication tables so that the tables ran both horizontally and vertically. With the help of this tablet, he found results relatively quickly. With the tablet in his hand, he pointed to the multiplicator, say 6, then to the multiplicand, say 8; then he drew a horizontal line through 6 and dropped a perpendicular line from 8; at the conjunction of these lines was the number 48. He would then give this number as his result. If he had to find an answer in division, he traced the horizontal line along to the left side and thus found the multiplicator. He acquired a visual image of the whole tablet and in this fashion found the result on the visualized picture. With time, his calculations became so rapid with the help of these tools that it was easy to overlook his defect. Certainly, this procedure was possible only because the man had particularly good visualization.

In cases of *central motor aphasia* we usually meet a more complicated picture, a combination of motor disturbances of calculation, and disturbances due to the defect in intellectual functions—corresponding to the underlying process (see p. 208). In these cases, where the motor series may not be impaired to such a degree, the patient may be able to give some correct results on the basis of these patterns.

It was assumed (Oppenheim, 1913, and others) that for dealing with numbers, the other (minor) hemisphere is of particular importance. There is no proof for this. Indeed, performances gained by the other hemisphere may, in defects of the dominant one, help calculation by the support through visual or motor patterns. Disturbances of calculation are more frequent in lesion of the dominant hemisphere than of the minor (Peritz, Henschen, Goldstein), probably because for the intellectual ability underlying calculation the dominant hemisphere is of greater importance.

K. Disturbances in Gestures and Pantomimic Performances in Aphasic Patients

Patients suffering from different forms of aphasia vary as to the appearance of changes of gestures. If we are to understand these changes in their clinical significance, we have to consider carefully the differences between the various phenomena which are generally all termed gestures, or, more or less indiscriminatingly, by words such as gesticulation, mimic, pantomimic, etc.

Gestures are not only facial movements but movements more or less of the whole body, particularly also the arms and hands. It depends on the personality, the cultural condition, the particular situation, as to what degree gestures accompany the language of an individual. One should distinguish two groups: those which *appear with emotions*, expressed with language or without; and those which *represent means of communication of ideas*, facts, etc. We are able to demonstrate some ideas or some objective things by gesture. Critchley recommends distinguishing gestures and pantomimes in a similar way as Jackson has distinguished, in language, emotional utterances from propositionizing ones, and it may be useful to call the first ones gestures and the last ones pantomimes. As much as I agree in general with his distinction, I have some objection to it, the same which I expressed in the discussion of the distinction between emotional and propositional language (see p. 59). Certainly, gestures belong mostly to "concrete" situations, concrete actions, and are executed without an active, voluntary, abstract attitude; pantomimes represent something, and presuppose the attitude of abstraction.

But we are able voluntarily to perform the movements which occur in expressions and gestures. We can show how to threaten, to wink, even how one laughs, etc. In testing apraxia, we ask our patients to show how one threatens, etc. In apraxia, the patients may have lost this capacity, while in a natural condition these movements may occur about normally; here alone they are concrete performances. On the other hand, pantomimic performances may not always occur with abstract attitude, they can be automatized and accompany speaking in an immediate way. Thus, both forms of "gestures" can appear as expression of the two attitudes which we have distinguished in human behavior in general (see p. 5). It is not at all easy always to distinguish in an individual case whether one or the other attitude is present. But only if we make this distinction shall we be able to understand the behavior as to gestures of aphasic patients. If we neglect it, we may be confronted with a confusing variety of pictures. With our supplement, the distinction of Critchley is very valuable. In general, one will agree with Critchley when he says that verbal speech suffers considerably more than gesture language, particularly if one considers the cases with pure motor and sensory aphasia. But this statement is not valid for those cases where the abstract attitude is impaired and this impairment is more or less the cause of the aphasic symptoms. Under this condition, particularly the pantomime may be disturbed severely, too, while some gestures may be better preserved. But even the latter may not be the case, the patients possibly showing a lack of the expressive movements in face and body; they may appear rigid even when they are emotionally excited. It seems that also the normal expressive movements can be impaired in brain defects, particularly in lesions near the frontal lobes.

In general, one will agree with Critchley that gesture suffers less than panto-mime in speech disturbances.

In some cases, in which we consider impairment of abstraction as the basis of the language disturbances—as in amnesic aphasia—the patients show an *exaggeration* of expressive movements which might appear like pantomimes. This could be considered to be in contradiction to the as-sumption that pantomime is a propositional behavior. I think we are not obliged to correct this assumption on the basis of these observations. What appears here is not *intentional demonstration but occurrence of learned movements which become abnormally manifest* if the words to which they belong cannot be uttered. In other cases of aphasia where the abstract attitude is preserved, gestures and pantomimes are often very much exag-gerated. As Critchley says, the jargon aphasia is "usually accompanied by an excessive range of facial and manual gesticulation" (see 40, p. 26). In some cases of motor aphasia, the use of gestures and pantomimes alone may allow the patient to communicate with the world, in spite of loss of speech, in an excellent way, as long as abstract attitude is not impaired.

It is a particular problem whether in deaf-mutes with an apoplexia the sign-language may be lost like verbal speech in speaking persons. Jackson wrote: "No doubt, by disease of some part of the brain the deaf-mute might lose his natural system of signs which are of some speech-value to him." Indeed their movements do not correspond to the gestures we have in mind. Critchley has published a case of a partial deaf-mute patient "whose ability to finger speech became impaired after a stroke."

L. Disturbances of Language in Polyglot Individuals with Aphasia

As long as the concept of circumscribed brain centers was dominant in the doctrine of aphasia, it was natural to attempt to explain the difference in disturbances of the various languages of polyglot aphasics by the assump-tion of differences in the localization of the underlying lesion. Indeed, Pitres (1895) had pointed to the inadequacy of such an endeavor and stressed that only a functional consideration can clarify why a patient loses one language to a higher degree than another, and why in improvement of the condition one may reappear earlier than another. His experiences taught him further that the rule of Ribot—that in a damage of the memory the oldest material remains less affected than the later acquired—cannot be valid in general and that other factors are also responsible for the symptomatology. He emphasized particularly for preservation of a lan-guage the significance of the factor of its longer use directly before the in-sult, the "fluency" which the individual had attained as to this language.

However much I agree with Pitres in both respects from my general point of view, I think, nevertheless, that stressing simply the functional significance in general means merely the presenting of the problem and not solving it. There are a number of other functional factors besides fluency which are of importance: the particular framework which determines the speaker—the outer world conditions, particularly the language milieu in which he speaks, the differences of the relation of the various languages he used for various speech performances (e.g., for expressions of his emotions, for speaking in everyday life, in situations of teaching, etc.), and other factors which were observed by various authors. But all this knowledge does not help us understand the patient's behavior if we do not know why the patient is determined in a special situation by one or another factor. This is still more important as we observe that the same patient may appear to be determined now by one, now by another factor. His behavior seems to be determined by a kind of selection. And what determines this selection? The answer to this question can only be the same which helped us to understand the performances of aphasic patients with only one language. Why a language performance occurs can be understood only from the situation as a whole. Only from the total situation can the influence of any factor be evaluated correctly. The patient uses that speech material which is most appropriate to help him, by means of language, to come to terms with the problem with which he is faced at a particular moment in his trend for self realization. If our standpoint in general is correct, it should be suited to clarify the behavior of polyglot aphasics.

The following survey of the observed phenomena which I have compiled is guided by this point of view and should prove its use for the interpretation of these phenomena.

1. First, there are those cases where the patient uses only (or mostly) his mother tongue. Indeed, as far as I can see, the other language is hardly intact at all. The published literature does not allow us to decide whether the other language was not always affected, too, and whether it did not appear so much better because of the particular circumstances. Certainly, a difference will depend upon differences in the relations of both languages to the total personality, and further, upon the kind of underlying aphasic disturbance and the situations in which language was observed.

The patient will, in everyday conversation, stick to his mother tongue, particularly to dialect (see p. 143), because it may appear to him as the best means of expressing himself. But that this is not always the case is demonstrated by some observations of Minkowski, to which we shall return later.

The problem whether and why a patient uses one language alone should be investigated with new material. If one language is preserved, or at

least is prominent, it must not be the mother tongue.   Usually the factor
of "fluency" shows its great influence.

One of the oldest published cases showing that the mother tongue is not
preserved best is the patient reported by Hinshelwood.

An Englishman, 34 years old, acquired, with an apoplectic insult, total
aphasia and alexia.   After improvement of speech, the disturbance of reading remained persistent.   The patient could read all letters and some words
when he was allowed to spell them aloud.   He was an educated man, who
knew French, Latin and Greek.   Astonishingly, he read Greek, though
slowly but with only a few errors which he could correct; Latin showed a
poorer performance but was better than English and French; his reading
in English was particularly bad.   Even after improvement, the relationship between the languages in respect to better or worse reading remained.
We do not know enough about the patient to deduce the reason for this
behavior.

2. Very often, more than one language is preserved, the patient using
all of them—although all are more or less disturbed,* and all in the same
way apparently, corresponding to the form of aphasia which the patient
suffers.   Indeed, a patient may not use all his languages under all conditions.   A closer consideration of the condition in which he uses one or the
other one is suited to clarify the problem in which we are interested.

It may be that the functional defect disturbs one language more than
the other—according to its different structure—and some speech performances in one language more than in another; this would explain a
number of differences.   The patient will try to use that language which
appears the best for his purpose.   Naturally, this means the use of different
languages in different situations.

The cases differ not only as to the greater or lesser prevalence of one
language, but also as to a more or less easy alternation between the languages.   Poetzl has tried to bring the differences into relation to different
localizations of the lesion.   Patients with lesion in the tempero-parietal
region—according to Pick, in the region between parietal region and speech
area—are assumed to be particularly fixed to one language; less fixed are
patients with purely temporal lesions (as the case of Kauders).   Stengel
and Zelmanowicz bring the easiness with which their patient changes from
one to the other language into connection with the localization of the lesion

---

* In this respect (and in others), the case of Weisenburg and McBride is particularly interesting because the very intelligent patient spoke, beside his mother
language, English, seven other languages, and he was disturbed in all of them, not in
one exclusively (see p. 177).   The greater or smaller disturbance of one or the other
language corresponded about to the greater or smaller fluency which he had possessed
in the various languages, and improvement occurred in about the same way in all of
them.

in the anterior region of the speech area. This is hardly in agreement with all the facts. There are very few cases to offer as proof of this assumption. I have known cases where alternation was not possible in anteriorly located lesions. I think we cannot simply distinguish between anteriorly and posteriorly located lesions; it depends upon whether the lesion is so extended or located that it is suited to produce one or another form of expressive or reactive aphasia.

However this may be, distinction of the cases according to the anatomic differences cannot give a real understanding of the symptomatologic differences. A comparison of the differences in the ability to alternate between the various languages with the mental condition of the patient in general is more promising. Such a comparison makes it probable that alternation occurs in such cases where the capacity of abstraction—which is presupposition of shifting in general—is not impaired, and it is not possible in cases where it is impaired. In lesions of the anterior as well as posterior part of the speech area, this capacity may or may not be disturbed.

In the case of Stengel and Zelmanowicz, one can discover from the other symptoms no reason to assume that this capacity was not intact; it was a "peripheral motor aphasia" (see p. 190). In the case I have observed, the capacity was disturbed and the alternation between languages was more difficult.

In order to avoid an erroneous interpretation, it must be stressed that not every appearance of the other language is real alternation. One should speak of alternation only if it occurs voluntarily. Frequently, passive alternation is to be observed. A patient may name an object in one language, but suddenly utters a name in the other language (see Weisenburg and McBride, 313, p. 157); or he may suddenly use this other language, which he possessed before, when the people around him converse in it. This may explain why the patient of Bychowski who, before the lesion, knew the foreign language rather insufficiently, preferred it nevertheless in an environment where this language was spoken. The desire to be in contact with the people determined his attitude and he spoke the "other" language. Even an imperfect use of the other language may appear a better means of communication.

An intelligent patient of mine with a definite defect of abstraction seemed to shift from one language (her mother tongue, Swedish) to the other language (English) which she had spoken since she came to this country a number of years before. She changed to English when somebody addressed her in it. But she was certainly not able to shift voluntarily from one to the other language. She changed particularly in everyday conversation when she had not to think what to say. But she could not change when she had to explain something which needed more active use of language.

This difference in the capacity to shift finds its expression in differences in the patient's capacity to translate from one language into the other. A slight defect in the capacity to translate may show in the fact that a patient can translate from the less preserved language to the better preserved one, but not the opposite.

The same difficulty was present with the patient of Weisenburg and McBride, who had previously been very much accustomed to translate. According to the results in the tests mentioned by the authors, it is to be assumed that he was impaired in abstraction (see 313, p. 177).

Our patient, to whom we referred a few paragraphs back, might sometimes repeat words or even sentences—first spoken in English or Swedish—in the other language. But this was not the effect of translation, as became evident when one asked her to translate a word which she understood into the other language. She was totally unable to do so; she did not understand what one meant, even if one tried to explain it to her by examples. While, in examinations as well as in conversations, she often repeated in English, in emotional situations she often reverted to Swedish. From this observation we may conclude that translation demands active shifting. Appearance of words of the other language concomitantly with those of the spoken language cannot always be evaluated as translation. These words may be associations which are not based on voluntary translation. This corresponds to the phenomenon, which shows in many performances of the patient, that she puts together two things, though she does not know why (see 113, p. 12).

The less difficult a performance was, the less interferences between both languages occurred; thus, for example, less difficulty in the association experiment in which her language was particularly good than in spontaneous speech.

The complexity of the situation can be shown by the phenomenon which a patient, like that of Stengel, may present: less interference in counting backward than in counting forward. One would certainly expect the opposite to be the case inasmuch as counting backward is ordinarily considered the more difficult performance. However, it is not simply more difficult, but differently performed. In counting forward we are accustomed to speak more automatically, in counting backward more voluntarily and to paying more attention to the individual act. The automatic performance was deteriorated in the patient, but not her voluntary activity. This finds its expression in the first very peculiar phenomenon that she could count backward better than forward. For her, the former performance was apparently the easier, and so it becomes understandable that interferences were not so apparent.

In another case with central motor aphasia where the voluntary activities were particularly disturbed, the opposite phenomenon can be observed. The patient shows greater difficulties in backward series and more interference in this performance. The patient displayed much similarity with the behavior of a normal individual who, emigrating to another country, must learn a new language for finding new contacts with the world and a new adequate existence. The individual still has a preference for his mother tongue but experiences more and more that he can come to terms with the world only by shifting to the new language. This changed attitude improves his talking in the new language and makes his talking in his mother tongue worse. He then mixes words and phrases, often being unaware of it. In a situation where people speak his mother tongue he immediately speaks the latter fluently. If words of the new language are acquired in relation to a special situation, occupation, etc., they are predominant in this situation; the words of the old language do not come to his mind. There is scarcely a better occasion to show how facts fit our interpretation than the situation of the emigrant.

3. The disturbance in language of patients who speak a *dialect* in addition to a literary language confronts us with a particularly complex problem. Dialect language is *not simply any other language*. It does not differ from others simply by being only a spoken language which is not read or written. No matter how much influence this factor may have on the structure of the language and how much it has to be considered for an understanding of the deviations in pathology, it does not of itself hit the point. The main difference is the much closer relationship to the total personality of the speaker and to a definite environment. As dialect is a product of a particularly intimate communication between the individual and the world around (a special group of people) the individual in speaking dialect experiences himself as embedded in this group, immediately belonging to it. Because of this well-established background, the "Unausgesprochene" (understood but unspoken part) of language plays a still greater role here than in other languages. Dialect is much more "concrete," more passively emerging out of the situation than voluntary. By all these characteristics it is a more adequate means than the literary language for coming to terms with the environment. But, on the other hand, it is more restricted, it fits only a definite environment. The use of reading and writing enables the individual to comprise a much greater and even more flexible world. Therefore, dialect is spoken naturally and freely only in an adequate milieu. In a milieu where the individual is doubtful as to whether he can be understood he is afraid to use it, feeling he may even appear ridiculous, and he may refrain from using the dialect, or speak a mixed language. All these factors have to be considered to understand the differences of the cases.

Those cases which concern aphasic patients who spoke dialect are infrequent.   Minkowski, living in a country where dialect is spoken generally even in conversations of sophisticated people, had thus much occasion to observe polyglot aphasics and says that the dialect "Schweizerdeutsch" (Swiss German) is usually earlier and better restituted than "Schriftdeutsch" (literary German), or at any rate not later.   Of more importance, it would seem, are his careful examinations of two patients who apparently represented exceptions to this rule.   Therefore, I should like in the discussion which follows to refer particularly to this author's publication (see p. 145).

The first patient, a 32 year old mechanic, had little formal schooling, but had a great urge to educate himself.   He learned the Swiss-German dialect as his mother tongue.   Later he read many and good books in "High German" and in this way and by writing many letters acquired the literary language.   For several years just preceding his injury, he had much occasion to speak "High German" and spoke it so well that he could pass for a German.   With his landlady with whom he was particularly close, he spoke dialect, which she did not speak well and usually mixed with "High German."   He knew a little French and Italian.

After an accident, a severe injury of the skull, he was unconscious, had a transient right hemiplegia, disturbances of sensation, was disoriented, could not speak and had difficulty in understanding.   (In his improvement, the speech disturbances disappeared, first in German and Swiss German totally, not so much in French and Italian.)   For many months, it was difficult for him to speak (spontaneously and on repetition) and to read and write, but afterward the restitution was very good.   The picture and its restitution corresponded in general to those in "peripheral motor aphasia."   Minkowski assumed as cause a diffuse but not severe damage of Broca's region.   The motor defect consisted in some dysarthria and paraphasic distortions as we considered them characteristic of this form of aphasia (see p. 190).   Further, there were defects in grammatical forms, sentences were short and the "little words" and grammatical endings, flexions, articles were missing or wrongly built.   Understanding of reading improved particularly well, reading aloud was soon better than spontaneous speech, but even here, reading of the "little words" remained difficult, or the patient could not read them at all.   Writing, too, soon became better.   Naming and repetition showed about the same defects as spontaneous speech.

In general, the patient did not show any mental deterioration; he was somewhat changed in his personality, but it seemed that he did not have impairment of abstract attitude.

The most astonishing symptom was that the patient *in his recovery spoke only "High German"* and not his dialect, even in a milieu where he was accustomed to use the dialect.   Thus, one could assume that he behaved contrary to the rule.   Minkowski's analysis revealed that his speaking was not a recurrence of his previous way of speaking but that he spoke now with the help of the visual image of the written words.   He read, as it were, the imagined written words.

Considering the origin of this preference for German, the case, indeed, cannot simply be considered as one where non-dialect was preferred.   Both

languages were damaged, but by the use of reading the patient could cover
the defect and retain his motor speech only in "High German," not in the
dialect.   This is more apparent inasmuch as reading and writing improved
first and best, and he was taught by his teacher through reading and writing.   Thus, the performance of "High German" was more the effect of
special training than of simple recovery.   It is interesting that when later
his teacher tried to retrain dialect in the same way the patient also improved as to dialect.

Thus, the case—although, because of the retraining method, of great
theoretic and practical interest (see p. 328)—is not well suited to teach
us much about the intrinsic causes of the differences between dialect and
non-dialectical language in aphasia.   However, Minkowski made some
further observations which are also of value in this respect.   It was remarkable that the patient never improved as well in dialect as in "High German."
Minkowski points to various reasons which all show the relatedness of the
recovery to the total personality.   There was the affective trend to learn
"High German" because his close friend, from whom he had learned to
talk again and upon whom he was, in general, dependent, preferred this
language.   There was a general factor effective in the same direction: the
patient, severely damaged in his social standard and isolated by his defect
from his normal environment, could expect by use of literary German to
give himself a higher prestige.

The second case of Minkowski concerns a Professor W., born in Zurich,
who spoke the Swiss German dialect as his mother tongue, and besides that,
literary German, French and English.   Until the age of 30 he spoke Swiss
German with his family.   At this time he became professor in Neufchâtel,
where he spoke French also in everyday life.

At the age of 54 an aptopleptic insult occurred.   At first there was total
aphasia, with, however, quick recovery of understanding in all languages.
Only slowly and with great effort did he learn to speak, at first French,
"like a schoolboy," with the help of books and training by his daughter.
Then the German came back, apparently without special training, and
some Italian.   But, living another ten years, he never reacquired his mother
tongue, the dialect.

Minkowski sees as the main cause for this lack of recovery of the mother
tongue the fact that the dialect was the language the patient had not
spoken for a long time, or only occasionally, while French was the language
which was related to his personal and professional life.

I should like to stress the following point in respect to this case and to
the problem of the preference of non-dialect language.   In peripheral motor
aphasia, the motor automatisms are particularly damaged.   The patients
lose especially the fluency of the motor act, while they may be able to pro-

duce motor performances, e.g., series, with effort and will, although somewhat imperfectly. This voluntary procedure may help in regaining a language which usually is more voluntarily, "intentionally" spoken (like the literary language) but cannot (or to only a lesser degree) be applied to dialect, which always is a less voluntary activity. For recovery, a restitution of the motor activities is necessary.*

We then come to the conclusion: *There are a number of factors determining which language is preferred in a polyglot individual if he acquires an aphasia. No factor, however, can be considered isolatedly as a cause of the individual picture, but only if one evaluates it in respect to the total personality (premorbid and after insult) and to the environment in which he lives, in respect to the trend of the man to use language as a means for the highest form of self realization which he can achieve under the circumstances.*

M. DISTURBANCES OF MUSICAL PERFORMANCES

Disturbances in this field are not rare in brain damage. They are of different kinds. Some belong to the field of apraxia, as, for example, loss of the capacity to play an instrument; or visual agnosia, e.g., loss of recognition of the musical signs. Closer to the aphasic symptoms are the modifications of the capacity to sing. I shall not consider them here in detail, as this would necessitate an extensive discussion of the musical functions in general, a difficult task which space does not permit us to undertake here. However, in this respect, Feuchtwanger's work should be especially cited ("Amnesie." Berlin, Springer, 1930).

Singing can be disturbed concomitantly with speech, or isolatedly. On the other hand, it has been known for some time that singing can be preserved in severe motor aphasia, either without the patient producing the words in singing the melody, or, in many cases, even retaining this ability. Liepmann, Marburg, Henschen and others observed such cases, and I have seen the same in a number of patients. I should like to restrict myself to some general remarks concerning the interpretation and examination of the behavior of patients in this respect.

An attempt has been made to explain the maintenance of singing in spite of speech incapacity as an effect of preservation of a localized anatomic structure. Regardless of the authority of Henschen, who assumed that a "motor singing center" is located in the pars triangularis of the third left frontal convolution anterior to Broca's area, one cannot say that the anatomic findings give definite evidence for this. It is more probable that the difference between singing and speaking is due to the different physiologic and psychologic structures of both performances. According to the more

* For another interesting case, see Weisenburg and McBride, 313, p. 160.

primitive character of singing and the close relationship of singing to expressive movements and to emotional language, it can be assumed that in a brain damage, singing will be preserved longer than language. Whether it is—in spite of a language defect—preserved or not will further depend upon whether singing was nearer to the total personality of the concerned individual, to his emotional life, and upon the degree to which he had developed automatisms in this field. If singing had always been more a phenomenon of "representation" than an emotional outlet for someone, he will be more disturbed after a brain damage than an individual with a more "concrete" attitude toward singing. Till now, no observations have been made which show definitely how the individual whose singing was or was not preserved behaved in this respect. Careful observation of the conditions under which the patient is able to sing would be of great significance. From my own limited experience with this particular question, patients are able to produce singing only as expressions, not as singing before somebody else does; they can sing with somebody, continue if somebody begins, but are not able to begin themselves.

If this is correct, the preservation of singing would be explainable in the same way as the better preservation of emotional language (see p. 57). In this respect, there is significance in the frequent parallelism between preservation of singing and other emotional expressions, such as the Lord's Prayer (see, e.g., a case of Oppenheim whom Henschen mentions; 139, p. 149).

There is a possibility that this automatized performance may be guaranteed by the function of the minor hemisphere.

Concerning the localization of the motor disturbances of the motor musical performances, particularly of singing, there was a tendency—since an observation of L. Mann—to bring the defect into connection with a lesion of the right second frontal convolution. This assumption seemed to be enforced by observations of K. Mendel and Max. Mann. Henschen and Marburg have stressed that these cases are not very conclusive. In the case of L. Mann, the possibility of a lesion of the cortical area of the larynx musculature cannot be excluded, as Henschen has pointed out. Henschen came to the conclusion—on the basis of a larger amount of material—that the most significant area for the defect in singing is located in the lower part of the pars triangularis of the third left frontal convolution, a region which corresponds, or is situated somewhat anteriorly to, that region the electrical stimulation of which produces movements of the vocal cords (according to Horsley and C. and O. Vogt).

Concerning the disturbances of the sensory musical functions, the situation is still more complicated. Not even the relation of acoustic perception to grasping an interval, a melody, etc., is clear. There may be a number of disturbances in the acoustic sphere which may impair hearing of melodies, while other kinds of hearing (voices, language) may remain preserved.

Henschen has stressed that the disturbance of elementary acoustic perception has not yet been considered carefully enough in respect to recognition of melodies. I should like to refer the reader for further information to Feuchtwanger's book. Certainly also here, the attitude of the patients toward the phenomenon of musical perceptions should be considered more than it has in the past.

Usually, disturbances of perceiving and recognition of music occur in cases of word-deafness; however, there are cases of word-deafness without musical disturbances. For the opposite observation, see Henschen, 138, p. 164.

As to the localization of the disturbances on the perceptive side, Henschen and most of the other authors assume that perception of language, music and noises is related to different parts of the temporal lobe. I am inclined to assume that the symptomatologic picture may be determined by the general factors I mentioned before (the attitude of one who listens to music) and by the fact that a definite dedifferentiation of the function of the acoustic sphere may mean a different functional disturbance for various performances related to it; thus, different effects on these performances may occur. It should further be considered that damage of perception of some tones may be disastrous for the hearing of music; damage of perception of others may not show the same effect. In this respect, it is noteworthy that Pfeiffer, in cases of musical deafness, has observed damage of definite parts of the acoustic radiation in the subcortex. Musical sounds, according to Quensel and Pfeiffer, are perceived by patients with perceptual defect in musical performances as disordered noises, and hence experienced as very disagreeable. It may be pointed out finally that disturbances of perception of rhythm, which is important for perception of music, can be disturbed also by lesion outside of the temporal lobe. The importance of lesions in the area "of non-language mental processes" for disturbances of the musical capacities, impairment of abstraction, of simultaneous function, has not yet been taken into consideration.

N. Nomenclature

Nomenclature in the field of aphasia is somewhat confused as a result of the use of different points of view from which the symptoms are considered. Disturbances of speech are biologic phenomena. As such they can be considered from two different aspects: as modifications of performances of the patient, or as modification of the anatomic structures, and their modified functioning (the anatomico-physiologic aspect). The anatomico-physiologic approach usually appeared in the form of localization of separate performances and their disturbances in circumscribed areas of the brain cortex. As I have explained (see p. 45), the results of this approach are very ambiguous in general.

It would be preferable to differentiate definite clinical pictures and to call them with definite names according to the changes of performances. This is possible, however, only in a very gross manner; the clinical pictures appear clear-cut enough for such a purpose if one considers only certain outstanding symptoms. Thus, one can distinguish motor and sensory aphasia, global aphasia, amnesic aphasia, transcortical aphasia, alexia, etc. Such distinctions are sufficient for some purposes, e.g., for comparison of the symptom complexes in respect to localization of the underlying lesion, as, for instance, for determination of the place where the surgeon should make the intervention, etc. This nomenclature does not at all do justice to the complexity and variation of the modifications of language found in patients. Thus, the more clinical and anatomic facts were collected, the more it appeared not only insufficient but confusing. The authority of such a man as Kennier Wilson, who has supported the anatomic point of view, should not prevent us from seeing the facts. A nomenclature based on an analysis of the characteristic picture of performance disturbances promises more success; this means analysis by psychologic means. Opposition to this approach was raised long ago. Men like Wilson and Nielsen are not much in favor of it. But this opposition overlooks the fact that all clinical distinctions of aphasic symptom complexes are finally based on psychologic analysis (see 96, p. 8).

The difference is not that of using or not using psychology, but of using a more or less adequate psychologic procedure. The primitive psychology often used by clinicians, which goes back to earlier theoretic concepts of the organization of the mind, is unsatisfactory indeed. Thus, for instance, the theory of images, their significance for normal speech and their destruction as cause of speech defects, is not useful as a basis for nomenclature because it is not an adequate concept (see p. 26). There do not exist symptom complexes which could be understood as due to damage of images.

Which psychologic concepts should be used is certainly difficult to decide. I know only too well that it is impossible to demonstrate that one psychologic theory is right and the other wrong. However, I think that from the organismic approach it is possible to find more or less useful concepts about organization of speech and the origin of speech disturbances. This approach deserves preference because it is in principle much more cautious in respect to generalizations and enforces a much more empiric procedure. It involves a much more detailed analysis of the condition, psychologic as well as biologic. It does not allow any phenomena to be omitted in our attempt to understand the condition. It proves very useful in discovering new facts and hence in creating a possibility of differentiating superficially similar symptoms. Thus, it seems to me better suited also to form the basis of a rational nomenclature.

I am aware that from this approach, the development of a nomenclature which should do justice to the great variety of modification of behavior revealed by this procedure will be a difficult task which can be fulfilled today only to a certain degree of perfection. Our analysis is not at all sufficiently developed, but progress is to be expected if analysis is no longer hindered by theoretic bias and corresponding nomenclature. Names are dangerous and often prevent disclosure of facts. Therefore, we cannot be too careful with them. We should maintain different names as long as we are not sure that we are dealing with the effect of the same underlying functional disturbance. Only when we *are* sure of this should we use a common name. But the presence of a few similarities only should not induce us to do so. For some time there has been a tendency to consider certain symptoms in the field of speech and other mental performances as similar with regard to the nature of the underlying defect, and thus to designate speech disturbances as special forms of apraxia and agnosia. But this seems to me a little dangerous when we know so little about the structure of both symptom complexes, and it may prevent detailed study of each. In spite of similarities between visual agnosia and sensory aphasia, there are characteristic differences. Visual experience is essentially a simultaneous phenomenon, whereas acoustic experience is essentially successive. Perception and recognition are set in both fields before very different tasks. Destruction of function in each field should not be considered as having equal effect, as is suggested by the use of the same name—agnosia. The situation is similar in the motor sphere. Certainly motor aphasia has some similarity with apraxia. This has been stressed time and again, but each of the respective performance fields has a structure of its own, and the same damage may thus produce different symptoms. Therefore, the name aphasia for the disturbance of speech should not be relinquished, etc.

In this state of affairs, our nomenclature cannot be very homogenous. Sometimes we may base it on anatomic findings, sometimes on psychologic analysis, sometimes on clinical experience. The main point is that the nomenclature should allow for such a clear characterization of symptom complexes that the names can be used for comparison and correlation. Thus, the following list of terms is considered only as a means of orientation.

We shall call all disturbances of language, *Aphasia*. We distinguish *disturbances of the instrumentalities* and those *due to impairment of abstract attitude and other non-language mental phenomena*.

In the disturbances of instrumentalities, we distinguish those which

concern the expressive side (motor aphasia) from those which concern the
perceptive side (sensory aphasia).

Disturbances of the expressive side of language due to cortical lesions:
   1. *Dysarthria* (see p. 74)
   2. *Peripheral motor aphasia* (cortical and subcortical aphasia of the old nomenclature, Broca's aphasia, pure aphasia) (see p. 80)
   3. *Central motor aphasia:* Disintegration of motor speech due to impairment of
abstract attitude and the function of motor instrumentalities (see p. 85)
Disturbances of language due to impairment of non-language mental performances:
   1. Those due to impairment of abstract attitude (see p. 246)
   2. Those due to impairment of the "basic function" of the brain (see p. 309)
Disturbances of the receptive side of language due to cortical lesions:
   1. *Cortical deafness:* disturbance of acoustic perception due to cortical lesion
   2. *Noise and music cortical deafness:* Disturbance of perception of the characteristic sounds of noises and music with maintenance of hearing
   3. *Sensory aphasia*
      a. *peripheral sensory aphasia* (pure sensory aphasia, "reine Worttaubheit")
         (see p. 217)
      b. *central sensory aphasia* (cortical sensory aphasia, combination of pure sen-
         sory aphasia and central aphasia, and more or less amnesic aphasia)
Central aphasia (see p. 229)
Amnesic aphasia (see p. 246)
Transcortical aphasias, characterized through better preservation of repetition than
   understanding and spontaneous speaking
   1. transcortical motor symptom complexes (see p. 293)
   2. transcortical sensory symptom complexes (see p. 297)
   3. mixed transcortical aphasias (see p. 301)
Agraphia:
   1. *Primary agraphia:* Inability to build letters without disturbances in the sphere
of speech and vision
      a. *Motor agraphia* (pure agraphia) (see p. 129)
      b. *ideatory-apractic* agraphia (see p. 128)
      c. *amnesic-apractic agraphia* (see p. 128)
      d. *amnesic-aphasic agraphia* (see p. 132)
   2. *Secondary agraphia:* due to defects in language or vision
      a. *motor aphasic agraphia* (see p. 132)
      b. *central sensory aphasic agraphia* (see p. 132)
      c. *central aphasic agraphia* (see p. 132)
      d. *transcortical aphasic agraphia* (see p. 132)
      e. *visual agnostic agraphia* (in patients whose writing depends on visual images)
Alexia:
   1. *Primary alexia* (visual agnostic alexia) (see p. 120)
   2. *Secondary alexia:* due to defects in language
      a. *motor aphasic alexia:* different disturbances in reading or understanding of
         read material in motor aphasia (see p. 125)
      b. *sensory aphasic alexia* (paralexia, corresponding to paraphasia) (see p. 125)
      c. *central aphasic alexia* (see p. 125)

d. *amnesic aphasic alexia* (see p. 246)

e. *transcortical aphasic alexia* (see p. 125)

Echolalia (see p. 303)

O. EXAMINATION

Examination should start in the form of an interview. The complaints of the patient should stay in the foreground in the beginning. The patient should feel that one is examining him mainly because one wants to help him overcome his difficulties.

If one sees that the patient is unable to follow a demand or to answer a question correctly, and that he is aware of this, one should transfer to something else, to tasks one has the feeling he will be able to react to in a normal way or in a way satisfactory to himself. This is to avoid catastrophic situations with their effects upon such reactions as perseveration, fatigue, etc. (see p. 10).

In the general interview, one should try to get information about the patient's personality, age, education, family relations, personal and family history, his orientation as to time and space, etc. It is fortunate if one can obtain knowledge about all these points without special examinations.

During the interview, one may be able also to recognize some of the special defects of the patient, which then will determine the task of special examinations. During the latter, one should try to reassure the patient as much as possible as to his condition. One should begin with physical examination. It will reassure the patient very much if he can be told that the physical examination does not show any severe defect and that from the findings by this examination it can be assumed also that the speech disturbances are not so severe and will improve. Reassurance will be reached particularly if one can demonstrate that he is able to do things which he thought he was unable to do; thus, for instance, if a patient is not able to utter any word spontaneously, it is significant for the success of further investigation and treatment that one let him become aware as early as possible that he may be able to repeat words or recite some series (e.g., numbers) and so on, and so let him experience that he is not completely unable to speak. This gives him confidence in his own capacities and in the capacities of the physician who has recognized so quickly what he, the patient, can and can not do. This confidence in the physician is a kind of transference which develops in the same way in organic patients as in neurotics and is of greatest importance not only for treatment but also for future examination. If this transference has developed, the patient will be ready to do whatever the physician asks him to do, he will meet difficult tasks without being afraid of catastrophic situations, he will not develop them to such a high degree (if at all); when he is not able to react in the correct way, he will take the risk. If we begin with systematic examination, catastrophic reactions may bring about a totally false impression concerning what the patient is able to do and what not.

Neurologic investigation will have given a general impression of the patient's condition and allowed us to make the diagnosis of a localized brain defect. From this and the knowledge gained in the interview, we will expect some changes in special capacities such as speech, reading, etc. Before we begin with examination of these special defects, we should study the *"mental capacities in general."* One can apply for this purpose the usual intelligence tests for adults, e.g., the Wechsler Bellevue battery. One may also determine the I.Q.; from this it may be possible to draw a conclusion as to the premorbid intelligence and educational level of the patient. The vocabulary tests are particularly useful in the latter respect. From the beginning, attention should be paid to the phenomenon of chatter, and one should try to find out in which subtests the patient is successful and in which not. A qualitative analysis of the way the patient comes to the result in each subtest should be performed. The patient's pathology often does not consist of a defect in performance but in impairment of a definite (normal) procedure to solve a task. If the result is correct at face value, one may overlook the defect if an analysis of his procedure is not made (see p. 2). This procedure will show us in a number of cases which of the patient's failures are due not to a defect in special performance fields such as speaking, reading, etc., but to impairment of so-called general mental capacities.

(1) *Examination of "General capacities"*

Usually one thinks in this respect of such capacities as attention, interest, memory. Of course, one should consider the patient's behavior in all these respects carefully; much of a patient's failure in a special performance may be due to impairment of one or the other of these general capacities. However, there is not much value in testing these capacities in special tests. They show their effect in all tests and whether a failure is based on them can be evaluated correctly only by analysis of the special performance in which the impairment of capacity appears. Observation will then show that in many cases it is not justified to speak in general of impairment of such capacities, because the patient may be attentive, have a good memory, etc., under certain conditions, but not under others. This variation may be due to the entrance of catastrophe in certain tasks (see p. 10) or to impairment of abstract attitude (see p. 5). Avoiding catastrophes and testing the patient as to this attitude is, therefore, and for other reasons, our foremost task (see p. 154).

We should—to avoid catastrophic situations as much as possible—

arrange the tasks in a way that the patient gains the impression that he is doing well, and should draw our conclusions as to the defect not so much from his failures as from the structure of the task set before him.   Certainly, this will be possible only to a certain degree.   Furthermore, we want to know the failures in their particular structure, also.

If we have come to the result that the patient is impaired in his capacity to abstract, we shall have to consider each task and performance from the point of view of whether a failure is due to this impairment or to a defect in a special performance or function.

The reactions of the patient should *never be protocoled in the form of plus or minus* (see p. 2).   One should always put down what the patient is saying and doing, as much as possible in all details.   There should further be recorded the general appearance of the patient before, during, and after every reaction, his behavior in general, expression of his face, body, gestures accompanying his speech, expressive movements as to fear, satisfaction, etc.   All this holds true also if one wishes to use the results for statistical comparison.

(a) *Tests of Abstract Behavior*

It is vital to determine whether and to what degree a patient is impaired in abstract behavior (see p. 5).   One can use various tests for this purpose.   The best tests are those which, on the basis of special tasks, permit a decision as to whether or not the patient's abstraction is disturbed. Such tests may reduce the need for other clinical, less-controlled methods and lessen the amount of qualitative analysis of each behavioral act of the patient.   If the results obtained in this way should be still ambiguous, further qualitative analysis is, of course, called for.   From my clinical experiences I find that the tests which we developed in examining aphasic patients are particularly useful for this purpose.   Their advantage is that the subject can perform them almost without the use of language, and hence the effect of speech disturbances is largely eliminated.*   They are all performance tests.   The tasks are so constructed that normal performance or failure permits a rather direct diagnosis of the patient's capacity to abstract.   In case of impaired abstraction, the specific type of concreteness to which the patient is limited can at the same time be determined. The degree of the defect can further be assessed from the following findings: (1) The patient is entirely unable to assume an abstract attitude; (2) the

---

* Regarding the difficulties which arise from the use of language in testing, cf. Goldstein and Sheerer, 115, p. 12.   In this monograph, the reader will find a detailed discussion of the tests described here, of the problem of abstract and concrete attitude in general, and of the pertinent literature.

patient is confined to the lowest type of concrete behavior (see 30, p. 7); (3) his performance range covers the lower and upper degrees of concrete behavior; (4) he is able to solve only some of the tests which demand abstract attitude; (5) he cannot learn the required procedures even if all helps are given and the solution is demonstrated to him (see 155, p. 30).

At present we are not able to elaborate a test series with a graduated scale which would correspond to definite degrees of the required abstract attitude and to definite degrees of prevailing concreteness. But this is not so important for our purpose here. We are chiefly interested in determining whether the abstract attitude is impaired or not.

In regard to the administration of the test the following points should be noted:

1. The instruction given should not "tie" the examiner in the same way as in the usual standardized tests. On the contrary, we recommend that the examiner, after having administered the tests according to instruction, should feel free to probe further by varying the experimental procedure according to his needs.

2. It is advisable that every subject be given the entire test series. Experience with numerous cases has taught us that a patient need not necessarily perform consistently in all tests: a partial success in the first given tests may be followed by failures in subsequent tests and vice versa. Comparative analysis of the different achievements of the subject in all tests provides a broader and sounder basis for evaluating the nature and degree of the defect.

Stick Test*

The patient is presented with different stimulus figures composed of sticks. The test is divided into two parts; first, the patient has to copy the model figure while looking at it; second, he has to reproduce the figure from memory after it has been exposed for from five to thirty seconds and then removed. The sequence in which the stimulus figures are given represents a scale of increasingly intricate configurations, in the numerical as well as in the geometrical sense.

The normal person may consider some of the figures pictorial presentations of concrete objects or of letter forms. Yet most figures are sufficiently unlike such realistic thing-like forms as to be generally perceived as mere configurations of spatial direction or meaningless forms in an abstract geometrical space, bearing no direct reference to a tangible life situation. The normal person may not be directly aware of the abstract geometrical

* The material for this test, including record blanks, can be obtained from the Psychological Corporation, 522 Fifth Avenue, New York City.

character of these figures when he later reproduces them volitionally from memory. While he unreflectively retains what he saw, the entire process is, at the same time, embedded in and guided by an abstract attitude towards space. He could not retain such an unrealistic spatial arrangement without having the capacity for mapping out "ideationally" a spatial system with coordinates largely independent of his own bodily orientation and manipulative experience. It is true, in our cultural setting, we have become habituated to handling purely directional features in space so that we hardly realize how much abstraction they involve. We can, however, become distinctly conscious of the role played by this conceptual frame of reference and of the fact that spatial direction, as such, is of highly abstract nature, when we try to retain a complex geometrical pattern for reproduction. We experience such a task as a challenge to our capacity to grasp diverse spatial relations and directions in one simultaneous act.

The fact that the entire procedure requires the abstract attitude becomes apparent when patients with impairment of this attitude (as proven by other tests) can copy the test figures but cannot retain them and reproduce them correctly. This phenomenon becomes particularly striking with those figures which seem to be very simple, such as one simple line, /. Such figures may cause the greatest difficulty for the patient because they may not represent a tangible object for him, being only abstract directions in an abstract space. On the other hand, if such a simple figure can come to represent a concrete thing for the patient, then he can retain and reproduce it. Some of the sample figures may be approached from either an abstract or a concrete attitude. Indeed, what may mean a concrete object to one person need not be of this palpable character to another. The nature of interpretation depends to a far-reaching degree upon the cultural background and the selectivity of the individual. Therefore, one and the same figure may be reproduced correctly by one patient with impairment of abstraction but not by another having the same defect in principle. Thus, we should not be satisfied with success or failure per se but try to determine whatever ideas the figures arouse in the patient or of whatever they remind him. The importance of this procedure may be illustrated by the following examples: one patient, presented with a stick model in the form of an angle pointing upwards, reproduced the figure promptly, but failed if the angle was presented pointing downwards. When shown each figure again and asked why he did one and not the other, the patient said, regarding the first figure: "This is a roof", and (pointing to the other) "this has nothing to do with the other one, this; I do not know what it is." Another patient could reproduce both angles. One was for her a roof, the other the letter V, both concrete objects.

Thus the failures of the patient with such figures which he cannot reproduce because he would need the abstract approach, and the successes with other figures where he can use the concrete approach, permits us to decide whether and how far a patient is impaired in abstraction. Using this distinction enables us also to explain why one patient may be unable to reproduce one stick presented in a definite direction, but will easily repro-

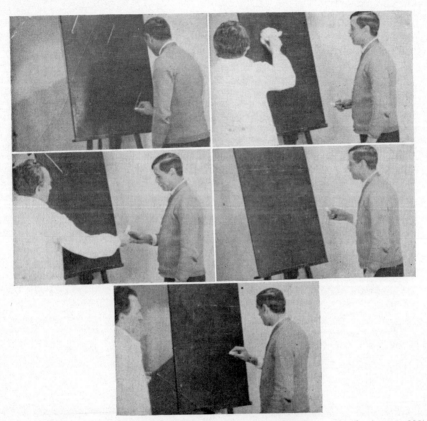

FIG. 1. Behavior of a patient with impairment of abstract attitude (see p. 208) in the stick test. He copies an oblique line correctly, but is not able to reproduce it from memory. Notice his expression of embarrassment here and in Fig. 2. (Figs. 1–4 are taken from a movie.)

duce a little house with a door, a chimney, etc., built of a number of sticks because this makes concrete sense to him. To consider a stick configuration, a concrete object is not simply an affect of familiarity or past experience in the sense of frequency. The patient *tries* to find in the stimulus figure something which makes tangible sense for him, because he can grasp only something concrete. This he finds sometimes only by certain modifi-

cations of the presented figure.   He may, for instance, reproduce a figure
like this □ as ⊞ because he considers it a window, as he says; and this is
confirmed by the fact that he inserts the cross into the square, converting
it into a window.   Or a patient may reproduce two figures like this | ○
as 10 because he sees it as a "ten."

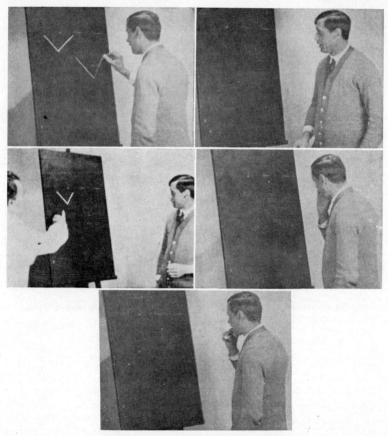

Fig. 2. The same patient as in Fig. 1 is unable to reproduce from memory an angle
pointing downward.   He says: "I do not know what it is."

There are possibilities of being deceived by a seemingly positive result.
One patient, while being presented with the sample figure, moved his hand
rapidly, outlining the contour of the figure, and then was able to reproduce
the figure after removal.   Evidently, he retained a motor image of his own
movement, on the basis of which he could reproduce the sample figure
correctly.   For, if the examiner prevented these movements, the patient

could not succeed.   Another patient, in the task of reproducing, kept his gaze fixed to the spot where the figure had been presented on the table. As long as this visual contact with the fixated visual image on the table was not interfered with, he succeeded in his reproduction.   If, however, the examiner forced the patient to change the position of his eyes, he was lost.   These two kinds of behavior, though they are not customary, may deceive the examiner by covering up the defect.

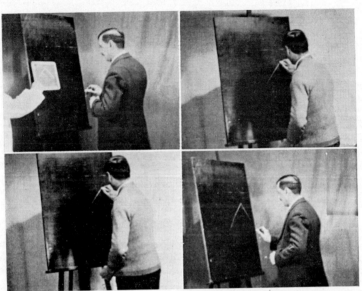

Fig. 3. The patient reproduces from memory correctly the same angle pointing downward.   He says: "That is a roof."

Administration of the Test

The stimulus figures are presented in the order in which they are numbered. Some of the figures are composed of two sets of sticks, slightly different in length. Others contain only sticks of the same length (length a, 3.5 inches; length b, 5.5 inches).   The patient is first presented with the stimulus figures with the instruction to copy them.   In the second part of the test, the patient sees the figure for five to thirty seconds (depending upon his condition) and then is asked to reproduce it from memory after the figure has been removed.   The patient is encouraged and induced to tell of what the figure reminds him, what idea the figure suggests to him.   In both parts, a record of the stick formations by the patient is made with pencil drawing and all spontaneous comments, questions and verbal responses as well as the examiners remarks, are recorded verbatim.   Particular attention is paid to the possible roundabout methods of the patient as described above so that they can be controlled and eliminated to see whether the patient can perform without them.   In case of doubt as to whether the patient performed by concrete or by abstract means, experimental variations such as use of other meaningless figures or of drawings can be introduced.

The test is particularly suited for cases with severe damage of the abstract attitude (see protcol case 6, p. 212).

Goldstein-Scheerer Cube Test

The patient has the task of copying colored designs with blocks. These blocks are colored cubes. Each of the cubes bears the same colors in

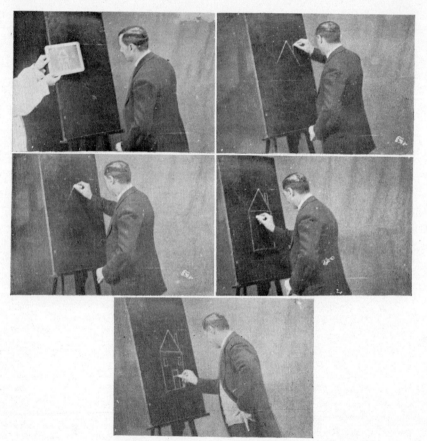

Fig. 4. The patient reproduces quickly and correctly from memory a little house with many details.

identical arrangement and distribution on all six sides. Each of four sides bears one of the following colors: blue, red, yellow, white ("one-color sides"). Each of the two remaining sides bears two colors, one blue/yellow, the other white/red in a half and half arrangement with diagonal partition ("two-color sides").

The task of reproducing the colored design models with the blocks may be attempted on an abstract or on a concrete level. Concretely, the subject

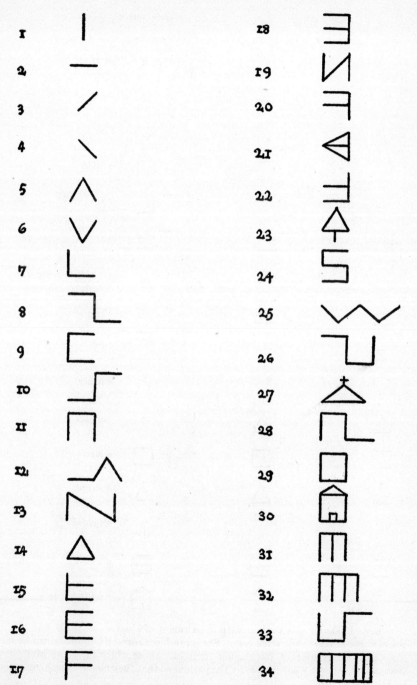

FIG. 5. The stimulus figures in the stick test.

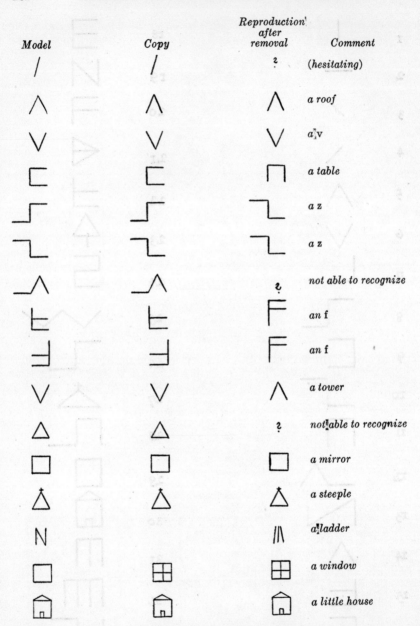

FIG. 6. Behavior of a patient with impairment of abstract attitude due to Pick's disease (see p. 113) in the stick test. She reproduces correctly those figures he recognizes as concrete objects, but cannot reproduce those which mean nothing to her. Note the changes in some figures by the patient so that they mean something concrete to her (see p. 158).

may try to reproduce his impression of the design model by arranging the block sides until he feels that they match the model design as a whole.

FIG. 7

The different design models of the cube test.

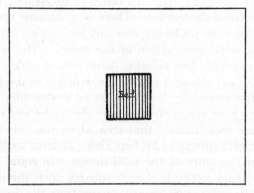

Model 1 on the card (¼ of original size).

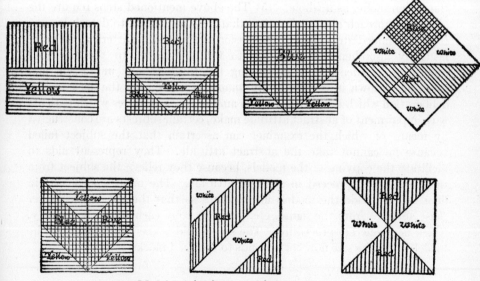

Model 2–8 (without cards), original size.

He follows the design model without a deliberate act of analytic reasoning and reproduces his impression of a unitary configuration by matching the block sides to it in a naive, unreflective manner. (The subject may not always carry through this matching procedure *in toto*, because he may be more impressed with the figure than with the ground or with a "sub-whole" of the figure. In these cases, a partial matching occurs which is, however, not piecemeal, but is guided from one unbroken sub-whole of the figure to another.) By this concrete procedure, only a few designs can be successfully copied. There is a definite turning point for the concrete approach: no longer can one, by turning up and arranging the block sides, build the pattern of the model. The relation between design and the required block sides has become too complex. The resulting confusion can be solved only by a shift in attitude to the problem. This approach consists essentially in the following abstracting operations: (1) To disregard the *given size* of the design of the model and to translate this size into a larger area, namely that area which the four blocks together occupy and which happens to be four times as large as the design. (2) To break down the unity of the total design into equal squares and to impose an imaginary network of such squares upon the design. (3) To translate the thus isolated imaginary squares from the design into squares composed of block sides. (4) To select the required block sides for these squares and to organize them into a pattern which corresponds to that of the design model as a whole. (5) The above mentioned steps require the abstract approach also in the sense that the patient has to detach his ego from the immediate, coherent impression of the design pattern as he unreflectively apprehends it; and has to willfully carry out the described procedures of ideationally destroying the total unitary impression and breaking it down into structurally *unnatural* units. On the basis of this deliberation which is confirmed by an analysis of the failures which patients with impairment of abstract attitude make, certain subtests are constructed by means of which the examiner can ascertain that the subject failed because he cannot take the abstract attitude. They represent aids to facilitate the copying of the models, because they relieve the subject from the necessity to proceed in abstract attitude. The main aid consists in lines which divide the models into squares so that the patient no longer must abstract from the figure, etc., and can copy each square separately, which is a concrete procedure. The second aid is the enlargement of the model so that its size now corresponds to that of 4 blocks.

Directions

1. The patient is given a standardized test of color efficiency, such as the Ishihara, in order to rule out color blindness.*

---

* The material for this test, including the prepared record blanks, can be obtained from the Psychological Corporation, 522 Fifth Avenue, New York City.

2. Examiner says: "Here are four blocks. Each of the four blocks bears the same colors, you see (*examiner takes a block in his hand and points with the other to the colored sides he names*) this side is blue, this side is red, etc., this side is half blue, half yellow, etc. The other blocks have the same colors in the same order. I want you to copy with these four blocks the design you see on the card." (*Examiner points to the model.*)

3. The patient is presented with the designs and their modifications in the following sequence. Each time the patient completes a step the examiner reshuffles the blocks.

Step 1: The original design. If the patient does not succeed:

Step 2: An enlargement of the same design which is the same size as the four blocks. If the patient does not succeed:

Step 3: The same design in original size, divided by lines which break up the figure into four squares, corresponding to the four block-sides required for copying. If patient does not succeed:

Step 4: An enlargement of the same design (as under Step 2) again divided by lines. If patient does not succeed:

Step 5: A model of the same design built of four blocks. If patient does not succeed: The correct block model is presented again, but each block separately and an inch apart. If patient does not succeed:

Step 6: (multiple choice): Three models each built of four blocks, two models are faulty and one is an exact reproduction of the original design. Patient is asked to identify the correct block-model.

4. Whenever the patient succeeds in Steps 2–6, the examiner at once presents the *original* unmodified design again and records success or failure.

After completion of each step, whether correct or not, the examiner asks the patient: "Is that correct? Is that right?" (pointing to his product). The reply is to be written next to the recorded design made by the examiner.

5. Throughout the procedure, a careful record is to be taken of all the comments, answers, and as far as possible of every move the patient makes with the blocks and of the stage the patient considers final or correct in his manipulation. It is advisable to use record blanks in which the model is drawn on top and six sets of lined squares are provided for recording the patient's procedure.

6. The criterion of success or failure should be derived from the following possible responses of the patient.

a. *Success.* The patient reproduces the design correctly and upon inquiry acknowledges his solution as the correct one. Any uncertainty on his part outweighs his correct solution. In this case, he has to be instructed to continue on the same design (if necessary, along further steps), until he reaches a reproduction which he considers exact, be it correct or not. The latter, of course, has to be scored as failure.

b. *Failure.* The patient's product is correct, but he persistently fails to acknowledge it. The patient's product is incorrect, but he insists on its being the exact copy. The patient's product is incorrect, but in spite of his realizing this, he cannot improve on his product and gives up. The patient's response is incomplete—no matter whether correct or incorrect—and he gives up. The patient's response is either incorrect or incomplete, but he does not give up and continues, although futilely. If this goes on for more than three minutes on the same step, it is scored as failure; this time limit may be exceeded according to the needs of the case (e.g., motor handicap).

Fig. 8

Different examples of wrong reproductions by patients with impairment of abstraction

Model 1
(¼ of original size)

Reproduction 1

Patient uses only one block, not all four, as he should. Inability to abstract from the size.

Reproduction 2

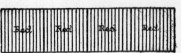

Patient built a horizontal row by 4 blocks

Reproduction 3

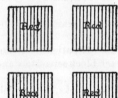

By 4 single blocks

Reproduction 4

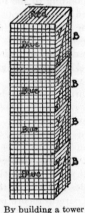

By building a tower

Reproduction 5

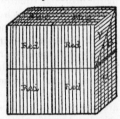

By a standing cube the vertical red sides facing the subject

Model 2

Different reproductions

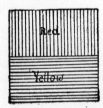

Only one color aspect realized in the required square

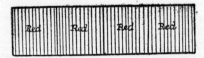

Only one color realized; built in a horizontal row

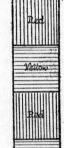

Both colors realized and put together alternately in one vertical row

FIG. 8 (*continued*)

Model 6   Different reproductions

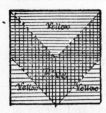 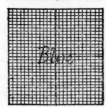 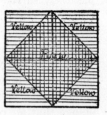

Only one color realized   The dominating blue impression is reproduced together with
in the required square   the yellow, using two color sides blue/yellow without grasping
                                 the blue arrow figure

7. There are cases in which the model presented with the line division (step 3) does not help to improve the patient's procedure. In order to ascertain whether he sufficiently realized the line division, the examiner may point out to the subject the lines on the model, and demonstrate how they might be used to determine the placement of the corresponding block-sides. He may, further, explain or even demonstrate the way the blocks belong and then proceed with the test.

Color Sorting Test*

The task in this test is to sort colors according to definite color concepts· Before the patient lies a heap of about eighty woolen skeins which differ sufficiently in hue and brightness so that each basic color hue is represented in at least ten different shades of brightness. The patient is given a red skein (or green, or blue) as a sample and asked to select from the heap all those skeins which can be grouped with the sample. There are two possible approaches to this task.

(1) When we are asked to do this we pick out all the various nuances of red even though we see that each has different individual attributes not equal to the other nuances. We can do this because we conceive of these various red nuances as falling under the same category, red; in other words, we proceed according to a concept. The differing shades of red are to us only examples of a common quality. We treat the skeins not as individual colored things as they are sensorially given, but as *representatives* of the basic concept, red. For the moment, we ignore all but the categorical character of the color hue requested. We supress or disregard all other attributes which may enter our attentive consciousness. We are able to do this since we can abstract from all these unique experiences arising from the varying nuances of red and can hold fast to the direction of procedure once initiated.

(2) There is another approach, however, open to the normal person.

* This test was first published by Gelb and myself in 1925.

When he starts with one particular skein and passes it over the heap, passively surrendering himself to the impressions emerging as he does so, two reactions will take place: (a) if any skeins resembling the sample in all attributes are present, these skeins will immediately cohere in a unitary sensory experience; (b) if, however, they do not match the sample in all respects, but only in some, the patient will experience a characteristic unrest concerning the heap and a varying rivalry between groupings according to the different attributes.   The characteristic in either case is the circumstance that *the coherence results from the sensory impressions* and occurs in an attitude of passivity.

There is an essential difference between the two kinds of approach, namely, *in the first, a definite ordering principle, a concept, determines the action;* in the other, there is no such principle and *the action is passively determined by the outer impressions.*   These two kinds of behavior correspond to the two attitudes toward the world in general which we have called abstract and concrete behavior (see page 5).

A normal person may begin with a concrete approach, but if he experiences that in this way he cannot solve the test, he shifts to the abstract attitude.   When we regard the behavior of the patient with impairment of abstract attitude in the light of this explanation, we may say: the patient's behavior is similar to the concrete approach of the normal person.   *He is determined by the present sense impression;* therefore, he selects only such skeins which are very similar, or he is determined by some quality of the sample, which is immediately impressed upon him, etc. (see behavior of the patient, p. 255).

From this interpretation, not only the failure in the test but also the various deviations from the norm which patients show becomes understandable.   They are all the expression of the abnormal concreteness in his procedure.

The patient, following the instruction to pick all skeins which can go with the sample, may choose only such skeins as are identical with or of a shade closely similar to the sample.   Though prompted, he will choose only a small number of skeins because there are only a few very similar ones in the heap.   Another patient matches a given bright shade of red with a blue skein of great brightness.   At first the patient may seem to be color blind, but his color efficiency is normal and he is even capable of discriminating very fine color differences.   More accurate observation discloses that the choice of the patient is determined by a particular color attribute of the given skein, for instance, in this case, by its brightness.   We observe further that the choice is decided now by one attribute, now by another one; by brightness or softness, coldness or warmth, etc.   However, the same patient who seems to be choosing according to a certain attribute is not able to carry out this procedure deliberately upon request. We note further that he seems unable to hold on to a certain procedure. He has chosen, for instance, some bright skeins. Suddenly his selection changes to the characteristics of another attribute, for example, to coldness or some other character, without the patient really shifting actively in this way or being able to do so deliberately. His proceedure is evidently always guided by the respective sense impressions governing him at the time. This is also the case when the patient seems to arrange the skeins as if following a concept of brightness. He may select first a very bright red, for example, then add a less bright red and progressively more neutral shades in this way. But if we ask him to place the skeins in a series according to their brightness, he shows himself incapable of such a performance, even if it is demonstrated to him. The patient never intended to form a series according to brightness, nor was he aware of forming the skeins in such an order. Moreover, closer analysis of his actual procedure reveals: the patient tries to find the red nuance which for his sample is the closest match and thereby finds skein *a* (a red skein one shade darker or lighter than his sample because no more completely identical skeins are in the heap). He deposits his original sample on the table and keeps the new skein *a* as a sample, now looking for a skein to match *a*, and finds skein *b* by the same procedure—a piece to piece comparison. Then he deposits skein *a*, keeps *b*, and continues in this same way with other red skeins. Thus, the last chosen skein always becomes the new sample and so it may appear as if the patient has formed a brightness or purity of hue series. (We call this effect a *"pseudo-series."*) It becomes clear that he does not form a brightness series if one takes the last chosen skein away each time and conceals it from the patient's view, or removes all the skeins already deposited. Then the patient is lost. He is either unable to continue at all or begins to pick out entirely different hues according to one aspect of the skeins by which he is impressed at the moment. (As to the details of the various ways the patient proceeds, see Goldstein and Gelb, 112, Goldstein and Sheerer, 115, and the protocols of case 14 and case 15, pp. 255 and 267.)

*Administration of the Test**

The patient is first given a standardized color efficiency test, such as the Ishihara, in order to rule out color blindness. He is then presented with a heap of woolen skeins placed at random before him. From the procedures described in the Goldstein-Scheerer monograph, the following are listed here:

1. The examiner asks the subject (a) to select a skein he likes (the sample skein) and to pick out all the skeins which he believes can be grouped together (go with,

---

* We used the wool introduced by Holmgreen for testing color efficiency. A somewhat different set, more adequate to our test, is in preparation.

belong) with the chosen one. If the number of skeins so selected is smaller than the number of skeins of the same hue in the heap, then the examiner picks up all the remaining skeins of that hue and asks, "Could they be included too?" "Do they not also belong to this one?" "Don't they belong to these too?" (pointing to the patient's selection). If the patient rejects the suggestion, the examiner presses further by asking, "Is there no way in which they all belong together?" "Is there no way in which they are all alike?" "Don't they all have something in common?" "Aren't they all alike in some way?" In every one of the above questions, the examiner records the answer and follows it up by asking the patient "Why?", again recording the answer. (b) The examiner himself selects the sample and asks the patient to pick out the skeins which can be grouped together with the sample. In all other points the procedure of (a) is repeated.

2. The patient is asked to select all reds, all greens, all blues, etc. (verbal instruction without sample). In each of the experiments, the subject is asked to state the reason for his groupings and the same procedure as in 1 (a) and (b), is followed as regards the presentation of skeins not included in his grouping by the patient.

Color Form Sorting Test*

The patient is presented with figures of different shapes and colors; four equilateral triangles, four squares, four circles, each of them in red, green, yellow, blue. The reverse sides of all figures are white. The patient has the task of "sorting" the figures presented at random in a way he thinks they belong together.

The task can be approached on a concrete or an abstract level. Concretely, the individual may respond to the various figures as individual things which consist of *colored shape* or *shaped color*, and in which shape and color are not separated but belong together in *one*. The sorting may be determined by the experience: (1) of a *color* variety in which congruent colors cohere and obtrude; (2) of a *shape* variety in which congruent forms cohere and obtrude. (In everyday life, a similar phenomenon occurs if one looks passively at colored patterns such as mosaics or tile floors and experiences a predominance either of like colors or of like shapes without any conscious effort.) (3) Or the individual may bring the figures into definite positions, building a pattern out of them. He will do that which is obtruded on his impression by the immediate sense experience.

A subject who is inclined to an abstract approach will transcend the immediate experience of each figure as one given thing. He will segregate the two properties, shape and color, from each other, and systematize each into a principle of classification: the category, the concept of form, or color. Adopting such conceptual frames of reference, he will take the single figure as a *representative* of a category, that of form or that of color hue. He will

* The material and Record Sheets can be obtained from the Psychological Corporation, 522 Fifth Avenue, New York City. The test was published by my pupil, E. Weigl (311), 1927.

therefore easily shift from one completed sorting to another if asked to do so and will also be able to account for the reason for each sorting in terms of verbalized concepts.   He will deal with the "categorically" selected figures more casually, throw them in heaps or pools of color or form, not being particular about spatial position of the individual figure.

A *patient with impaired abstract attitude* will, even if he has sorted according to color or form, *not be able to shift* to the other way of sorting.   He will, further prefer to bring the figures into a definite spatial pattern, thus building quasi-ornamental patterns.   The crucial difference becomes experimentally evident in the following: A patient has grouped according to the color.   Asked to group differently, he may either switch around the positions of the figures without changing their color arrangement or he may be at a loss.   Now the examiner turns the figures so that all are white side up.   Since here only the shape aspect can obtrude phenomenally, the patient usually has no difficulty in arranging the figures according to like shape, which indeed does not indicate a guidance by the concept of form. That this is not the case becomes evident if the examiner now turns the figures back, colored side up, and requests the patient to sort again.   If the patient, now impressed by the colored "things," groups according to color congruency, he is asked again to sort differently.   Since he has just grouped the *white* shapes according to shape he should be able to sort the *colored* figures also according to shape.   But such is not the case; he is unable to do so, cannot proceed in any other way than by sense impression, he cannot shift actively on the basis of categorical reasoning.

Directions

The Ishihara color efficiency or any other standardized color-blindness test is given to rule out defects in color vision.   The patient is presented with the twelve figures and told, "Sort those figures which you think belong together," or "Put those together which you think can be grouped together."   Variations of the wording are permissible to insure the patient's response to instructions.   A careful record is made of each grouping the patient makes (arrangement of figures, sequence by numbering the figures in the record, etc.).   All verbal exchanges between the examiner and the patient are recorded verbatim.

Experiment I: Sorting.   If the subject asks any questions as to how he should group the figures, the examiner answers, "That is entirely up to you."   It should be recorded whether or not the patient builds a pattern.   After the patient has completed his grouping, the examiner asks, "Why have you grouped them that way?" or "Why do they belong together?" or "Why do they belong together in this way?" etc.

Experiment II: Voluntary Shifting.   The examiner asks the patient, "Put the figures together in another way" or " . . . in a different way."   After the patient has completed his new grouping, the examiner inquires as in Experiment I.

Experiment III: Induced Shifting.   (a) If the patient grouped colors together in Experiment I and was unable to shift to form-grouping in Experiment II, the examiner turns the figures white side up and asks the patient to sort them (as in Experiment I). After the patient has completed his grouping, the examiner inquires as in Experiment I. If the patient has now grouped according to shape, the examiner turns the figures again back to the colored sides and repeats the procedure of Experiments I and II. (b) If the patient grouped shapes in Experiment I and was unable to shift to color-grouping in Experiment II, the examiner may present the appropriate color groupings to the patient and ask him, "Is this all right too?" or "Can it be done this way too?" etc., and "Why?" If the patient accepts, he is presented with the figures in random order and Experiments I and II are repeated in order to determine whether the patient can shift volitionally and "learn" from the helps given before.

The patient is scored as successful if he can sort and shift without difficulty and account verbally for the principle of his sorting in Experiments I and II. He is scored unsuccessful if Experiment III is necessary *and* he does not learn from the helps presented in Experiment III. Further control experiments can be found in the Goldstein-Scherer monograph.

Object Sorting Test*

In the object sorting test, the patient has the task of arranging groups from a variety of objects according to general concepts. The patient is first asked to group together all the articles which he thinks belong together. After completion, he is asked (1) to arrange the articles in *another* way; (2) to group the articles with an object which he has selected himself; (3) with an object the examiner has selected.

The following articles are used, one set for males, another for females. Of course, other objects may be used, but they should be selected according to the principles which governed the presented selection (see Weigl, 311). This selection allows the arrangement according to different aspects; the most important are as follows: (1) *Use* (tools, eating utensils, smoking utensils or material, edibles). (2) *Situation:* belonging together in a concrete situational context; e.g., all eating implements for setting a dinner table, all tools in one's tool case at home, etc. (3) *Color:* (e.g., brown, white, red; for instance, in each of the mentioned groupings, one object is of an equally intense red, as a red cardboard disk, a red apple). (4) *Form:* in each of the groupings at least one object is oblong and also one object is round. (5) *Double occurrence* in pairs: in each of the groupings an object is represented in two samples (e.g., two lumps of sugar). (6) *Material:* there are objects of metal, wood, rubber, etc.

A normal individual usually can produce any one of the mentioned groupings, and each grouping can be reached by the concrete or the abstract attitude. In the abstract attitude the subject brings objects together according to general class-concepts, categories like metal, wood, colors,

---

* This test was first published by Goldstein and Gelb (112), 1924. See also Weigl (311).

tools, toys, etc. The objects are then taken as representations of categories. The same grouping may occur via the concrete attitude as effect of an immediate, more passive impression. The objects can be organized together as belonging in a concrete situation, e.g. "things belonging to carpentry," etc. Such a situational context can be classified as to the following types.

1. *Actual manipulation:* Fitting the objects together according to their *factual usability* in the present situation, e.g., *eating* utensils or *smoking* utensils.

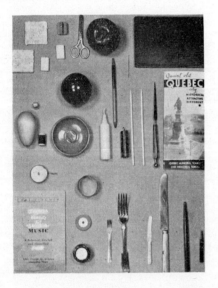 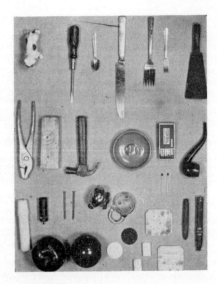

a   b

FIG. 9. Groups of objects used for the object sorting test. (a) Group for females. (b) Group for males.

2. *Personal context of action,* momentary or non-immediate. Fitting the objects according to the way one *subjectively* experiences their appurtenance to a personal situation; e.g., a patient sorts the piece of wood and the nail together with the hammer, because "*you* put the nail in the wood with the hammer"; he then adds the white candle "because *you* make a light when you hammer.'

3. *Familiarity:* Fitting the objects according to one's past experience with them; e.g., having seen all toy objects in a toy store or all metal objects in a hardware store.

4. *Sensory cohesion:* Fitting articles together according to the way they cohere together sensorially in a concrete experience of like form or color;

e.g., the redness of two or more articles obtrudes perceptually. This redness is a unitary "Gestalt" and comprises the two objects, both being members of that embracing color whole. The subject does not have the primary experience of two *separately* apprehended objects with two similar colors in juxtaposition, thereafter abstracting a common property, the color red. Rather, he surrenders to one immediate unitary color impression, and the two (or more) articles are parts of that sustaining totality as one experimental whole.

Restriction to concrete behavior is indicated by the following groupings:

1. The grouping is confined to narrowly realistic aspects of use or manipulation of the individual articles in their uniqueness, factual usability in the present situation. Objects not directly belonging to the situation are rejected. Therefore, only *a few are grouped together*, e.g., the cigar and the matches, while the cigarette is rejected.

2. A less realistic level of concreteness is present when the patient groups according to use, but is not oriented towards the present situation; e.g., the patient may bring together all tools "because I have them all in my tool chest."

The subject in this attitude may be disturbed by missing something which belongs to the concrete situation: for instance, he groups together the pipe, the matches and the toy spoon, "for cleaning the pipe," but indignantly "misses" the tobacco.

Or the subject may bring together a number of objects which belong in some definite place, e.g., in a store. After having done this, he may make other groupings determined by some other belongingness issuing from some of the objects. He *shifts, determined by some sensorial experience*. This is a passive shifting, in contrast to abstract deliberate shifting (see active shifting, p. 175).

3. Sorting as to *sensory characteristics*, such as color, form or material, usually *needs abstraction*, because the subject has to disregard the use and all other properties of the objects.

But under certain conditions, such a grouping may occur even if the abstract attitude is impaired, namely if a special color or material is precisely *impressed upon the patient by the arrangement of the objects*. Thus, if all red articles are presented in one group and all others in another group, then the patient *may* choose objects which all have the same colors. This is not a volitional sorting as to a concept, but on the basis of immediate (concrete) sensory cohesion. Outside of this situation, the patient will not understand that one can bring objects together as to colors (see p. 178). Even if different objects are presented together which have the same color, the patient usually will not grasp that they can belong together in this way.

4. Preference for pairs: If only the other member of a pair is selected,

e.g., fork with knife, this indicates that the selection is based on immediate experience of a specific "mate".   The objects are not taken as representatives of a class; if this had been the case, more objects belonging to this class would have been chosen.

The mentioned *characteristics of concreteness* can be considered as pathologic only if the subject proves unable to *shift volitionally* within the concrete realm and from that to a conceptual frame of reference.   Thus, the *question of shifting becomes the center of the experiments*.   It should always be tested whether the patient is able to shift, and determined whether he goes over to another grouping determined passively by impressive sense experiences, or by active shifting.

There are some peculiarities in the behavior of patients with impairment of abstract attitude which may *indicate the defect:*

1. If the individual presents or accepts *only a small amount of objects* in a group; if the individual presents only *one or very few groups* and leaves a number of the presented total of objects ungrouped; if he rejects other presented groups.

2. If the individual *does not show any shifting* or if he is shifting only passively.   A greater number of shifts does not speak for preservation of abstract attitude without further test for volitional shifting.

3. A decision should never be based simply on the fact that the patient *likes* to proceed concretely, but *whether he can or cannot shift to the conceptual attitude*, i.e. can assume the latter at all, or is restricted forcibly to concrete groupings.   From this it is evident that each grouping must be analyzed from the viewpoint of whether it was performed in the one or the other attitude.

Administration of the Test

Before the subject is asked to sort the articles, he has to identify them, to make sure that they are familiar to him.   Unknown objects are explained.   Defective color vision is to be ruled out.   In all experiments, a record is kept of the instructions given, the subject's procedure, and sequence of the objects selected; all his answers, questions, and spontaneous comments should be reported verbatim.

Throughout the test, whenever the subject asks whether his performance is correct or not, he should be reassured that there is no correct or incorrect response, but that every person has a different way of putting the things together—or that the examiner just wants to see the way the subject puts the things together.

Experiment I. Handing Over

(a) Examiner instructs subject: "Select any one of the objects you like and give it to me" (object of departure).

Examiner then says: "Give me all objects which you think can be grouped with this one."

If subject does not seem to understand, examiner says: "Give me all objects which you think belong together with this one," or, "What belongs together with this?"

Each article handed to the examiner is removed from the subject's view.   Prompting should take place only if subject selects less than two more objects. When subject indicates that no more objects can be grouped with the initial object, his sorting procedure is considered ended.

Now the examiner presents the selected articles to subject and asks: "Why do they all belong together?" or, "Why did you group them together?" or, "Why did you put them together?"

If subject proceeds to name the chosen articles in turn rather than to give the basis for their all belonging together, the examiner may say: "But in *what* way do they all belong together?" or, "But in *what* way are they all alike?"

From the groups formed by the subject and his verbal responses, it should be tentatively determined whether or not the subject has sorted concretely and if so, whether predominantly or exclusively.

(b) After completion of the first experiment, the examiner himself selects the initial object. Presenting it to the subject, he instructs the subject as in Experiment I(a) ("Give me all objects which you think can be grouped with this one," etc.), and continues with the same procedure as in I(a).

This experiment has to be continued by varying the initial object chosen. The examiner's selection of objects should serve the purpose of eliciting abstract groupings from the subject in case the subject had preferred concrete groupings. For instance, the examiner selects the red disk with which it is hard to group concretely. Other suitable objects of departure are: bicycle bell, rubber ball, white candle, chocolate cigar, cracker.

The sortings made by the subject have to be sufficient in number to warrant an estimate whether or not the subject sorts concretely, and if so, whether predominantly or exclusively.

Experiment II. Sorting

Examiner re-establishes the original random order and says: "You see these objects lying on the table. I would like you to make order out of this hodge-podge. Place those objects which you think can be brought together, into separate groups; but sort *all* articles!"

If subject does not seem to understand, examiner repeats instruction, modifying the two last sentences: "Put those objects together into separate groups that you think belong together," or "Make groups of those articles which belong together."

Examiner prompts and encourages the subject to accomplish a grouping which will leave no object unsorted. After subject has finished his sorting or indicates that he cannot group any more objects, examiner asks: "Why did you group them in this way, why did you put them together in this way?" or "Why do they all belong together?" (pointing to each group).

If subject should attempt to use objects from a group which has already been established for another group, examiner should ask the above question before the established group is destroyed. Using objects from established groups for forming new ones should, however, be forbidden as long as subject has not explicitly exhausted his trials to form groups of *all* the given articles.

From these groups and the subject's verbal responses, the examiner should tentatively determine whether or not the subject has sorted concretely and if so, whether predominantly or exclusively.

Experiment III. Shifting

(a) After the subject's reasons for his own groupings have been determined as far as possible, examiner says: "Are there perhaps other possibilities of grouping the articles?" or, "Can you sort the articles in a different way?" or, "Make other groups of the articles," etc.

If the subject denies any other sorting possibility, and in spite of prompting, refuses to sort differently, one may conclude that subject is unable to shift volitionally and is therefore abnormally concrete.

(b) If the subject complies, the same directions are followed as under II(a), regarding procedure and inquiry. After completion, the examiner repeats the experiment, instructing the subject again to sort according to still *other* possibilities, etc. This procedure is continued until subject has exhausted his sorting attempts. From subject's groupings and verbal responses the examiner determines: whether the subject's sorting is *confined* to a concrete basis of pertinence, or whether the subject has given sufficient evidence that he is able to shift volitionally and according to abstract frames of reference. It is noteworthy that normal subjects easily tend to discontinue rearranging the experimental objects and spontaneously begin to *enumerate other sorting possibilities verbatim*. In this case, the subject deals rather with *the names of the articles in a categorical sense* than manipulates with them existentially. If he thereby evolves true class concepts, this fact strongly suggests that the subject was able to adopt an "attitude toward the conceptually possible" and therefore sorts in the abstract, independent from the real nature of the objects.

Experiment IV. Coercive Conditions of Sorting

(a) In spite of being prompted, the subject may either reject any other grouping possibility or show paucity of shifting to the extent that is suspect of rigid concreteness. In both cases, the examiner *himself* presents new groups to subject. After removal of all articles from the subject's view, the examiner presents such groups which the subject has not yet formed and which represent "categories" or "classes" from a conceptual point of view; e.g., the following classes of objects are placed one after the other before subject: all metal, all round, all red, all oblong, all double occurrences, all toys (including toy dog), all brown, etc. Each time, the examiner asks: "Do these objects belong together?" If subject fails to understand their belongingness, he should be prompted by saying: "Isn't there any way in which they could belong together?" or "Isn't there any way in which they are alike?" If subject answers in the affirmative, examiner asks: "*Why* do these objects belong together?" or, "*Why* can they be grouped together in that way?"

(b) There are five possible responses.

1. Subject accepts the group on the basis of a genuine class concept or generalization.

It has to be ascertained whether subject's responses are in concordance with his performances in Experiments I–III; if not, his response in Experiment IV should be scored doubtful.

2. Subject rejects the belonging together of the articles in any sense, spontaneously or upon inquiry. This response should be scored as abnormally concrete, but for safety is to be corroborated with the performances in Experiments I–III.

3. Subject accepts the groups, but spontaneously or upon inquiry gives reasons, which do not have the demanded categorical nature of a class concept; instead they are definitely concrete (situational, etc.). Subject should be urged to find out whether there is not another way in which the articles belong together or are alike. If subject persists in his non-abstract response, the performance should be scored abnormally concrete, but also corroborated with the performances in Experiments I–III.

4. Subject complies with the suggestion of the experimenter that the articles are alike in some way, etc., but he cannot offer a reason other than to comply (e.g., to please the examiner). This response is scored doubtful.

5. The subject accepts the group, but offers such "abstract" reasons that they

either contradict his performances in Experiments I–III or are doubtful as to their genuine abstract reference, or both.

Experiment V.   Control Experiment

In any case of a doubtful response, the following experimental variations are indicated.   It is, of course, difficult to exhaust in these instructions all possible criteria for a doubtful response.   A well-trained observer will be less uncertain than one who has no experience with the application of the test and with patients.   Therefore, it is advisable to administer the experimental variation in most of the cases.

One ambiguity, however, is to be pointed out in principle: the ambiguity of verbalization, which contains potential pitfalls.

It may happen that a subject has accepted the groups and accounted for them by saying, "They are all red," or "long," or "metal," or "toys," or "round," or "They all have the same shape," or "same material."   The examiner should be cautioned against concluding prematurely that this verbalization is a univocal proof of an abstract approach, especially in the case where the use of these seemingly abstract terms contrasts with concrete performances in other experiments.   The subject may have uttered the words without actually having meant them as names for class concepts (see p. 61).   He used them only as description of his concrete palpable experience of the shift in phenomenal organization or situational context, in which the articles cohered for him under more forcible experimental conditions.   Therefore, the subject's acceptance and verbalization may just as well be an expression of his sensory cohesion with regard to, e.g., all long or all red articles, etc.

In order to ascertain whether subject has accepted the experimenter's grouping on a *conceptual* basis, the examiner should perform the following control experiments:

1. Establish the original order and ask subject: "Group the objects according to the principle of (a) size, and subsequently (b) form, (c) color, (d) material," etc. Naming of the specific color-name or name of the material should be avoided.   This experiment is to be continued until it is clear whether subject has sorted according to a principle and can account for the principle verbally.

2. Establish the original order and ask subject to sort the articles into two groups, one according to "material," the other one according to "color," etc.   After subject has completed the grouping, ask: "How did you do that?" or, "Why did you group this way?"   Prod subject on to formulate the principle of his sorting.

3. If there is any difficulty in subject's understanding the instructions of experiments 1 and 2, the experiment may be varied as follows: Present two groups, one according to color, the other according to material, and ask: "Does this kind of arrangement make any sense to you?"

If patient answers in the affirmative, ask: "Why?"   Establish whether his reason for acceptance is due to a conceptual reference or to an unreflective apprehension of the two groups, as two experiential wholes on a sensory basis.   If this question needs further clarification, destroy the presented order and ask subject to sort the articles according to (1) the two principles of color and material, (2) two other principles which you think are appropriate (e.g., size and form).   Vary the groups as follows: (a) remove consecutively several objects from either group and ask the subject each time whether "this makes any difference" to him, whether the group still "makes sense."   Such changes do not, of course, affect the normal subject's class concept but do easily upset the concrete "togetherness" or belongingness within the respective groups as the abnormal subject experiences it.

4. Re-establish the original order and ask subject to sort the articles into three groups, two according to different forms (round, oblong, but do not name) and the

third according to use, or any other class in which the articles partially overlap with the characteristics of shape.

This experiment can be varied in any desired way. Its purpose is to confront the subject with a task of sorting, in which he has to keep in mind *at least two different principles simultaneously* (shape and any kind of use). At the same time, he must make a decision, whether the article, e.g., the chocolate cigar, could be placed with either group, i.e., with that of oblong or that of edibles, etc.

Patients with impairment of abstract attitude will encounter the greatest difficulty and manifest extreme discomfort at such "crucial" decisions, or they cannot follow the instructions at all. (See a characteristic protocol of a patient, p. 262.) There is definite indication of impairment in abstract behavior if the patient cannot profit by the aids introduced in steps 2 to 6, i.e., the facilitating modifications and simplifications of the model. This fact becomes unmistakably clear when the patient succeeds with any one of the aids, but then fails again on the standard design which is immediately afterward presented. From our experiences, we submit that whether or not a patient can learn from the aids given is a reasonable measure of his disturbance.

Any learning which occurs is indication of a lesser degree of disturbance. There is definite evidence that patients who improve in their mental status also show improvement in their performance on the test. Therefore, retesting at certain intervals is feasible for checking up on possible recovery or progressive impairment. Because patients with impairment of abstract attitude are incapable of reacquiring this abstract attitude through learning or experience alone, this test may be repeatedly administered without any risk of training effects, which otherwise might conceal an existing defect.

Experimentally verifiable criteria for different levels of abstract and concrete performances on this test have not yet been developed. However, the experimental findings in this test suggest that there are *degrees* of lesser and stronger concreteness in a given patient, which correspondingly require more or less concrete aids. A patient who needs only the aid of step 2 for overcoming the difference in size between total area of the blocks and of the design model is in all probability less concrete than a patient who fails with this help and requires the line division of step 3. Likewise, a patient is still more concrete if he can succeed only with the block models (step 5), etc. In turn, these degrees may offer a measure of the degree of deterioration.

(b) *Other Recommended Tests*

I. The Manikin and the Feature Profile Test (see description in Pintner and Paterson, and in Weisenburg and McBride, p. 590). Often useful in testing of impairment of abstraction (see behavior of the patient described, p. 283).

II. Gestalt Completion Test of R. F. Street.

III. The Test of Rashkis, Cushman and Landis. A test similar to our object sorting test. Instead of objects, printed cards are presented which have to be sorted according to the meaning of the words printed.

IV. The Clock Test (see Head, p. 155): The patient has, on a model of a clock, (1) to place the hands in an exactly similar position to that of another model, set by the observer (direct imitation); (2) to set the clock according to oral and then to printed commands (the time may be given as: 20 minutes to six, or past six, or 5:40.); (3) to give various times set on the model by the observer.

Analysis of the procedure, not simply protocoling, is necessary.

V. *The Bourdon Test.* In this test the subject is presented with a printed text, easily understandable for the average individual. He has the task of crossing out as quickly as possible one letter, say *a*. The number of crossings made in five minutes is recorded. This test is usually considered as a measurement of attention; but it tells us only something about attention in this specific condition, i.e., under the experimental condition, with which the patient is able to cope. Modifications may be useful for testing special capacities. Patients with defect in abstraction may be able to fulfill the test in the usual way, but not if they are asked to cross out each second *a* (see p. 109).

In some cases, such as those mentioned on page 109, the test may give different results, depending on whether the text is understandable for the patient or senseless. Results may be better in the last case (see case 6).

VI. *Sentence completion test* (Ebbinghaus). The patient has the task of finding the words which are missing in sentences. The following sentences which Weisenburg and McBride selected (see 313, p. 586) fit the purpose of the test and cover a sufficiently wide range of difficulty. (They are selected from Kelley-Trabue material.)

1. I see you. Can you see — ?
2. The boy has — book.
3. Men — older than boys.
4. When two persons — about — which neither — they — almost — to disagree.

We can choose sentences which present different degrees of difficulty insofar as they can be completed with concrete or abstract attitude. Thus, patients with impairment of abstraction may be able to fulfill the test if the text concerns their own personal affairs or situations concrete for them, but not if the text demands the imagining of a strange situation (see case 6).

VII. *Analogy tests.* All analogy tests are somewhat ambiguous. They are supposed to be solved with "higher mental" capacities, in my terminology with the abstract attitude, and a defect, therefore, could be recorded as a lack of these capacities. But they can be solved—one example more than another—by roundabout "concrete" ways. An often successful way is by the use of language. The individual does not think about relations, etc., but searches for a word which fits the presented ones. The presentation of the task in the form of *x is to y*—, results in an attitude which frequently brings forth the correct association. Only if such procedure of the patient can be excluded may the test results reveal a defect in analogic thinking. The following samples selected from Weisenburg and McBride (see 313, p. 584) may be used as test material:

Horn is to blow as bell is to — ?   (ring)
Rain is to summer as snow is to — ?   (winter)
Vinegar is to sour as sugar is to — ?   (sweet)
Iron is to heavy as aluminum is to — ?   (light)
Year is to month as week is to — ?   (day)
Foot is to leg as hand is to — ?   (arm)
Front is to back as top is to — ?   (bottom)
Box is to wood as bottle is to — ?   (glass)
Man is to legs as carriage is to — ?   (wheels)
House is to door as field is to — ?   (gate)

The same comment we have made concerning the ambiguity of the analogy tests holds true as to the proverb test (see p. 111).

VIII. In *Head*'s hand, ear, and eye test, the patient has to imitate movements which the examiner performs, who brings once his left, once his right hand to the ear or eye. The test consists of five parts:

(1) The patient, seated opposite the observer, has to imitate a series of movements which consist in touching an eye or an ear with one or the other hand.

(2) The patient is placed in front of a large mirror and is asked to imitate the reflected movements of the observer standing behind him.

(3) The patient has to imitate the same movements by looking at cards each of which represents a human figure carrying out the same movements.

(4) The patient has to carry out the same series of actions in response to oral and to printed commands read silently. Here he reads aloud each order and executes it under the reinforcing influence of the words said by himself.

(5) He is told to write down in silence the movements of the observer sitting opposite him or in other instances the same movements reflected in a mirror.

Head states that only in the fifth part may normal persons fail. One of the commonest pathologic mistakes was the lack of appreciation of crossed movements in the first subtest. The aphasic patient is liable to become confused even over the simple task of the second subtest. In the third subtest the patients make the same kind of mistakes as when seated opposite the observer. When they are allowed to see the reflection in the glass, every movement may be executed rapidly and correctly.

Head means that the defects are due to the impairment of "internal verbalization," such as "opposite," etc., which are necessary to fulfill some of the tasks, and which the aphasic patient cannot fulfill.

Unfortunately, this ingenuous test is not very useful because the assumption of Head is not correct, as the investigations of Quadfasel, Gordon, and C. Fox have shown, and which I can confirm from my own experiences with normals and aphasics. The different subjects perform these tests in varying ways; the result does not depend at all only upon verbal formulation but also upon other processes, visualization, kinaesthetic cues, etc. Therefore, the test cannot be used without careful analysis of each performance and this makes it less simple for testing language failures than Head has thought.

Also, the other tests of Head largely do not fulfill the intentions from which they originated. Head wanted to find means to determine differences in the severity of disturbances. From what we have said in general about the use of tests, it will be doubtful whether in patients in whom we are dealing with qualitative changes, such a procedure can be successful. At any rate, it has always been supported by qualitative analysis of each reaction.* That concerns particularly the disturbances of the so-called higher mental functions.

IX. For "intelligence" testing, the Wechsler-Bellevue Test is to be recommended (see p. 110).

(2) *Special Examination of the Defects in Language*

We examine the patient according to the different reactions we distinguish customarily, indeed somewhat abstractively: motor speech, comprehension, etc. In the examination of each of them, modification of performances in the other realms will become manifest which we add to what we have found in special investigation of them. The general interview will have led us to know whether the patient hears, understands our language in general, and is able and willing to cooperate. If a defect in the perceptive sphere becomes apparent, we first study in detail the anomalies in this realm. If this is not the case, we begin with examination of the expressive part of language.

(a) *Examination of Motor Speech*

We protocol as carefully as possible everything which the patient says to us and let personnel or patients with whom he lives and who seem to be suited and reliable to do this write down what he says in their presence.

---

* See, concerning this comment on Head's tests, the similar criticism of Weisenburg and McBride, 313, p. 86 ff.

It is fortunate if the patient is not aware of the protocoling. In the protocol, attention has to be paid to the following details:

I. *Spontaneous speech:*

(A) As to the *occasion* in which it occurs and as to the *contents.* Does the patient speak spontaneously at all? Does he speak in the form of communication with others or only as expressive utterances? Are the contents of these utterances of descriptive character or always expressions of emotions? Does it occur in reaction to outer world events and to which? Does he begin conversation with others, or does he only speak in answer to questions? Does he speak little, or does he like to speak with others? Is he easy to interrupt when speaking or not?

(B) As to the *form:* Does he speak fluently or slowly, hesitating, stammering or in a more accelerated way than normals, quick, compulsive? Does he make pauses after some words? Does he pronounce the sounds badly, and which?

Does he leave out letters in words or misplace them? If there appears a similar sound in the word a second time, has he difficulty in speaking the second, does he assimilate it to the first one (see p. 78)?

Does he use wrong words? which? Does he speak only words or sentences? Does he want to express with the words he utters a statement, a desire? How many words does he speak in one sentence? Does he leave words out in sentences? the "small" words (see p. 68) or nouns (see p. 60)? Is he able to speak the small words in reading, repetition (see p. 68)? Is he able to write them on dictation? Does he speak in telegram style? Are the sentences, in spite of the omissions, understandable? Does he utter the words in a wrong order or put in words which have no relation to the rest? Does he often use the same stereotype phrases, as "I do not know," "Goodbye," etc.?

Does his speech *differ in different situations?* In expression of emotions or in statements or in reactions to outer world events or questions by the co-patients, in naming, etc., or in conversation which grows out of a special situation?

As to all the properties mentioned before, is his speech better in the conversation with the examiner than in conversations with other people? Does his speech differ in a conversation with the physician, in which he progresses casually with no definite aim, from that in intended conversation, and if so, in which respect? Has he difficulty in beginning to speak and does he speak better after he has started? Does he become very easily tired in speech? Does his speech get worse after a somewhat longer conversation? In which respect?

II. *Reciting series:*

Can he recite the series on demand or only in continuation after the examiner has begun? Does he speak the series fluently as series? Are the words in a series spoken in a correct way, or do they show abnormalities? Are they spoken better than separated, or worse? Or does he speak the words correctly but separated, not in the series-like rhythm? Record the time till he begins and the interval between the words and the duration of speaking the whole series. Can he repeat the series in a rhythm other than that in which he performs it spontaneously, in a slower or quicker rhythm?

If he is not able to begin a series, the examiner may begin 1, 2, 3—the patient repeats and continues or is not able to do so. The same with the alphabet, days of the week, months, and other series which one would expect him to have known before. Can he recite some poems, prayers? Only after the examiner begins? Can he recite a series with omission of each second part, for example, numbers 1 – 3 – 5 – 7, etc.? Can he recite the series backward? Can he repeat numbers represented in a definite rhythm (6–5–3–0–9–7–8)? How many? Can he repeat them backwards? Is he able to recite some grammatical series? (naturally, only if one can expect that he was able to do this before): I am, you are, he is; they were, they will be; they will have been. Is he able to write down a series with which he has difficulty in speaking? Can he combine letters, heard or presented in blocks, to words, words to sentences?

III. *Repetition:*

(A) As to *form:* Does he repeat quickly or slowly, only quickly? Immediately, or a little later, apparently with intention, or parrot-like, passively, compulsively?

(B) As to *contents:* Isolated *sounds* (k, g, ch, sh, th, r, n, a, o, k, etc.) in seeing the examiner's lips and without seeing them. Names of the letters: isolated, or in alphabetical sequence, forward, backward.

Words: short ones, long ones, different categories of words (nouns, "small words," verbs, numbers); very familiar and strange words, words he has never heard, senseless combination of syllables.

List of words which should be tested: water, table, New York, United States, body, nose, eye, leg, mouth, brother, picture. Temperature, beautiful, answer, dress, watch, administer, scrupulous, engine, justice; kindred, smooth, lovely, true, present, zero, poor, hard, red, black, Africa, Constantinople, atom bomb, today, yesterday; drink, carry, take, show, measure, disturb; until, on, an, one, in, up, it, what, third, the, whether, beneath, nothing, under, upward, there, these, and similar small words in familiar combinations, e.g., in the street, he went up the hill, something is under the table, etc.

Does he omit a letter in repeated words or bring the letters in wrong order, or does he speak the single letters with dysarthria? Does he speak the letters in a word better than isolated? Does he speak words isolated different from speaking them in a sentence?

Sentences: short, simple ones and longer, more complicated ones. Does he leave out some words, are the repeated words understandable, concerning meaning of the sentence? Is he able to repeat letters, words or sentences which he does not speak spontaneously, or is the opposite the case, particularly every-day phrases?

Examples of sentences and familiar phrases (see Weisenburg and McBride, 313, p. 570): Today is nice weather. It is dark outside. I am married. Today is (day of the week). Goodbye. How do you do. Are you well? Good morning. You are welcome. All right. Thank you. What time is it?

Is the patient able to use the just repeated words directly afterwards for other purposes, e.g., in a conversation, in answers to questions, or reaction to outer world events, a situation, as naming of objects?

Has one the impression that the patient does not simply repeat the words, etc., but tries to get the meaning and then utter the word voluntarily? Does he utter words which have relation to the presented word as to sensory or motor similarity, as to length, rhythm, similarity of some parts, characteristic vowels, consonants, etc.? Or as to content? (verbal paraphasia, see p. 312). Do they belong to the same conceptual sphere, as, for instance, God, instead of church, child, instead of mother, etc.

IV. *Word-finding*

Does the patient have difficulty in finding particular words or word categories (nouns, verbs, abstracta, concreta, color names, proper names, names of letters, for which he may know the sound)? Has he experienced greater difficulty in finding these words in conversation or in spontaneous utterances, or in answering questions, or in naming objects? Does he simply omit the words, or does one have the impression that he tries to find the word, but does not find it; does he utter parts, or another word (verbal and literal paraphasia). Is he able to repeat words which he has difficulty in finding? Has he particular difficulty in naming objects? Test a great number, at least 40–50 objects of everyday life, and more rare ones (as compass, flashlight, tape measure, different kind of watches, etc.)—those parts of the body the names of which are not so generally known. Test all colors. Has he difficulty in finding words for abstraction?

Does he use *circumlocutions* (see p. 248) which show that he knows what is meant, e.g., that he recognizes the object he has to name, etc.? Is he able to repeat the word he cannot find? Is he able a certain time later after he has accepted a word, particularly after he has answered another question, to name the objects he could not name before, or has he the same difficulty? If he does not find a word, can he say with which sound or letter it begins, or whether it is long or short, can he give some outstanding letter, vowel, consonant? Does he bring a word which shows verbal paraphasia (see p. 66)? Does it help him if one presents the first letter or part of the word? Is he able to write down a word which he cannot find orally?

Is there a difference in naming objects as to whether they are presented with the one or the other sense? Visual, tactual, acoustic, etc.? Does it help whether we allow him to perceive the object with another sense too? Is there any regularity, any preference to one sense? Test many objects in this way which are usually recognized with one sense or with another one. Test objects which are perceived with the auditory sense (noises produced by shaking a bunch of keys, or hammering on metal, etc.), or smell or taste.

Can he name the parts of the body to which the examiner points, nose, eye, ears, etc.? Can he name the objects we use in a kitchen? Or animals, streetnames, names of persons, first names of females, etc.? Pay attention whether he utters the names in a chance way or as if in relation to a certain situation which comes to his mind (see p. 311)? Ask him about his procedure. Does it help if you say some words, for instance, horse, dog, bird; is he able to name other ones belonging to the group?

Does he use words in sentences which he does not find in naming? Does he name the letters which he cannot name if presented separately, in spelling words?

In all these tests *does he find the object among others if the word is presented?* Does he recognize the correct word if it is presented in a group of words? For example: fish: is it a house, door, dog, bird, fish? (Do not accentuate the right word). Use words which belong together to a group and those which do not; use words which sound similarly and which do not.

Determine the time between presentation of objects and naming. If the interval is long, or if he presents a wrong word, ask him what was in his mind in the interval: ideas, words? (see p. 66).

V. *Auditory comprehension*

Testing of *sound perception* with tuning forks, the distinction between different sounds and the duration of the stimulus necessary to be heard; particularly tones which are important for hearing language. Let him repeat sounds, sound combinations, words (different word categories), sentences. Pay attention to whether he makes mistakes which point to a wrong perception and to wrong understanding (be sure that the cause of his failure is not a defect in motor speech). Can he distinguish between correctly and distortedly presented words? Can he simply find out which are wrong, or say in which respect they are wrong?

VI. *Responses to everyday questions and comments*

Does he understand them under all conditions, or only if they belong to a situation, if they concern his own personality, his interest, etc.? (Be careful that he does not comprehend what is meant from accompanying gestures.)

Does he understand better full sentences or if only characteristic parts are presented? For example: "Today is beautiful weather," or: "Beautiful weather"; "Please show me your tongue," or: "Show tongue."

Does he understand words belonging to a group better when other parts have been understood? E.g., does he understand "Show pink finger," after he has shown hand, leg, eye, etc.?

VII. *Following directions*

Close your eyes, open your eyes, mouth
Point to your nose, point with your hand to your nose, point with your right (left) hand to your nose
Point with your hand to your eye
Point with your hand to your left (right) eye
Point with your left hand to your left eye (ear)
Point with your right hand to your right eye (ear)
Point with your left hand to your right eye (ear)
Point with your right hand to your left eye (ear)
Where is the right side in the room?
Where is above?
Where is below?
Where is the ceiling?
Where is the floor?
Make a fist. Lift your foot. Cross your hands.
Stretch out your arms.
Stretch out your arms over your head.
Stretch out your fingers.
Stretch out the index finger.
Stretch out the index finger of your right hand.
Put your hand on your mouth and close your eyes.
Put your hand first on your mouth and bring it then on your head.
Put your right hand first on your mouth and bring it then on your head.
Put your right hand first on your mouth and then to the left eye.
Knock on the door, bed.
Go into the other room (or to the table), take the bottle of ink, and bring it to me.
Put the key in the door, shut the door, and bring the key back.
Paper test: There are on the table three pieces of paper, a big one, a middle-sized one, and a small one. Take the biggest and rumple it up, and throw it on the ground, give me the second. Put the smallest one in your pocket (Marie's paper test).

Examination of capacity of calculation has to discover first whether the patient has the concept of the value of numbers, and second whether his learned automatisms are preserved.

(1) the capacity to count (see p. 133). Can he begin at the command:

"Count!" Or does he need to have the first members presented? Forward and backwards. Oral and written counting.

Starting at one or another number, can he continue when interrupted? Counting by twos, by fives, tens.

(2) Which is greater, 5 or 6, 8 or 4, etc., 89 or 98?

(3) Counting coins. Names of coins. Equivalent in cents or nickels of a quarter, a dime.

(4) Oral and written tasks of addition, subtraction, multiplication and division. Use the words familiar to the patient. Multiplication table.

(5) Try to find out whether the patient uses, in calculation, visual, motor or written images.

(6) Memory for numbers; of his life experiences, historical dates, etc. Determine span of repeating numbers.

(7) Reading and writing of numbers.

(8) Reading and understanding of the signs of counting, $+$, $-$, etc.; whether he can use them in tasks and understand their meaning isolatedly.

(For specialized instruction in examination of all factors having to do with numbers, see Goldstein, 189, p. 126 ff.; and W. Benary, 8.)

Part Two

CASE REPORTS, PATHOLOGIC ANATOMY, TREATMENT

THIS second part will present a number of cases. The selection among the material published in the literature and among my own cases, some previously published, some as yet not reported in the literature, was made from the point of view of illustrating typical clinical pictures, the investigation of which was performed carefully enough and communicated in great enough detail that interpretation is possible. It seems to me more valuable to give the reports of a few detailed individual cases than of a great number of cases which do not do justice to these postulates. However, this detailed description had to take into consideration the space limitations of such a volume as the present work. For important cases which are not reviewed, specific references are made to the bibliography.

The characterization and interpretation of the clinical pictures have been, in most instances, given in Part One, while in this second part the detailed description of the observations will be presented; thus, for instance, in the presentation of motor aphasia. In some instances, the interpretation is given in this second part together with the description, as, for instance, in the presentation of the transcortical aphasias. This arrangement was chosen as appearing to be best suited for making communication of the facts possible. Instead of rigidly adhering to what might be considered a strictly systematic procedure, it seemed a certain liberty might make the presentation simpler, and so an organization more expedient in respect to our purpose has been arranged for the material which follows.

CHAPTER V

Pictures in which Disturbances of the Expressive Side of Language Are in the Foreground

A. PERIPHERAL MOTOR APHASIA

Case 1

The first case illustrates the simplest form of motor aphasia. A business man, age 50, who had suffered from hypertension for years, had a stroke which paralyzed his right arm and left him speechless. He was not unconscious. He complained of headache in the anterior part of his skull on the left side and of some dizziness. He was oriented in every respect, understood what was being asked, followed directions. His intelligence apparently was not changed. He was in normal contact with his family, interested in his business, etc. His writing seemed to be normal and he tried to express his wishes adequately in writing.

The paresis of the arm improved, he had no sensory disturbances, there was slight right facial paresis, otherwise no paretic or apractic symptoms in the muscles of the face.

Examination of his mental capacities revealed no abnormalities. He behaved in the abstraction tests normally. He was very cooperative and interested in the effort to help him through exercises.

The only defect was the inability to speak any word or sound voluntarily. Only occasionally, some words such as "yes," "no," "oh God," might be heard. He was not able to repeat them voluntarily. He was able to indicate what he wanted to say by knocking with the fingers of the right hand on the table as to how many syllables and letters the word had which he had in mind.

Repetition and reading aloud was totally lacking, understanding of written material intact. Writing with the right hand was impossible. With the left hand, he was able to write spontaneously, better on dictation; copying was prompt.

The patient moved the lips, tongue, etc., correctly, also on demand or in imitation of presented movements. He could not imitate movements corresponding to sounds, or only very inadequately.

All attempts to help the patient by exercises of different kinds were without success. Even a year later, no progress was observed.

Diagnosis: Typical peripheral motor aphasia which did not improve. Cause for this consistency of defect was not clear. See, regarding this problem, the general discussion, p. 203.

Case 2*

Lieutenant A. C. A., aged 22, university education, was wounded October 1915 by a fragment of shrapnel; he was unconscious. First examination was three weeks

---

* Case 1 of Head (see 127, II, p. 1).

later: two wounds on the left side of the head.   The missile entered in the frontal-temporal and made its exit in the temporo-parietal region.   The wounds healed completely in fifteen weeks.

Right hemoplegia was observed, in which face and tongue participated.   His mental state was excellent.   At first he was completely speechless except for yes and no, which he could use in their proper sense, or if he made a mistake, he corrected it.   He could not repeat these words when asked to do so.

His speech improved rapidly and after some weeks he spoke as follows: "I don't know," "please," "good night," "just so," "to tell you the truth," "I want something," "dressing has moved," "breakfast," "lunch," "tea," "dinner," "pineapple," and his address.   He could repeat "I don't know," "dressing is moved," (instead of dressing has moved), "tea," "breakfast," but not any of the other utterings, including his name.   He tried vainly to count on demand.   But sometimes, suddenly, he burst out: "One, two, three, four, five, six," after a pause he began "one," "two"—to twelve.

He was unable to articulate, to write or to copy the name of any of the common objects, but he pointed to the written name immediately when the name was spoken. He had some difficulty in understanding language.

He was *unable to read*, although he could point to the word on the list beside him which expressed the thing he desired.   If he was shown an object he could not find the name on the paper, but he could point to the name of an object he wanted.

He was right-handed, learned rapidly to do everything with the left.   There were signs of apraxia.

Writing: At first he was unable to write anything except his surname and a scrawl which somewhat resembled one of his Christian names.   He could not copy.

He improved rapidly.   Thirty to thirty-one weeks after he was wounded, he presented the following picture:

He could walk with characteristically hemiplegic gait.   He could not use the right hand.   He became extremely clever with the left hand.

His memory was excellent.   He was well oriented.   He was able to describe the exact position of his bed, etc., the colors of the uniforms, etc.

Speech: He talked slowly and with obvious difficulty, but the pauses gradually became less frequent, the words were emitted in larger groups and more perfectly pronounced.   Asked what he was doing, he said: "Walking a little...talking difficult a bit...five or six times in the...that's all I think."   He describes his bed: "This bed in the corner...opposite the door... er...facing the...er...door...It's a big room...picture...over fireplace," etc.

He recited the alphabet rapidly, but omitted U and V.   He had difficulty in writing the letters in due sequence and made mistakes.   He knew it was wrong but had difficulty to correct it.

Understanding: He understood what was said to him and could execute even the complex hand, eye and ear test to oral commands without mistakes.

Reading: He could read with understanding.   Orders were better carried out when he was permitted to say the words aloud than if he remained silent.   Speaking was a definite help for understanding.

Writing: Spontaneously written words were very poorly spelled.   Writing on dictation, the mistakes were less frequent.   He wrote the alphabet to dictation generally without mistakes and corrected errors.

The next case is particularly interesting because the detailed description of the treatment shows the influence of treatment on improvement of such cases, as well as it reveals many details of symptomatology.

Case 3*

The patient was a high school teacher, very intelligent, a lieutenant in the German army, 28 years old. He was injured by shot in the left side of the skull, fronto-parietal region. Right sided hemiplegia was observed; *at first there was total loss of speech*, including loss of abilities to repeat, to name objects, and to read aloud. *Understanding was slightly preserved.* Shortly after operation, he said, "My God." For a long time, this was the only speech preserved. Later he occasionally uttered "yes," or "no," but not appropriately. The facial paralysis and the paralysis of the leg improved. The hand did not improve; it became more and more spastic. *After operation, there was no real improvement of his speech. He communicated with other people by using an alphabet which he had written down, pointing to the single letters in the sequence they follow in the word which he wanted to express.* At the start, he had some difficulty in placing the letters in the proper order but this defect corrected itself spontaneously. He was able to *read silently*, not only newspapers but also some books. He gave the impression that he *understood* what he read and that his mental condition, as revealed from tests not requiring speech, could not have been seriously damaged. But one *never* heard him say *spontaneously* any other words than those already mentioned. Some exercises which he himself tried with the aid of his fellow patients were unsuccessful. *Three and a half months after injury,* he came under my observation. He was in good general condition; the wound was healed, but had left a pulsating scar, and a remarkable defect of bone. He had remnants of right hemiplegia. He was a little depressed but very attentive, very interested, and eager to be helped.

A protocol about his speech at that time revealed the following: *Spontaneous speech: totally missing.* In emotional conditions, single words were uttered such as "Hans," his first name, "mother," "My God," "Yes," "No," "You." *He could neither produce sounds nor repeat them. Repetition was totally lacking,* including the words just mentioned. *Speaking of series was totally missing. He was able to sing,* but only the tune, not the lyrics. Reading aloud was absent. Understanding of speech was nearly normal. Writing was somewhat paragraphic, particularly agrammatic (typical telegram style). *However, the patient could express his opinion by writing.*

One example is the following: "Dear Professor: Language is improved. Scar feels pressure. Hairs stick together. Restlessness evening, anxiety attack. Sleeplessness. In last time bad. Before better. Best greetings, respectfully, Hans."

Because the way in which he acquired his lost motor speech capacities gives such a good insight into the character of the defect, we give, in our further presentation of the case, a detailed description of the procedure of retraining.

As the patient could produce no sound, we had to begin training with the *formation of sounds. Repetition of heard sounds was without effect;* therefore, we taught him to *watch the lips* of the teacher and to repeat the movements. He was also allowed to touch the moving lips of the teacher. By this abstract procedure, he learned most of the sounds.

First day. We began with the letter *m.* The patient looked at the teacher's lips and tried to repeat the sound. He was not successful. At the same time he pointed

---

* Published first, 1919, by the author (89); published in English, 1942 (108, p. 176).

to the letter in his alphabet. He was then given an explanation about the way to proceed in building the *m* sound; we called this the "humming" sound. In a similar way he learned the sound of *p*. He pointed to the *p* in his alphabet and understood the name "expeller." He was unable to pronounce *b*, so we postponed the training in that sound. As he was not able to learn *n* by simple lip reading, the way to build the sound was demonstrated. He got the name of the sound, the nasal quality. After several trials, he was able to say *n*, but easily slipped into pronouncing it like *t*. This first training lasted only ten minutes. It was terminated because of fatigue.

Second day. The sounds learned the day before were repeated. The patient had to repeat a sound with the aid of lip reading, and then produce the sound upon hearing the name. Pronunciation of the heard sound was, at first, not good. But at the end of an hour he was able to pronounce *p*, *m*. Similarly he learned *t*; *d* was very difficult, so it was postponed. He could not repeat the sound of *f* upon hearing it, nor produce it with the aid of lip reading. It was demonstrated that it is similar to *p* in the use of the lips. After some trials, he succeeded. At the end of the lesson, he wanted to repeat all the sounds. However, he was so fatigued that he mixed up the various procedures, having particular difficulty in distinguishing *f* from *p*.

Third day. The sound *k* caused the greatest difficulty. He made the sound *ch* (hard, as in German). The making of the *k* sound in the posterior part of the palate was demonstrated. After some trials, he pronounced *k*. The *f* sound was still difficult. If he saw the position of the mouth, he succeeded. In the attempt to speak the broad *a*, he pronounced it with an aspirate, as *ha*. He realized this, but was unable to change it. The *h* sound before vowels remained for a long time.

Fourth day. He produced the sounds in response to the above-mentioned names. In learning *l*, he often repeated the *n* sound; *k* still gave difficulty. The teacher demonstrated that the tongue remains unmoved on the palate. The teacher held the patient's tongue while he made the sound. After some trials, the *k* was spoken quite correctly. He was so glad to be able to pronounce it that he repeated it again and again.

Fifth day. The sounds learned in response to the names, and with the aid of lip reading, were repeated. The patient thought that he might learn the sounds, but never combinations of sounds; therefore, we tried the combination *pa*. He was glad that he could repeat it, also *ta*. *Ma* was a little difficult.

Sixth day. He reads *papa* and *ta*. He repeated *o*, *n*, and *i* by lip reading. Before *o* and *u* he again emitted aspiration. He learned the difference between *o* and *u* from the difference between the two positions of the lips. He was unable to produce *e* because he could not quite grasp the position of the tongue. The similarity between *i* and *e* disturbed him. After some trials he was able to repeat *mu*.

Seventh day. He repeated *who* (hu) but was unable to produce the sound *u*. He said, "Hans, no no."

Eighth day. On occasions when he disliked something he said, "Be-be." After that, he was able to repeat the *b*. Then he learned *t* and *ta*. The sound *f* was still difficult. At times he repeated "Hans" instead of a sound with which he was having difficulty.

Ninth day. He read aloud all the sounds he had learned. He could not produce *w*, but could pronounce *why*. Then he was able to make the *w* sound, but *g* was difficult. He was able to say *f*. He could not say *l*. The forming of this latter was demonstrated—how the tip of the tongue touches the anterior part of the palate. He pressed his tongue on his palate with his hands, and finally succeeded in saying *l*.

Twelfth day. He was able to produce nearly every sound, partly by repetition of the sounds heard, partly in response to the names called. Some sounds he repeated upon hearing them once; he did not have to learn them. He was so eager that he practiced alone with aid from his fellow-patients, and was, therefore, very tired in the evening.

About fourteen days after beginning the exercises, the patient was able to *pronounce the majority of the sounds and to speak some words.* All the sounds which were not practiced he acquired by himself. Usually he trained himself in the following way. When he wanted to learn a sound, he tried to find out how the sound was formed by the mouth, tongue, and so on. When he tried to learn a new word, he used the sounds he had learned and combined them into words. Usually he separated the letters in the written words or wrote each letter separately, spoke the individual sounds, said them together, and became more and more acquainted with the word. In a few weeks he learned a great number of words without special training. The training had to be interrupted for external reasons.

A protocol *six weeks after starting training* revealed: He produced all sounds, often emitted an aspirate before the vowel. He had some difficulty with some combinations, such as *sn* or *sw*. From then on, speaking of words was practiced particularly. He had to answer questions; thus the single word might represent a whole sentence. He had to name objects. He was now able to sing entire verses of songs he knew. He still had great difficulty in repeating numbers. Training did not seem to help at all. One day he began to tell a story in his imperfect way of speaking, and during this performance, had to count, "one, two, three, four, five, six, seven." Suddenly he was able to do it. After thus unintentionally uttering the numbers, he was able to repeat numbers and to use them, but it continued to be laborious for a long time.

In the next week, he acquired a large number of words with the aid of a picture book. The *construction of sentences*, even simple ones, remained *especially difficult.* He usually said only one word, generally the essential word of a sentence. He scarcely ever used transitive verbs, or if he did, he used them in the infinitive.* He very often omitted suffixes and prefixes. It is interesting to note that *he wrote in the same way as he spoke.* Sometimes his letters expressed very well what he wanted to say, though they also consisted of words put together with no regard for correct grammatical construction. Because of his difficulty in this respect, *practice* was begun in *building sentences grammatically.* Each word of a short sentence was written down on a small sheet of paper. He now had to place the words in order to form a sentence. In the beginning, he had very little success. He tried to use a grammar by himself, and tried to construct the sentences on the basis of the rules. It is interesting that this man, who, as a school teacher, knew Latin grammar very well, preferred the Latin grammar book to the German for his own retraining. Although reading aloud helped him to learn the pronunciation of a word, he had *difficulty in understanding the meaning of the word when reading aloud.* In time he learned to speak such simple sentences as, "I don't know"; "Do you know that?"; "It rains"; "Do you like bread?"; "Sit down."

A summary of the patient's performance *half a year after the training began* is as follows:

Spontaneous speech. He spoke much, but preferred to say only those words which were essential for expressing his thoughts, mostly nouns, few verbs, and those mostly in the infinitive. Usually he omitted the little words (prepositions, articles, adverbs, etc.). He said a number of correct short sentences, such as those instanced above.

---

* A one-word form in German (the patient's native tongue).

Reciting of series. He placed the words of a series in the right sequence, but said them *very slowly* and always *with much deliberation.* This included number series, the days of the week, months of the year, etc. He could sing the words of a song he knew.

Repetition. He could repeat almost all words, but still had the inclination to lip-read.

Reading. Very good.

Understanding. Greatly improved, even in reading aloud.

Writing. He could write all letters, and many words. He still had difficulty in constructing sentences. He showed the greatest defects in mathematical performances, even in the simplest addition, multiplication, etc.

The continuation of the training was as follows: first, exercises to acquire a better articulation; second, exercises in reciting series, particularly those combinations of words which we need as a basis for correct, grammatical speaking; third, reading aloud; fourth, spontaneous reports about things, repeating stories, etc.; fifth, writing letters and compositions.

His speech showed a general improvement. Pronunciation steadily improved. *Grammatical forms improved.* The little words appeared more frequently in sentences. Later he was *able to construct even complex sentences,* consisting of main clause and dependent clauses. He could carry on a conversation very well.

Two years after beginning the training, during which time he did not have continual lessons but constantly and eagerly practiced and tried to train himself, he spoke a great deal in quite well-constructed sentences. His speech was only a *little hesitant.* As he said himself, he spoke with *too much consciousness* of each word, rather than mechanically. He had a hard time finding words. His difficulty was not so much with motor performance of the word as with combining words in a fluent sequence; consequently, pauses appeared in his speech, very often before a conjunction or an adverb. He frequently did not know which conjunction he should use in a sentence. He pondered, recited several ones to himself, and experimented with each one until he found the right word. He then immediately said it aloud. For instance, if he wanted to say, "This gentleman is interested in me," he said, "This gentleman—is interested," and then, silently, "up-with-in" and then aloud, "in me." As he had further difficulty in *declining* nouns and conjugating verbs, he would always experiment with them. His approach was very scientific, since he had a great deal of scientific knowledge of words.

The *principle defect* was the *difficulty to speak automatically.* Expressing his thoughts in writing had improved extraordinarily, but the structure of the composition remained simple (particularly in respect to the fact that he was a very educated man). A few sentences (translated from the German) may illustrate this. Writing about his injury, he said:

"It is far from my intention to write a novel, therefore I go immediately to the heart of things. I found myself lying on the ground, lying on my back. I didn't feel any pain but had a dull feeling. I didn't know at all what was the matter with me. My subordinate sprang to my rescue, and I heard him cry, 'Lieutenant, what has happened to you?' I felt him put my head on his shoulder. Then I felt that everything went black. In the afternoon I was wounded and during the night awoke to find myself in the first-aid place. I was tucked in a cot and the orderlies took me away from the front line."

When the patient went home, his training was not considered complete. He still had to acquire a more mechanical way of speaking, which could best be accomplished by systematic training of his motor capacities, through speaking series, sentences, etc. He also required special attention in regard to improvement in grammatical forms and saying the multiplication table.

This is a typical case of *peripheral motor aphasia* due to an injury. The intellectual functions were damaged in no way. The patient was a highly intelligent and educated individual. It is interesting that his spontaneous recovery and also self-administered training did not bring about any essential progress, but that the *response to systematic training was excellent.*

The procedure in training, its failures and successes illustrate the general aspects we shall explain later (see p. 329), particularly also the usefulness of the so-called "unnatural" abstract ways in which learning becomes evident. It may be that the intelligence of the patient was responsible for the particularly good results in this respect.

The end effect was characteristic for cases even with especially good improvement. The remaining defect consists in a *lack of the mechanical ways of speaking.* The remaining grammatical difficulty is interesting; it clearly shows the dependence of grammatical forms on motor performances.

The next case shows a similar motor defect but in general a much more severe picture. The patient is *impaired mentally* and also in other than motor speech performances. But the *motor speech defect is in the foreground.* The case is interesting because it demonstrates how successful treatment can be even in such more severe and complex cases.

Case 4*

W. M., 21 year old male, of average education, was injured at the left parietal bone. Total paralysis of right arm and leg, and *total loss of motor speech* resulted; prolapsus cerebri. After operation, improvement of the general condition and healing of the wound was noted.

Observation began six months after operation. Over the left parietal bone was a defect of about 5 cm. in diameter, and a scar without signs of inflammation. There was severe right hemiplegia and hemihypesthesia.

Mentally: The patient was quiet, oriented but dull and showed no interest in the events in the surroundings; *he was somewhat dejected, sometimes sat several hours in the same place without attention to anything. He was not inclined to respond to questions, and, in general, not very willing to undertake exercises.* Examination of his mental capacities revealed *some impairment of his abstract attitude.* His memory for previous experience was not definitely diminished.

The condition of his speech capacities was as follows:

Spontaneous speech: He said spontaneously only "mama," "papa," "anna"— which he produced as reactions to any request for speech. He could not speak his own name.

Repetition: He could repeat: a, o, u, i, m, n, but not b, p, d, t, f, g, k, l, s, v, w, x, z, h, r, ch, sp, st.

Speaking of series was totally missing, even when the first parts were presented. *Naming of objects was totally lacking,* as names in spontaneous speech.

---

* Published in German, 1919, by the author (89); in English, 1942 (108, p. 183).

Understanding: Single words were mostly understood; sentences usually not.
Reading: The patient could read neither written nor printed letters.
Writing: Spontaneously absent. He was able to *copy* letters and short words, written as well as printed ones. He could write on dictation. Sometimes without being able to name them, he could write down numbers in digits. He could not write on dictation the symbols + or −, but used them correctly in addition, for instance, 3 + 3 = 6. He did not understand what multiplication and division meant. He also did not know the symbols. He could do addition or subtraction only by counting on his fingers.

Because the defect of motor speech was in the foreground and its improvement particularly important for the patient, training was started with *exercises in building up sounds.* Speaking of those sounds he could not repeat at all could *not be improved even by influencing him to imitate the heard sounds.* Therefore, we started with *imitation of the movements* of the lips, etc. Pictures which demonstrated articulation of particular sounds were shown to the patient. He was further aided by being allowed to touch the lips of the teacher. The sensations he experienced during the production of sounds were pointed out to him. He learned names for sounds, as previously described (see p. 193). Sounds which he produced in emotional situations were also used for training.

The following method proved to be very useful. The *similarity between familiar movements and movements used in the pronunciation of specific sounds* was pointed out to the patient. Later, when asked to pronounce the sound, he would perform this familiar movement, thus learning to pronounce the sound. For example, the teacher would sit opposite the patient, with a cigar in his mouth; the patient had his pipe. The teacher made the movement of smoking and the patient imitated him. Now the teacher took the pipe in his hand and made the movement of blowing out smoke. The patient repeated it. The teacher now pointed out the similarity of this movement to the pronouncing of *b.* The patient repeated the sound of *b,* and soon was able to repeat it upon being shown the pipe. Later he could recall the pipe without having it shown to him and pronounce the *b,* and finally he was able to repeat it, without even recalling the pipe.

In this way, he learned most of the sounds in a few weeks. Soon he was able to pronounce some words better than sounds in repetition. He was even able to say short sentences, as, "I shall go out tomorrow."

About three weeks after starting the exercises, the man appeared totally changed. He was much more active and interested. He performed the exercises with pleasure; he was hopeful of improvement. He was able to express the fact that he had never thought he would be able to speak again. He still found it very difficult to speak spontaneously, being generally limited to a few simple words such as "good," "this woman," etc. However, he was able to repeat a great number of words, although he still had difficulty with sounds.

Because the patient spoke words better than sounds, words and short sentences related to real situations were emphasized. The patient might name objects, describe events, recite series, describe pictures, and even carry on a conversation.

After the patient's speech had progressed, it became evident that his reading had not improved. Therefore, this defect had to be treated separately. He recognized the forms of all letters, and was able to place the individual letters of the various types of alphabets together—capitals and small letters, printed and written. However, he was able to *name only a few letters, a, i, m, f,* was uncertain about *b, d, o, u, l, n,* and was unable to name the others. As all attempts to rebuild directly his capacity for reading failed, we tried first to improve his writing.

The patient was *not able to write*. Analysis revealed that he did not remember the movements by which a letter is produced. As it became evident that he was not able to regain his capacity in a direct way, it was necessary to develop *indirect methods* here also. He acquired the movement of making a letter by forming an association between the spoken letter and the name of an object which has a form similar to the form of the required letter. For example, *f* awakened association with the word "flag," the form of a flag suggesting the form of the capital *F*. Asked to write an *f*, he remembered the flag, traced the visual image of it, and thus produced the capital *F*, and later, from that, the small *f*.

The letter *b* was acquired by association with the form of a pipe, which was evoked by the association with the blowing movement "be" in smoking. As another example, he learned to associate *m* with three fingers placed on the mouth, representing the form of the letter. If he was supposed to write *m*, he brought three fingers to his mouth and imitated the form of the fingers by written lines; in the same way, *n* was made with two fingers.

In this and similar ways, he learned to write all the letters, and later the writing of syllables and words. Besides this indirect method, exercises consisting of copying letters were performed, which later substantially helped to improve his writing. In the beginning, however, all attempts at copying were without success.

Ten months after beginning the exercises, the examination report was as follows:

In general the patient was very much improved. He was more interested in what was going on in his environment. He was gayer, and much more eager to improve his language.

Spontaneous speech. He was capable of speaking very little, only single words, at most two, a noun and a verb (in infinitive form). His answers also consisted of only one or two words, but were understandable. This impairment of spontaneous speech was one expression of a general lack of spontaneity. In order to do anything he had to be asked.

Repetition. He repeated *sounds* correctly with the aid of lip reading, but without such aid he was a little uncertain. *K*, *g*, *ch*, were especially difficult. He repeated words consisting of two or three syllables exactly, but repeated longer words haltingly, broken up in pieces. He repeated *sentences* of two or three words promptly, but not sentences of more words.

Reciting series. This was still very much disturbed, at times totally lacking. He sang songs, even with the lyrics, astonishingly well. He had the greatest difficulty in reciting some words of a song without singing the tune.

Naming of objects. He was still impaired but showed improvement. Understanding of language was intact, if the sentences were not too long and were composed of nouns and verbs. He did not understand prepositions and other "little words" (articles, expletives, adjectives, and adverbs) so well.

Apraxia. None.

Reading. He was still very slow and needed the help of associations. He read words usually by reading the letters, then combining the letters into words.

Writing. He copied promptly. Dictation was uncertain, accomplished partially with the help of associations. Spontaneous writing was very poor. He showed no inclination for it.

Thus we see that *ten months after beginning the exercises, the patient showed great improvement*. He was in general more eager and interested. His spontaneous speech was still impaired but, however, much improved, especially responsive speech. Repetition was very much improved, even without lip reading, for sounds and words and sentences. Recitation of a series, such as days of the week, numbers, months, was good. Naming of objects was prompt and certain. Understanding was fairly well retained. By articulating each word, he could read, scarcely ever depending upon associations. He could read some poems in the correct rhythm and understood them. He could write short sentences without mistakes, the letters usually without associations. His dictation was also almost normal. His grammatical performances had improved very much.

Summarizing, we can say: the patient had a typical *severe motor aphasia of peripheral type*. All other speech functions were not essentially disturbed, his mental condition showed some impairment of abstraction but was, in general, not bad, as was evidenced particularly by the ingenuity with which he followed the procedure in training and the progress he made in this respect. His mental condition, in general, improved during retraining.

(1) *Anatomic Consideration of Peripheral Motor Aphasia*

The anatomic localization of the lesions of this type of aphasia corresponds to the classic area of Broca, though not in the limited sense of the foot of the third frontal convolution as it is usually assumed.

Morgagni was probably the first (1762) who observed a defect in the left frontal part of the brain in cases with impairment of motor speech. He failed to recognize, however, the constancy of this relationship. Gall's attribution of the localization of language in the frontal lobes did not originate from pathologic findings but he supported his hypothesis by pointing to a series of cases with motor disturbance of language and lesions in the frontal lobes. Similarly, Bouillaud and Aubertin, who tried to prove Gall's thesis by means of anatomic findings, regarded the lesions of the frontal lobe, and perhaps especially the foot of the frontal lobe, as the crucial ones.

Broca approximated this view in the demonstration of his first case which showed extensive lesions in the second and third frontal convolutions. In his reports of further cases, he spoke of the great likelihood of localizing articulate speech in the third frontal convolution.

Further observations led him to localize aphemia in the posterior third of the third frontal convolution and hence to name it "circonvolution du langage," without emphasizing the importance of the left hemisphere. Even later, when Broca stressed the location of the crucial area, his statements remained rather indefinite, probably due to his extraordinary cautiousness. It seems, according to Niessl von Mayendorf, that only his followers attributed to Broca this very definite relationship of aphemia to the foot of the third frontal convolution which eventually was designated "Broca's area." Originally, according to a suggestion by Ferrier and Charcot, the whole third convolution was called Broca's convolution, probably because Broca was the author of the first detailed morphologic description of this convolution. We distinguish now, primarily on the basis of Broca's observations: the foot (pars opercularis frontalis), the pars triangularis (designated as 'cap' by Broca) and the pars orbitalis. Later investigators have sometimes used synonymously the expressions foot and posterior third of the third frontal convolution.

For a long time, the foot of the third frontal convolution was assumed to be the place lesioned in cases of motor aphasia. Ferrier added the neighboring parts of the Insula and the pars opercularis centralis, other investigators also the pars triangularis and orbitalis. Later, particularly after the critical discussion of von Monakow, the crucial area was *extended in anterior and caudal direction*. Monakow's delineation of Broca's area includes: the third frontal convolution, the anterior part of the Island of Reil, the small gyrus connecting the third frontal with the operculum of the precentral convolution, and the operculum itself. Numerous authors adhered to this description; there were a few exceptions, e.g., Pierre Marie and Niessl von Mayendorf, who regarded a "more extended" area as essential for motor speech. There is, however, disagreement with regard to two points: (1) The belongingness of the pars triangularis and orbitalis to the motor speech area; (2) the significance of the foot of the third frontal convolution and pars opercularis Rolandi.

With regard to the first point, Henschen, after critical analysis of many "positive" and "negative" cases, came to the conclusion that the pars triangularis does not belong to the motor speech area. This is supported by an observation of Bonvicini. He describes a patient with "injury of the pars triangularis and orbitalis of the third frontal convolution, both sides, as well as their subcortical and commissural fibers, who died nine days after the injury without having shown any language disturbance or symptoms of aphasia." (See 20, p. 62, the German reprint. This author's translation). As von Monakow has indicated, there can be no doubt that a lesion affecting this convolution (in the absence of injury to the foot of the third frontal convolution and the operculum of the central convolution) can produce a transient speech disturbance. But this does not prove that this region itself is crucial for aphasia. Aphasia in these cases is certainly not caused by this lesion. The aphasia is a secondary effect of the lesion in adjacent convolutions. Therefore, it should be excluded from the "motor aphasia area" proper.

Pierre Marie and his co-workers denied any significance of the third frontal convolution for aphasia. This view stems from Marie's refusal to regard certain speech disturbances as aphasia which usually are considered as such. He named them anarthria in opposition to most authors. If one takes this different terminology into consideration, there is no disagreement between Marie's view and the more generally accepted opinion as to the significance of lesions in this region for motor speech disturbances.

The same cannot be said as to Niessl von Mayendorf's concept. According to him, the essential locus of motor speech is not the third frontal convolution, but the *operculum of the precentral convolution*. He thus stressed the great significance of this operculum for motor speech which Monakow and Liepman had indicated. According to him, there is a gradual transition from pure word muteness to dysarthria. He therefore holds that there can be only one location for sound formation and that is in the operculum Rolandi. He sees no reason to assume a special locality for word formation in the operculum frontale. The disturbance in word formation is regarded as an effect of impairment of inner speech, unrelated to the motor aspects of the speech mechanism, and inner speech, in his opinion, is a function of the sensory speech cortex. Niessl v. Mayendorf here agrees with Pierre Marie's theory. It must be admitted that word muteness is in principle the same as a dysarthric defect since we are dealing here with an impairment of the *formation* of sounds, and not with a disturbance of the meaning of sounds (see p. 80). However, there is in this respect also no difference between sounds and words, just as a sound or even a sentence or a series is either a motor activity or a linguistic structure.

But I think we cannot deny that there are differences as to the complexity in the motor formations and I do not see why for the more complex formation a function of a more extended substratum should not be necessary. I agree with Niessl v. Mayendorf about the character of the disturbance in pure motor aphasia and the great importance of lesions in the operculum Rolandi for appearance of motor aphasia. But I cannot overlook that the facts show that lesions in this *region alone cannot be made responsible for the occurrence of this form of aphasia.* The cases where this region is affected should be distinguished from those where the lesion is located in Broca's region in the frontal lobe.

In order to understand the variety of syndromes observed in lesions of the extended area of Broca we have to consider the relationship of the third frontal convolution to the operculum Rolandi and to other parts of the brain. From such a survey, we come to the following conclusion:

Without any doubt there are in the *operculum Rolandi* the *foci for the musculature of mouth, tongue and larynx.* The injury to this substratum produces impairment of the use of these muscles with regard to non-linguistic as well as linguistic activities, e.g., sound formation. *We assume that the more complicated a given motor activity, the larger the area of its representation: in the case of language activity it includes the third frontal convolution.* Indeed, this is probably a very essential part, since in cases of lesions exclusively in the third frontal convolution, with intact operculum Rolandi, severe motor aphasia has been observed, occasionally even of permanent nature. This can hardly be explained by assuming that the focus in the third frontal convolution causes the aphasic symptoms by affecting secondarily the neighboring operculum Rolandi, which is free of primary defect.

Subordinate to this extended motor speech area—one could speak also of extended motor area in general—are the subcortical and bulbar areas; there is no full agreement as to how the relationship is mediated. We are certain only about the pyramidal tract running from the foci in the anterior central convolution to the bulbar nuclei. It is uncertain whether or not there are also direct or indirect fiber connections running downward from the whole region including the third frontal convolution, with synapses in the basal ganglia. Mingazzini assumes that there are direct fibers to the basal ganglia from the operculum Rolandi as well as the third frontal convolution, the former passing through the basal ganglia, the latter ending there but making synaptic connection with new neurons which transmit impulses to nuclei in the medulla oblongata. This view, however, lacks anatomic support. Niessl von Mayendorf has subjected it to a thorough criticism and refuted it. In any case, we do not know of any long tracts extending from the caudate or lentiform nucleus down to the bulbar nuclei (cf. von Economo, 51). Yet, irrespective of this, even if we assumed that shorter paths connecting the individual divisions of the subcortical apparatus could conduct the stimulus from the basal ganglia to the bulbar nuclei, we find that pathology does not support the attribution to the basal ganglia of such a significant rôle with regard to sound formation as Mingazzini proposed. No doubt, lesions of the basal ganglia impair the speech—as Mingazzini was the first to point out—but in a way different from the characteristic motor aphasia. When the lesions are very extensive with severe speech defect, it is difficult to decide whether or not the language impairment is due to direct or indirect injury to structures in the vicinity which may be important for the sound formation.

No matter what the rôle of the basal ganglia in the formation of sound, I do not believe that the crucial pathways from the "speech cortex" to the bulbar nuclei run through the basal ganglia. Rather, as other voluntary movements, it follows the pyramidal tract. I agree with Niessl von Mayendorf that this part of the pyramidal tracts originates from the anterior central gyrus. On the basis of pathologic findings, we can further assume that *each central convolution has connections with oblongata nuclei of both sides.*

The above does not yet complete the picture of the structure of the motor speech area. Even though there can be no doubt that, for the right-handed person, the left hemisphere is of paramount significance for language, it must be noted that for the *formation of sounds the corresponding area of the other hemisphere may play an important part, different in individual cases.* In our discussion (see p. 51) of the function of the right hemisphere in bilateral synchronous (non-speech) movements, the conclusion was drawn that with regard to these movements each hemisphere has retained its own special significance. The case is different, however, and more complicated with regard to the bilateral synchronous speech movements. No doubt, there is a *close relationship between the two motor speech areas.* But if in the adult there is a definite functional differentiation of the two hemispheres, lesions of the fibers connecting the projection area of the speech musculature with the motor nuclei of the medulla oblongata produce paralysis of these muscles but not aphasia. There can be two reasons for this: either the left hemisphere has connections with the motor nuclei of the oblongata in both sides so that impulses are transmitted directly to the motor nuclei of both sides; or, the homolateral motor speech area stimulated activates the motor speech center of the other side. As a matter of fact, if there is destruction of the projection fibers of the left speech motor area as well as the corpus callosum, aphasia appears. It is difficult to decide, however, whether in such cases only the corpus callosum fibers from the motor speech area are affected, or also fibers of the remainder of the hemisphere. It seems more probable that the destruction of the former is the cause of the aphasia. Such an interpretation would assume an intimate connection between the two motor speech centers and that the most important connections of each hemisphere to the homolateral nuclei in the oblongata pass through the motor area of the other hemisphere. Such an arrangement would best guarantee the exact coordination of both motor speech areas, but the *activity of the right area would be depending upon the activity of the left.* Such a cooperation seems to be supported by the fact that destruction of the "left motor speech area" almost always produces motor aphasia. This would seem to show that there is no other direct relation between the left hemisphere, e.g., between the "central speech area" located in the left hemisphere, or if such relation exists, it becomes unavailable, at least in the beginning, if the left "motor speech area" is destroyed. There remains the question of whether the relation achieved through the fibers of the corpus callosum concerns only the motor areas "proper," i.e., the anterior central convolutions, or whether it includes also the region of the third frontal convolution. The fact that occasionally the aphasic symptoms recede in spite of lesions in the anterior central gyrus (cf. case of von Monakow, 206) *supports the assumption of connections between the frontal convolutions.*

However, we do not always find such improvement. There are two possible explanations for this: (1) The function of the right-sided part of the apparatuses cannot always be guaranteed by the corpus callosum fibers of the FIII; or, (2) the apparatus may have an individually differing independence from the left one, or at least may be able to function after it is set out of function only temporarily by the lesion of the left side (see p. 9). This could produce a different effect of the lesion of the left side. We are scarcely able to come to a definite decision about this point in an individual case.

The *connection of the two motor speech areas through the corpus callosum is not the only means guaranteeing the cooperation of the muscles of both sides for the speech movements.* There is a still deeper association mechanism, situated in the subcortical ganglia and the medulla oblongata, but the function also of this part of the apparatus seems to be dependent on the function of the speech area in the left hemisphere. This explains the continued *normal activity of the muscles cooperating in speech in cases of disruption of the corpus callosum fibers,* which eliminates the connection between the two motor areas as well as the activation of the right motor speech area by the left hemisphere. With regard to any concrete case, we face the difficulty that *we never know for certain to what extent previously, in the given patient, the right motor speech area was relatively active and independent,* to what extent it is thus capable of taking over the activity of the whole apparatus (see p. 51). It is for this reason that our views concerning the significance of the single divisions of the left motor speech area are of such problematical nature.

If we try to understand why, in cases with similar lesions, the motor aphasia sometimes improves, sometimes does not change at all, we must remember that *restitution does not depend only on the locus of the lesion* but, as indicated above (see p. 48), also on the general physiologic condition of the whole brain, the age of the patient, the blood supply, other lesions, etc. Diaschisis recedes much less in a poorly nourished brain; lesions in the other hemisphere, which did not produce any symptoms previously, begin to produce marked disturbance after any further insult to the left hemisphere also, reducing the possibility of restitution, etc. Schematically, we may represent the relationship between symptoms and focus of the lesion in the following manner:

Large lesions in the "motor speech area" (operculum frontale and operculum Rolandi) produce in general motor aphasia. The aphasia is the more permanent the more extensive the focus, the more it involves the operculum Rolandi and the greater its depth. On concomitant destruction of all fibers through the corpus callosum, there is usually no restitution (for exceptions, see further).

In cases *with a lesion limited to the left third frontal convolution,* we sometimes find no aphasia at all, or there may be aphasia of a rather transient nature, either because there is a large enough remainder of functionally active tissue, or because the corresponding area in the right hemisphere has taken over the function of the whole apparatus. This is the more likely to happen the more the operculum Rolandi is intact and for two reasons: (1) Because in that case, the connections between the left central speech area and the right motor speech area via the remnant of the left motor speech area are retained, and thus the normal way of activating the motor area in the right hemisphere is guaranteed at least to a certain degree. (2) Because in the case of such lesion, the connections between both central speech areas as well as those between the left "central speech area" (see p. 244) and the right motor speech area remain preserved, which may be of importance if these connections were functioning normally and would explain why restitution is the poorer the more the left operculum Rolandi is involved.

Lesions deep in the third frontal convolution usually produce severe motor aphasia, since they affect both the function of the third frontal convolution and the connections through the corpus callosum to the motor speech area of the other side. This probably also explains the great significance of lesions of the supra-prelenticular region for the appearance of motor aphasia. Mingazzini was the first to make such observations. Even though his explanation of the findings may be questioned (cf. Niessl von Mayendorf's critical discussion, 216), he was probably correct in his assumption that such lesions produce destruction of homolateral fibers as well as corpus callosum connections. However, with regard to the latter it is more likely that connections to the speech area are affected rather than fibers to the lenticular nuclei.

In some individuals with *extensive lesion of the left Broca's area, we do not find a motor aphasia at all,* or, if present initially, good *language returns very rapidly.* We assume that in these individuals the left area of Broca has always cooperated very closely with the corresponding area in the right hemisphere (see p. 9); in order to activate the latter, however, the connections through the corpus callosum between the operculum Rolandi and the central speech mechanism of both hemispheres must be preserved. We frequently observe in these cases a transient motor aphasia. This is probably to be understood as a result of a functional elimination of the right Broca's area by the lesion in the left hemisphere (see p. 9). In such cases, language may return *rapidly* and without special practice or exercises. *On the other hand,* there are cases which do not improve without exercises, but *with them* in a very satisfactory way (see p. 192). In these cases, we cannot contribute the effect of exercise to a new learning with help of the "other" hemisphere but to an improvement with utilization of the remained defective function of the left hemisphere. Only thus can it be explained that improvement occurs in such a relatively short time and shows such a high degree. But there are cases where this may be different —cases with complete initial word muteness in which the *return* of motor speech is *very gradual* and very incomplete, even with exercises. To be mentioned here are the observations of *Monakow, Bastian, Liepmann, Quensel, Niessl von Mayendorf* and of myself. I have observed brain injured patients in whom the return of language was extremely slow, laborious, requiring months or years of special exercises and practice and even then remained poor.   This, then, is obviously *not* a result of *restitution of language through improved function of the left area*; nor can it be explained as a result of a taking over by the right corresponding area of an activity it had previously shared.   We are probably *dealing here with an entirely new activity slowly acquired by the right area.*   The assumption of a return of speech due to a recession of the diachisis is untenable here, since the time elapsed between insult and restitution is much too long and the influence of practice is too clearly marked.   This is supported not only by the fact that speech does not return spontaneously but also by the observation that it never regains its normal premorbid promptness; it continues to maintain marked motor difficulties.   The laborious, voluntary character and certain special particularities determined by the respective exercises point in the same direction.

We should be careful about the implications of this view of the significance of Broca's area in the right hemisphere for restitution of language. It does not mean that any dysarthria appearing in the course of restitution is a function of the right hemisphere, an expression of "ataxia of the unexercised right speech cortex" (Niessl von Mayendorf).   In my opinion, there is no reason that a lesion of the substratum in the left hemisphere, should not be followed also by dysarthria.   This dysarthria can only be looked upon as due to the function of the right hemisphere in those rare cases where the substratum of the left side has to be regarded as altogether out of function (see p. 51).   We discussed above that even then we might be dealing with a taking over of the whole mechanism (normally including both sides) by its right part; even this does not essentially mean a total substitution through the activity of the region in the right hemisphere. In any given single case it is always very difficult, if not impossible, to decide just what the particular facts and functions represent.

Finally, observations have been made on cases with large lesions of the left hemisphere in which the only aspect of motor speech preserved or restituted is a certain type of repetition.   As I have shown in greater detail on another occasion (87), this oral repetition is characterized by poor articulation, inadequate sound formation as well as lack of understanding by the patient of the content repeated, and may be regarded as an activity of the right hemisphere.   (Cases of *Bischoff,* case 1; *Noethe; Monakow,* case 4.)   Apparently, these cases are rather rare.

Surveying the above considerations, the following becomes evident: *There are numerous anatomic components involved in the structure of motor speech and, in any given case, we have the greatest difficulty in attempting to determine the significance of the various defects for the impairment of motor speech, for restitution or absence of restitution;* similar lesions can produce very different symptoms and we can only speculate about the reasons therefor.

I have treated the question of the *localization of peripheral motor aphasia* in such detail because this is a problem which has been investigated extensively by many eminent scholars and with the help of all available methods and means. Yet, no satisfactory results have been achieved. There is no better example to show the weakness of the commonly accepted theory of brain localization (see p. 45).

Attempts have been made to differentiate pure word muteness from cortical motor aphasia on the basis of presence or absence of a disturbance in writing (Wernicke, Lichtheim, et al.). The first defect, so-called subcortical motor aphasia, was thought to be related to a subcortical lesion which does not affect the "motor images of words," leaving intact writing which was assumed to depend on these images. The destruction here was supposed to concern only the connections between Broca's area and lower centers. On the other hand, with regard to the cortical motor aphasia, the locus of the "motor images of words" itself was presumed to be destroyed, thus involving also writing. The incorrectness of this view can hardly be questioned any more. These two forms cannot be localized in the cortex and the subcortex respectively. Subcortical lesions can produce cortical motor aphasia; on the other hand, not all lesions of Broca's area result in this defect (cf. previous discussion, p. 203). Nor is it correct to differentiate these two types only on the basis of presence or absence of a writing disturbance. There are a variety of origins of writing disturbances (see p. 125). It may be a result of a concurrent destruction of the second frontal convolution, i.e., a defect which has nothing at all in common with motor aphasia (see p.127). Or it may simply be the result of the inability to speak, which in some people produces impairment of writing (see p. 132). In the latter case, the locus of the lesion is, of course, identical with that underlying pure word muteness. Finally, it may be the result of an impairment of inner speech.

(2) *Transcortical Motor Aphasia Due to a Lesion of Broca's Area*

Cases of transcortical motor aphasia are reported in greater detail in another section (see p. 000). I should like to set forth here an example of one type of this aphasia because it is close to motor aphasia insofar as it often represents a state of peripheral motor aphasia. In these cases, the transcortical motor aphasia is the effect of an increase of the thresholds in this sphere (see p. 82). As an example, I refer to a case published by Bonhoeffer (18).

Case 5

A 56 year old man underwent injury of the head and brain by shrapnel; he was examined thirty years later. After the injury, changes of character, periodic psychotic conditions with catatonic symptoms were noted. Attacks of headaches, paresthesias, central facial paresis, right side, were present. The increase of the symptoms thirty years after injury induced operation because depression of the skull was considered the cause of the symptoms.

Before operation, no other neurologic symptoms besides the mentioned ones were observed. *Language was intact in every respect.* In the operation, a part of the bone was eliminated. The brain did not show anything definite. *Directly after operation*, the catatonic symptoms disappeared. *Right facial paresis increased;* slight paresis of right hand and right-side epileptic fits were noted. *The patient could not speak at all.*

Five days after operation, the patient improved in general, did not have any epileptic fits. The right hand was improved. The patient understood single demands, followed directions, but understanding of longer sentences was lacking.

Spontaneous speech was totally lacking, as was also repetition. In conversation he used a great number of words which he uttered with some motor difficulties.

Repetition was about normal, as well for short and well-known long words as for rare words.

Reading aloud was now possible, with some (motor) paraphasic distortions. Spelling was correct, but the patient had difficulty in combining the presented letters into words.

Understanding in reading was improved, the patient particularly understanding Polish.

Writing was limited and produced only with great difficulty, the patient spelling before he wrote a word. "I cannot bring it together." He spoke much better than he wrote.

Dictation revealed most letters to be correct, also his name. The digits were given correctly.

Ten days after operation, spontaneous speech was missing. Repetition improved. He spoke certain words correctly *with some amount of interruption.*

Twelve days after operation, spontaneous speech included t—tu—a—to—toto, but *no other combinations of sounds.* Vivid gestures and mimical expressions, abnormal opening of the mouth, attempts to get the right position for producing sounds were all noted. The rhythm of the intended word might come to the fore without correct pronunciation.

Repetition showed him to be able to repeat a number of known words and even senseless syllables.

Naming of objects was severely damaged for the German language. He found, however, some names correctly in his mother tongue (Polish). He was able to choose objects according to the presented names.

Singing: Correct melodies without words.

Writing on dictation: Missing, also his own name.

Sixteen days after operation, he said to the doctor: "Gu-ten Mor-gen Herr Doctor." (Good mor-ning, Doc-tor), slowly.

Twenty-five days after operation, spontaneous speech was as good as repetition. Writing was much improved, as was reading also.

Six weeks after operation, there was nothing definitely abnormal in his language. Reading and writing were not very good, but evidently at about the same level as before. "Ja," however, was repeated as "j-a."

The case shows the characteristic effect of a superficial damage of the motor speech area, the picture of the first type of transcortical motor aphasia: at the beginning, complete inability to speak at all (total peripheral motor aphasia); with recovery of the substratum, first recovery of repetition, while all other speech functions remain disturbed, especially understanding of reading and writing—least understanding of speech. Singing was possible at an early stage, although without words.

Speech was recovered: repetition became normal in all respects, but voluntary speech was still severely disturbed, being better in conversation than spontaneously; reading aloud improved but showed motor paraphasia. Understanding of written material also improved. Writing was longer disturbed than spontaneous speaking, which slowly improved.

Six weeks after operation, all language performances were normal.

B. Central Motor Aphasia

In our discussion of the disturbances of the expressive side of speech we have distinguished the peripheral from the central motor aphasia. A case of the latter type is described below.

Case 6*

L. R., 24 years old, a bricklayer, was wounded by an infantry bullet. The bullet entered the skull at the right side of the forehead, close to the midline, left the skull in the left temporal bone, 1½ inches above, 1 inch before the ear.

Little is known about the period directly following the injury. The patient said he was unconscious and could not speak for a long time. He had understood what was said to him. In a hospital, his defect was diagnosed as transcortical motor aphasia and amnesic aphasia of severe degree.

He was examined by myself ten years after injury. In general, he was in good condition. He had no paresis, no changes of the reflexes, no disturbances of sensations. He suffered from epileptic seizures, which started with twitching of the right side of the tongue and then affected the whole right side of the body, later also the left side. Sometimes in the beginning, there was twitching in the left eyelid. The patient was unconscious, bit his tongue, lost urine. The attacks became less frequent after eleven to twelve years. When he could not fulfill a task set before him, it was often observed that he interrupted what he was doing, stood up, made a peculiar movement, began to yell. After two minutes, the rigidity passed away, his face became again more vivid, he looked around as if awakening from sleep (catastrophic condition). Sometimes under this condition, there was a typical epileptic seizure.

The man was, in general, a little slow; his face was rather immobile and rigid. His attention was strictly directed to what he was doing. Suddenly addressed, he would be somewhat startled and give the impression of one awakened from sleep. He would look astonished, then smile and gives the adequate replies or perform the task as far as it was within his capacity.

As to the tasks which this patient could perform and those he could not, there seemed to be, at first sight, no regularity which would make it possible to speak of his showing a lack of capacity for any specific performance. In fact, it would seem at times as if the patient had no defect at all in performance, except perhaps a degree of slowness. He seemed to be oriented in time, space, and the attributes of his person. He gave correctly the date of his birth, the ages of his children, etc. He could count, and was able to solve simple problems in arithmetic. He could reproduce the elements of his schooling and report the events of his more recent experiences.

I would tell him a simple story, and he was able to recount it after some interval. He could draw simple designs, a house or human face, copy a simple drawing, and

---

* The case is partially reported in Goldstein, 1923 (91) and (97), and further in the publication of my pupil, Sieckmann (271).

he recognized pictures known to him. His language showed a somewhat simple structure. Frequently he seemed to be hunting for words, but when the right word was supplied he usually recognized and adopted it readily. He could read and write. He did very well in simple reaction tests—for instance, in a test requiring him to withdraw his finger from a reaction key whenever a light was shown. Whatever fields of performance I tested, and I tested a great many, *I may say that in nearly all I found apparently normal responses.* As I have said before, the patient was *slow;* at times he appeared to make a *great effort to respond;* he perseverated; yet, up to this point, he revealed no grave defects.

But, in the same patient we might also encounter *a totally different behavior.* In tasks which on the surface seemed closely similar to those he had performed quite well, *he suddenly failed completely.*

Careful investigation revealed that he *was disturbed when the execution of a performance demanded the abstract attitude* (see p. 5), while he might perform well if it could be done in a concrete way.

This change of the behavior in general has to be considered if one wants to get an insight into a patient's *speech performances.* Here we also observed *great variation.* In general—even at the patient's best—he spoke slowly, abruptly, but somewhat fluently and lively; while at other times he stammered, hesitated, was in great tension and seemed unable to utter the words he apparently wanted to say. In this case, he uttered *definite phrases which he repeated again and again* in a stereotype way; his speech then was more fluent. He *might fail totally if he searched for a definite word or if such a word were asked of him.* In this condition, he gave the impression of a severe motor aphasic. In an other concrete situation, he might utter the same words without any effort. He did *not show paraphasia* of the type we observe in central aphasia, nor such distortions as we see them in motor aphasia (see p. 83). He spoke *spontaneously very little.* His speech was *better in conversations* but also here it showed severe abnormalities.

The following may illustrate his language in a conventional situation where he had to answer a definite question (the answer is translated as well as possible into English):

(How do you sleep?) "If I then...ah!...evenings...so at ten thirty (he wants to say: 'If I go to bed,' but is not able to do so; he points to the bed beside which he is standing) ah...ah...go...do not ask, doctor...ah...the m-a-a the Jacob (his room 'mate') (he wants to say 'snoring'; he cannot find the word and produces noises like snoring) do not ask, doctor, o God. ('Herr Doktor, o Gott,' this phrase he utters always in excitement)....The J-ah-ah (he looks to the bed and moves the hand quickly back and forth in a way as if he holds something)...bed...and so... Jacob, do not make noise. (He puts his hands over his ears and says): "Don't ask, doctor."

This example shows that he was *able even with his poor language to make himself understood,* indeed, very much supported by expressive and other movements.

Reciting series: The patient *could not recite the series of numbers on demand.* If one presented the first digits, he *continued till 10.* Sometimes he hesitated and could not find the next number. He might *begin again with 1* and then proceed better. He was much better if he had to *count objects,* coins, cigarettes, also if he were allowed to use his fingers. He then proceeded in the following way: He put the little finger of the left hand on the margin of the table and said *one,* then the fourth finger and said *two,* etc. Then, using the right hand, he began with the thumb and said *six,* etc., until he reached ten.

He was unable to say the series from 10 *backward*. He was more successful when he used his hands. Then he proceeded as follows: he put both hands on the table and lifted the little finger of the right hand. Beginning to count, he would start with the little finger of the left hand and thus come to the number 9.

If he were asked to continue to count up to 10, beginning at 4, he could not do so. If he started at 1, he was successful. If he had to continue to count, beginning at 5, he would put the left hand on the table, saying 5 and continuing 6, 7....

He was not able to recite the alphabet. Occasionally, he would want to say O, but he could not say it. Instead of that he would begin to recite the alphabet, continue fluently till O, and then say O. Shortly afterwards, he was unable to recite the alphabet on demand. If one urged him he would say: "Wie, Herr Doktor?" (What, doctor?) (I would say: Please try: a...b...c) He would say (German) "a...be...ce...de...en...r...el...ka...en..." Even urged, he could not say more. He was shocked by his bad performance.

Naming of objects: He had the *greatest difficulty in naming an object* on demand, while he found the concerned word in a situation to which it belonged without hesitation. It was very difficult for him to repeat voluntarily the words he had just spoken.

Repetition: Simple repetition was a *difficult task* for the patient. He stammered, uttered different words, which were similar in respect to certain sounds of the presented word, but was usually not successful with the whole word. Often one observed that he was not able to find a word; presented with it, he immediately caught on and repeated it fluently, showing by his gestures how grateful he was. "Yes, that I meant, doctor." *He uttered under this condition even long and motorically complicated words.* He was often *not able to repeat the same words on demand.* He then became excited and entered a catastrophic situation which hindered the continuation of his examination. Apparently he could *repeat a word voluntarily only if it belonged to a definite concrete situation.* In respect to this incapacity to repeat intentionally it was often astonishing to see that *his lips were moving in a way which corresponded to the pronunciation of the demanded word which he could not repeat.* He was not able to repeat these mouth movements on demand. They apparently occurred *involuntarily.*

A similar behavior was observed in his *reading.* Confronted with a text, printed, or written, *he moved his lips,* thus frequently reading even sentences correctly, although he did not understand what he was reading in this way. He had the greatest difficulty or was unable to read the same words *aloud.* Understanding of written material was fair, but only if he were allowed to accompany his reading of letters and words with movements of his finger on the table. If one hindered the movements of his hand, the patient tried to move his arm or the whole body. Without the movements he could not read any word. He recognized the letters apparently by these movements. Seeing of the letters did not elicit understanding, but apparently tracing did, and from these movements, understanding was elicited (see, regarding the problem of tracing, p. 123).

The patient could not name *any seen letter if he were not allowed to trace,* to "write" it.

The patient *did not write anything spontaneously.* But he was *very able to copy,* even long words when they contained contents he wanted to communicate to somebody.

On dictation, he could write only if he spoke the words repeatedly in a low voice. However, he did not simply speak the words but *sounded them out;* e.g., the word Taunus, the name of a mountain which he knew very well, he spoke: t.t.t.t.a.a.a. u.t.au.tau.tau.n.n.n.u.s.us.

Understanding: In a conversation which did concern a concrete situation and where he was not required to "shift" (see p. 6), he *understood quite well*. He did not understand if such shifting were necessary. He could not understand if two people spoke to each other, if somebody recited something, as, for instance, the prayer in church, etc. He understood stories only if simple activities were presented and such things were reported which were in his *concrete reach*. Therefore, he might, for instance, understand very well when one spoke with him about the thunderstorm which had occurred on the day before and a number of events which happened then, but he seemed to be totally at a loss if one reported a simple event at which he was not present or which he could not bring into relation to his personal experience. He grasped the things better when they were illustrated by simple drawings, but here also he was able to understand only if it concerned a concrete situation.

He *followed simple directions* and was able to fulfill such a task as: Go to the second floor and bring me the book from the table. However, he was not able to continue, if interrupted, or to give an account of what he was doing or had done.

Examination of the *intellectual functions* revealed the following: As we said before, his *knowledge of old material was not bad*, the same was true concerning his attention, interest and judgment; but all this was *possible only if he was confronted with concrete situations*. Therefore, he often appeared dull, but one could see from his behavior that he had grasped a great number of events occurring in his environment, apparently more in a passive way than intentionally

Concerning *memory* we find that under certain circumstances the faculty for reproduction of facts acquired long ago might possibly be normal. For example, school learning, etc., might be recalled very well in some situations, but not in all.

He was *incapable of recollection when he was asked to recall things which had nothing to do with the given situation*. But when it was possible to put him into a situation to which the material inquired for belonged, recollection appeared suddenly. The patient was also unable to remember if the required answer demanded an abstract attitude or whether it demanded that he give an account of the matter in question. Therefore, the patient *failed in many intelligence tests* which might seem for us very simple, and he was *amazingly successful in apparently difficult ones*.

Observation of the patient in other situations demonstrated clearly that memory failures were not caused by an impairment of memory content but that the *lack of memory was caused by faultiness in the attitude or approach* which was requisite for the specific test. The patient had the material in his memory but was unable to use it freely; he could use it only in connection with a definite concrete situation to which it must have seemed to him to belong. In the same way, he was able to learn new facts; he might be able to learn numbers, syllables, or movements by heart; he was able to hold in memory situations, facts of environment, etc., but he *was able to learn these only in a concrete situation and to reproduce them only in the same situation in which he had learned them*. In the specific situation, he might be very well oriented, but he was unable to give an account of some place he had visited. Therefore, the acquisition of new material remained scanty.

Thus, we come to the conclusion that there was no real defect in remembering, but that reproduction and new acquisition were defective because the normal basis of reproduction and acquisition was not given. Therefore, the patient's performance constantly varied according to whether the task were embedded in a concrete or in an abstract situation. In the first, the patient performed well; in the second, he failed. Since, in normal memory, the abstract situation plays an important rôle, for reproduction as for acquisition, the memory of the patient seemed to be feeble.

As to *attention*, here, too, one found wide differences in the facts. At one time, the patient appeared inattentive; at another, even abnormally fixed in attention. Attention was usually weak in the special examinations, particularly at the beginning of them, before the patient had gained the real approach to the whole situation. Then he appeared much distracted. However, once the patient became part of the situation, his attention might be satisfactory, might even be abnormally fixed. He might be totally untouched by other stimuli from the environment to which normal persons would react unfailingly. Thus, he might appear distracted in some tests, in others attentive, depending upon whether he were equal to the test or not. In some tests he would always appear distracted, for example, in those which demanded a change of approach (a choice reaction), because he was incapable of making such a reaction. Thus it was not correct to speak of a change of attention in the sense of a plus or minus of attention. The patient's state of attention was but an expression of his total behavior and could be understood only in connection with it.

Behavior of the patient as to space: He was, for practical purposes, well oriented in his room, in the house and garden where he lived. He seemed to behave about like a normal. But he was unable to describe such ways; he had *no understanding* for what we mean by *direction in space.* He might point to a noise coming from a place behind him in the room correctly, but was unable to say whether it was right or left, or how near. With *eyes open,* he could show where was up, down, right, left. With eyes closed, he was unable to, or made definite mistakes which revealed his way of procedure in his correct and wrong reactions. He did not show the direction at all, but the ceiling, floor, the writing right hand (making writing movements); left was the other hand, etc. If this kind of orientation were impossible he failed and sought another way to fulfill the task, namely, his only means, orientation on his own body. Up was for him where his head was, etc. Hence he pointed to a wrong place if he were lying on a bed, etc.

These results showed that he had *no idea what direction in space meant.*

This lack of having direction became manifest in his behavior with the simple test which we call *stick test* (see p. 155). The patient has the task to copy different simple forms, e.g., different angles, composed by two small sticks. He was able to do this *only* if he were allowed *to trace the lines of the angle.* Then he repeated this movement. Without tracing, he was unable to copy the angle. He could not even copy the position of a single stick presented in a definite direction if it were taken away so that he could not trace it. When two sticks were presented in the form of an angle he might produce an angle but not the right one. This is more astonishing in that the patient could copy quickly a little house with a door, a chimney, built of a number of sticks after he had looked at it for only a short time.

At first sight these differences may seem totally incomprehensible. Further examination clarifies the situation. We have seen that the patient failed in the test with two sticks joined together in the form of an angle with the opening upward. It appears amazing at first that if we composed the same angle with the opening pointing down, the patient would reproduce the figure very well at the initial trial. When we tried to ascertain how this were possible, when we ask the patient how it happened that he could reproduce the second figure, but not the first, he said, "This one has nothing to do with the other one," and "this is a roof."

These two replies lead us not only to an understanding of the patient's behavior in these tests but also of the fundamental change undergone by him.

His first reply made it clear that the two objects with which he had to deal in these two tests were to him totally different from one another. The second answer showed that the angle pointing downward was apprehended by the patient as a concrete object of his own visual experience, and he constructed a concrete thing with the two sticks. A concrete apprehension and concrete behavioral action were sufficient to meet the condition of this test. In the former test, the two sticks did not arouse in the patient an impression of a concrete thing. He had to conceive of the positions of two meaningless sticks in a meaningless connection, one with the other. He had to regard the sticks as mere representations, indicating directions in abstract space. Furthermore, he had to keep these directions in mind and re-arrange from memory the sticks as representatives of such abstract directions.

In the first test the patient needed to deal simply with a known object; in the second one he had to give an account to himself of relations in space, and act on the basis of abstract ideas. His action was not determined directly by a given concrete thing, but by a representative of an abstraction.

The disturbance of the patient, it was apparent, *lay in the circumstance that he was unable to assume an attitude towards the abstract, but was able to act in a concrete way.* Therefore, he was unable to perform tests the execution of which demanded the abstract attitude. The angle, with the opening pointing down, did not demand it and the patient was able to execute it perfectly. For the same reason, he was unable to place a stick in a definite direction but was well able to imitate the con-structing of the little "house," which would seem to be much more complicated.

How important it was for success or failure whether the patient could act directly or had to give account to himself about the activity before he acted may be seen in the following simple example:

The patient was to throw a ball into boxes successively situated at a distance of 3, 9, 15 feet from him. He did it quite well. When he was asked how far the several boxes were from him, he was not only unable to answer this question, but even to say which box was nearer, which farther. However, he might give correct replies if he were allowed to walk over a definite distance and to count his steps, knowing that each step covered 1 foot. He could tell by counting how many feet there were for each distance and thus could infer as to which box was farther and which nearer.

In the first task, the patient had only to deal with objects in a behavioral fashion. It was unneccessary for the patient to be conscious of his act and of objects in a world separated from himself. In the second test, however, he had to separate himself from the world and give himself an account of his actions and of the space relations in the world facing him. Therefore, he failed.

The patient's *behavior as to time* was similar. He spoke about time but did not really know what time meant; he could not distinguish between different durations, which was longer, which shorter. He was apparently able to use the watch in a concrete situation. When he had to be at a definite place at a definite time, he looked at his watch and when he found the hands at the place corresponding to their position at the concerned time he concluded it was this time. But he was unable to say where the minute hand was at a certain time, for instance at 13 minutes past four o'clock. He could give a description here only if he was allowed to point with his finger at the minutes from 60 to 13. All times were moments combined with definite concrete behavior: 12 was lunchtime, 3 o'clock when his mate left the room, etc. He could not grasp anything which was only imaginary, only a possibility, or where he had to shift because during the activity the situation had changed. Therefore, he was often totally at a loss when he was interrupted in his activity, even such a simple thing as counting from 1 to 20. He could not do anything where he had to pretend. He seemed to be apractic if he were asked to show how to threaten, but he might do this in a situation where he was angry at somebody, quite normally. He showed seemingly a great lack of "Antrieb," of initiative, but in other—concrete—situations he could become very active, even violent. He usually appeared dull, but might sometimes be greatly excited.

If we analyze precisely the situations in which the patient appeared emotionally inert and those in which the contrary was the case, we ascertain that the presence or absence of *emotional expression* corresponded to his entire behavior in the given situation, and that the emotional behavior was at best inseparable from the rest of his behavior. The fact seems to be this: If the patient did not react emotionally in a satisfactory way, it was in situations in which he also failed to comprehend the essentials to which a definite feeling attaches. The patient appeared emotionally inadequate when he was in a situation in which that feeling which we regard as belonging to it could not be aroused. He might have grasped only a part of the situation to which that affect which the patient showed was appropriate. It appears to us inappropriate because we regard the whole situation and not merely a part of it. If we regard the behavior of the patient from this point of view his feeling does not appear abnormal to the situation as it is experienced by the patient.

In the same way we have to understand the lack of interest in the next example. The patient never seemed concerned about his family, never spoke of his wife or children, was irresponsive when we questioned him about them and when it was suggested to him that he should write to his family he would show cool indifference. Thus, he appeared to lack all feeling. Now it was an established practice that he should from time to time visit his home, situated in another town, and stay there several days. While at home, the patient conducted himself, as we learned, quite as would a normal man in the bosom of his family, kind and affectionate to wife and children, interested in their affairs, in so far as his ability would permit. After his return to the hospital from such a visit and being asked about his people, he would smile in an embarrassed way, giving evasive answers. He seemed utterly estranged from his home situation. Unquestionably what ailed this man was not really a deterioration of his character on the emotional and moral side.

Another example: the patient had a friend who was his close companion. One day the friend went to a cinema with another man. He did not take our patient because the latter had seen the particular picture before and would not go to see it a second time. When the friend came back from the movie, our patient was in a state of great excitement and refused to speak to him. He was not to be quieted by any arguments. No explanation such as that his friend did not want to offend him, that his friendship had not changed, made any impression. From that time on, our patient was his old friend's enemy.

This reaction, at first so unintelligible, can be understood if we remember that the patient is able to make only a direct concrete approach to any situation. This is also the case in his approach to his friend. He saw only that his friend was friendly with another man and he felt himself slighted. He was unable to understand that his friend's conduct in no way actually affected their relations. He could not recognize why his friend went without him and he could not perceive the situation as a whole because he could not abstract it from his own concrete personality. He saw only the concrete separation between himself and his friend and from this standpoint his exaggeration was thoroughly understandable, particularly if we consider how difficult it is, in the case of a change of attitude, for a patient with a lesion of the frontal lobe to enter into the relation of friendship. The patient felt his loneliness and sank into a catastrophic situation of confusion and anxiety. He regarded his friend as its cause. This insight into the workings of his mind renders his behavior intelligible. Since many situations were not grasped conceptually by the patient, his total affective state must necessarily be more equable and the result was that he appeared emotionally blunted.

Summarizing the findings in this patient,* I come to the conclusion that he has, *on the one hand, motor speech disturbances similar to peripheral motor aphasia; on the other hand, he presents symptoms which are an expression of impairment of abstract attitude. This combination I call central motor aphasia;* (see p. 85), in contrast to other cases belonging to the group which show certain speech disturbances as secondary effects of damage of non-speech mental processes (see p. 293). Our patient shows similarities with these cases because in both, abstract attitude is impaired. He differs from them by the fact that the motor speech disturbances are primary and therefore show characteristics which the others do not show. I have observed a number of similar cases. To this group belong the important cases of Woerkom.

With this interpretation of such cases, one could consider it unjustified to speak of them as motor aphasia.

The situation is similar here as when we deliberated (see p. 277) whether certain cases should be called amnesic aphasia after the disturbance of word-finding has proved to be only one symptom of a more general mental modification. Here, as there, I like to maintain the names because the defect in motor speech and in word-finding is so much in the foreground that these patients are usually considered as motor aphasics or amnesic aphasics, and this with good reason. The dominance of these symptoms is due to the fact that they are not alone produced by impairment of abstraction. In amnesic aphasia, I have stressed the point that there exists also some damage of the speech instrumentalities which gives the picture its characteristics (see p. 291). The same is true with our patient. Here the characteristic picture is due to the damage of the motor speech sphere.

The difficulty in finding the right name for the cases reveals the close relationship between language and non-language mental phenomena. I think we should, for the time being, maintain the name for clinical reasons.

I would like here to add some remarks about the relation between central motor aphasia and amnesic aphasia. Both have in common the fact that speech shows modifications which can be considered due to impairment of abstract attitude. They differ in the following points: In central motor aphasia there exist motor difficulties, in amnesic aphasia

* The foregoing report does not give by any means all details investigated. For a fuller description, the publication of this case by W. Sieckmann (271) should be cited.

not. The patient with the first form speaks very little, the amnesic aphasic often speaks much. On the other hand, the defect in naming in amnesic aphasia is much more outspoken; the presented correct word is immediately accepted and repeated in amnesic aphasia, but not in central motor aphasia. Voluntary repetition, which is excellent in amnesic aphasia, is particularly disturbed in central motor aphasia.

The differences seem to be due to the difference of the localization of the lesion. In amnesic aphasia, the lesion in general is located in the posterior part of the brain, and thus damages the posterior part of the "central area of the cortex" (see p. 46) and to a certain degree the speech area itself (except the motor part). Disturbances of abstraction result, plus the severe defect in word-finding (see p. 290). In central motor aphasia, the lesion is located in the anterior part of the brain, damaging the frontal lobe and the motor speech area, and thus producing a picture in which, besides impairment of abstraction, motor speech phenomena are prominent.

CHAPTER VI

Pictures in which Disturbances of the Receptive Side Are in the Foreground

W<small>E CAN</small>, indeed with some abstraction, distinguish three symptom complexes:

1. The patient *hears* but does *not perceive the sound-complexes as known familiar phenomena,* is not able to "understand" and to repeat them. There are no other speech disturbances; particularly speaking, reading and wording are intact (so-called *pure sensory aphasia,* pure speech deafness, subcortical sensory aphasia, *"peripheral sensory aphasia"*).

2. In a second type of case, the patient has, *besides the perceptive disturbance, symptoms which show a damage of inner speech, particularly paraphasia* (so-called *Wernicke's sensory aphasia, cortical sensory aphasia, "central sensory aphasia"*).

3. In a third group, the patients are *able to repeat heard language, but do not understand the heard word.* Repetition is more or less echolalic (so-called *transcortical sensory aphasia*).

As to the second and third groups, I refer the reader to the discussion elsewhere (see pp. 88 and 293). Here I shall discuss only peripheral sensory aphasia, that form in which the sensory side of language only is disturbed and which, therefore, is particularly suited for study at this time.

PERIPHERAL SENSORY APHASIA

There was much discussion about this symptom complex, first described by Lichtheim; its existence was even denied by some authors, as, for example, Pierre Marie. But there is no doubt that it occurs, that there are patients who perceive all other acoustic stimuli but not the sound complexes which we use in language, without any other speech defect being present. Indeed, the picture does not appear frequently in pure form; particularly the differentiation from cortical defects of hearing is not always possible because such defects may exist simultaneously (see also p. 89).

In typical cases proved by exact methods, hearing appears undisturbed, particularly the perception of those tones which, as we said before, seem to be presupposition for perceiving language, or at least hearing is preserved to a degree sufficient for understanding language.

The patients are aware of the defect. They are unable to distinguish between similar sounds or sound complexes. The sounds appear strange, unfamiliar acoustic phenomena, not as language—possibly like words of a foreign language. Some patients hear sounds which may appear familiar, but they are not experienced as combined to words. The same sounds are repeatedly experienced (po-lo-lo, to-to-lo or momomo, or drub-drub-drub). Language may be differentiated from other noises, as foreign language, but, indeed, even then without recognition of the sounds as known speech sounds. Not infrequently a lack of attention exists in respect to all acoustic stimuli, also to those which do not represent language, or sometimes only to language.

In some cases, the patient shows from the beginning the typical picture, but often it develops out of a so-called cortical sensory aphasia, or it is the first stage of this. In cases of total defect, there is scarcely any improvement to be expected.

There are cases described where the defect is *partial*. A patient of Schmitt recognized vowels, not words, but if the words were presented to him slowly, then he would recognize them. In some cases (Ziehl, 330, and Henneberg, 137), the vowels, consonants were perceived, but not words. A patient observed by Bonvicini (121) recognized some vowels and a few consonants, but not words. A case of mine perceived some words, but it was particularly interesting that the vowels and consonants of which they consisted were not perceived. This shows that we cannot consider the perception of sounds as simpler than that of words, as it was assumed from such observations as those of Ziehl and Henneberg, and Bonvicini. With respect to the problem of which is more difficult, which less, the following has to be considered. For the child, each acoustic perception represents a word, even if it may be only a sound to the adult. Later, sounds recede into the background and the child perceives particularly sound *complexes*, corresponding to words. The direction is changed again when we begin to learn reading and writing. We become more and more aware of the individual sounds corresponding to the letters. This, naturally, does not occur, in the same degree in all individuals. For the educated individual, the letter becomes much more an independent phenomenon than for an individual who does not read and write much. This is enforced by the fact that for noneducated people, phenomena which have no particular practical significance are easily neglected, also as to perception. Words with abstract meaning are not well known, and, in like instance, the letters, too, which have little meaning in themselves. Hence the sounds of letters may, to the uneducated individual, appear like strange words. Their perception which, from the acoustic point of view, may be easier than that of words, loses much of this character because they are so strange.

From this point of view, the differences in the behavior of the patients as to letters or words may become understandable. The patient of Ziehl who perceived letters better than words was a businessman, my patient, a seaman of little education. In the future, adequate consideration should be taken of this point.

Lichtheim (185) and Wernicke (316) had assumed that the subcortical sensory aphasia is due to an interruption of the subcortical acoustic pathways which bring the acoustic stimuli to the Wernicke center in the temporal lobe, where the acoustic word images were thought to be deposited. There is no doubt that a subcortical lesion in the left temporal lobe can be followed by this form of aphasia. (Cases of Liepmann, 187, Wernicke, 316, van Gehuchten-Goris, 75, Henneberg, 137, Schuster-Taterka, 267). But it can occur also in cortical lesions in the first temporal convolution, as in cases of Henschen, Poetzl, Kleist, or in diffuse, usually symmetric atrophy or sclerosis or diffuse luetic processes, affecting more or less the whole temporal lobe (as in cases of Pick, 231, Dejerine-Serieux, 47, Veraguth, 303, Strohmeyer, 292, Stertz, 286).

The interpretation of the anatomic findings differs correspondingly to the differences of opinion about the organization of the temporal lobe, particularly whether there are separate areas for hearing and speech perception. There is agreement that the acoustic fibers end in Heschl's region and that its lesion damages hearing. There is, further, no doubt that in destruction of each hemisphere, disturbances of hearing occur on both sides, in the opposite much more than in the homolateral one. The defect consists not in a loss of perception of some tones, but in a constriction of the realm of tone perception, as investigations by Boernstein (17) and others have shown. All else we might say about the organization of the temporal lobe in relation to perception of speech is hypothetic. Wernicke had the opinion that outside of Heschl's area there exists a center where the acoustic speech images are deposited. Lesion of it is followed by the so-called cortical sensory aphasia. This region was later named Wernicke's center, and the form of aphasia which occurs in its destruction Wernicke's aphasia. Wernicke considered pure word deafness as due to a lesion of the fibers which go from Heschl's area to this center, which in itself had to be assumed intact, otherwise Wernicke's aphasia, not pure sensory aphasia, would occur. According to Kleist, there exists a special region, separated from the area for tone and noise perception, located in the middle and oral part of the transverse convolutions, the destruction of which brings about the pure word deafness. It destroys the acoustic speech images, leaving the general acoustic perception intact. The cases where this symptom complex is observed in subcortical lesions (as in the case of Schuster-Taterka, 267, one-sided subcortical lesion, or in the case of Burrett, subcortical lesion in the white matter of both temporal lobes) are explained by elimination of stimulation of this center, due to destruction of the pathways from the acoustic centers of both sides to Wernicke's center.

The interpretation of Wernicke and Kleist would make plausible the appearance of pure word deafness in subcortical, but not in cortical lesions, at least if one maintains that Wernicke's region is not only important for perception of speech but for the regulation of motor speech, as is almost generally assumed. The cortical defects should always be followed by Wernicke's aphasia (which is not at all the case). Henschen (139), Poetzl (245) and Burrett have published cases where in lesions outside of Heschl's region pure word deafness existed without defect of "inner speech."

Henschen, too, separated the cortical acoustic center from a region for speech perception. He observed a case where lesion in Wernicke's zone produced word deafness, not deafness in general. According to him, this is due to the lesion of a special place in the caudal-lateral part of the transverse convolution.

This difficulty of interpretation which exists because of the assumption of different centers for sound perception and speech perception, may be eliminated if one does not attribute to Wernicke's area a function different from Heschl's, but considers it as *belonging to the perceptual sphere*. While the *smaller part*—located in Heschl's region—*guarantees the simple acoustic perceptions, the intactness of the wider field is necessary for perception of the more complex acoustic phenomena of perception of language.*

Such an assumption would explain the appearance of acoustic defects in general in a lesion of Heschl's region, appearance of pure word deafness in conditions which set the wider acoustic sphere out of function but leave intact Heschl's region.

Lesion of one Heschl's region, even of that in the major hemisphere, does not hinder acoustic perception in general, and as long as there exist fiber connection with the intact acoustic sphere in the minor hemisphere, it does not disturb speech perception. Word deafness happens if a lesion in the left temporal lobe destroys the connection between this wider acoustic field in the major hemisphere and Heschl's region there *and* in the minor hemisphere. The intactness of Heschl's region in the major, even in the minor hemisphere alone, guarantees hearing in general. We know that only lesions in both temporal lobes destroy hearing totally. Whether word deafness can take place also in lesions of the wider acoustic sphere (Wernicke's center) in the major hemisphere alone, is not absolutely certain. It is very difficult to say how much in such cases the pathways to the other hemisphere's wider acoustic sphere are intact or destroyed. If both temporal lobes (first and second convolution) are destroyed with preservation of the transversal gyri of one or the other side, hearing may be intact, recognition and understanding of speech impossible. Speaking must not be severely disturbed (as in the case of Henschen, and in Burrett's case). Indeed, in the case of Henschen only the posterior part of the first temporal convolution was affected, so enough may be preserved to guarantee speech (particularly because the other part of the "region of inner speech" was not destroyed).

My interpretation of pure word deafness involves the setting out of function of the wider acoustic sphere, i.e., the effect of impairment of a cortical function. It is a defect of complicated acoustic perceptions of more complicated acoustic "Gestalten." The symptoms correspond to a differentiation of these. This interpretation makes it understandable that in cortical lesion outside of Heschl's region, sensory aphasia occurs, without any disturbances of inner speech. The Wernicke center has nothing to do with inner speech, or, more precisely, the damage of it with defects of inner speech. In Wernicke's aphasia, other regions are always damaged which must be intact if inner speech is to function normally (see p. 240). That cortical sensory aphasia is an expression of a more extended functional damage than pure word deafness shows also in the fact that the lesions in the first type of aphasia are mostly gross lesions of the cortex (see Stertz, 286), while to pure word deafness, smaller cortical lesions correspond.

Our interpretation makes it understandable also that pure word deafness appears in diffuse atrophy of the temporal lobes and usually in symmetric atrophy due to luetic processes (cases of Pick, 233, Dejerine-Serieux, 47, Veraguth, 303, Strohmeyer, 292, Stertz, 286). These affections may damage first and to a greater degree the complex function of speech perceptions, but leave intact the simpler acoustic perception in general. The same holds true for the case of Gehuchten and Goris (75), where in an abscess in the depth of the medial part of T. II, in which pure word deafness was observed, the word deafness disappeared after elimination of pus.

How complex the situation is becomes evident from the fact that from similar processes and similar localization of lesions, sometimes transcortical aphasia may result (see p. 297).

We come to the result: *"peripheral sensory aphasia" (pure word deafness) is due to incomplete damage of the area of acoustic perception which does not disturb acoustic perception in general, but dedifferentiates more or less the complex acoustic phenomena which correspond to language (acoustic speech "Gestalten").*

Which *special localization* of the lesion in the temporal lobe is particularly suited to produce this effect is not quite clear. The published material is not sufficient to come to a decision on this point. We may say: The *lesion must leave Heschl's convolution intact.* Wernicke's region is important. In the cases of Henschen, Poetzl and Burrett, where Wernicke's region was lesioned, inner speech was intact (an expression that it has nothing to do with inner speech). It seems that the *middle part of the left first temporal convolution is the place which must mainly* be taken into consideration: this is a region close to Heschl's area. It was affected in the two cases which are investigated best (Henschen, case Nielsen, and Poetzl's case). How much the lesion must be extended to produce speech deafness, and how much it must be restricted so that no other symptoms come to the fore—particularly cortical deafness and symptoms belonging to Wernicke's aphasia—cannot yet be decided. It seems necessary to me that the region between first temporal convolution and Isle of Reil (at least in the left hemisphere), the Isle of Reil itself, Heschl's convolution and the connection between T. I and parietal lobe must be preserved.

Our result concerning the interpretation of this form of aphasia corresponds to the interpretation which I gave years ago and which was given in a similar way particularly by Sachs.

My concept of the organization of the temporal lobe in respect to speech is not so much in contrast to that of Henschen as it may appear at first. He assumes that we have to distinguish three parts; one center for word hearing, one for perception of word sounds, and a word sense center. This corresponds to my dedifferentiation of a *smaller part of the area* sufficient to guarantee hearing in general, a *larger area* to guarantee hearing of word sounds and *another part* which belongs to the area for "inner speech." Indeed, I do not assume separate areas but more or less complicated functions of a great region.

Apart from the significance of this result for understanding this special form of aphasia, it is of general importance for the theory of brain function:

1. In so far as it brings an aphasic picture which was often considered as effect of interruption of pathways into relation with a damage of *cortical function*, and thereby considerably undermines the theory that destruction of pathways can produce aphasia—a theory which I have always rejected.

2. In so far as it makes the assumption of acoustic perceptions unnecessary and considers the perceptive speech phenomena only as complicated phenomena of these. This brings us to a standpoint similar *to* the interpretation of motor aphasia (see p. 80) which is, for our interpretation, also the effect of impairment of more complicated motor activities which do not differ essentially from the other voluntary movements.

There have been published a number of cases of *incomplete word-deafness* (e.g., by Ziehl, 330, Henneberg, 137, myself, 78), which need particular consideration because they show symptoms which bring to the fore some important factors concerning the relation of *speech perception to understanding and repetition*. The following case may serve as illustration for the behavior of such patients.

Case 7*

A 34 year old seaman suffered a fall from a boat into water. He could not speak directly afterwards, was disoriented, confused. After several days, general condition was reported as good, and the patient was oriented. Speech improved and remained in about the same state during my observation. History was without significance. The patient had never been sick before, no headache, no dizziness.

Physically, he showed no abnormalities except some arteriosclerotic changes of the heart; no paralysis, no other neurologic symptoms.

Sense organs: Visual perception, visual field and visual recognition were without disturbance. *Hearing, even by testing with finer methods, was without defect.*

Mentally, the patient was quiet, cooperative, aware of his defect. He often became excited and angry when aware of special failures. Judgment, memory for previous and recent events was normal. *Counting:* additions and subtractions corresponded to his poor education. Multiplications and divisions were impossible, although he was probably never capable of these performances.

Examination with the usual intelligence tests revealed no deviation from the norm, only that his education was on a low level. Attention in general was absolutely normal. In contrast to this, often a great lack of attention as far as speech was concerned was noted.

Speech: The patient did not speak much spontaneously, but answered in well constructed sentences, often somewhat hesitatingly. Outstanding was the lack of certain words, particularly nouns. He often uttered such phrases as "I know it, but I cannot say it." Only *very seldom was there literal paraphasia; no verbal paraphasia noted. Naming of objects:* Defects in naming concrete objects were observed, on visual as well as acoustic and tactual presentation. He never displayed defect in recognition.

No defect in perception of spatial relations was noted. While in the beginning he was unable to name most objects, later he was able to name a very large number of everyday objects.

Protocol from a later period:

Window +	Brush −	Teeth − ("also with H")
Finger +	Cork +	Wood +
Paper +	Handkerchief +	Metal −
Knife +	Nose +	Purse +
Key +	Shoe −	Thimble −
Pencil −	Cuff +	Cat −
Apple +	Chain +	Dog +
Boat +	Button −	Penholder −
	Hand − ("with H")	

---

* Published first by the author (78), 1906.

He was unable to write down a name he could not say.

Sensory speech function: This was seemingly not grossly disturbed in usual conversation. Here and there he seemed not to understand a sentence, but understood better if the question were formulated in another way. Following directions was often impossible; he showed wrong objects, wrong parts of his body.

Protocol of his behavior in showing objects to given names:

An earlier period		A later period	
Finger −	Cat −	Nose +	Button +
Key −	Dog +	Finger +	Cupboard −
Chair +	Knife +	Bottle +	Chair +
Table +	Pencil +	Pencil −	Cat −
Funnel −	House +	Funnel −	Thimble −
Paper −	Teeth −	Clock +	Window +
Chain −	Button −	Table +	Ship +
		Handkerchief +	Chain +
		Cake −	Fish +
		Paper +	Penholder −

If the object he was supposed to show were among some presented to him, *he made less mistakes* than when he had to look around and find it; he showed, by expressive movements, that seeing the object helped him to understand the word. He then repeated the word often, which he never did when he had apparently not understood it.

He was *unable to distinguish acoustically correct presented words from those presented in distortion.* He seemed not to recognize which was the right one.

Repetition was disturbed to a high degree: He was not able to repeat letters, although sometimes *u, o, t, a.* If one began to recite a, b, c.... he would say correctly a, b, c, and repeat letters correctly as long as one presented the individual letters in the series. He *did not recognize the fault if one omitted a letter or named a wrong one* and was unable to continue if one stopped speaking. He behaved in a similar way regarding digits.

Repetition of words:

Protocol I

Examiner	Patient repeats	Examiner	Patient repeats
Hund (dog)	+	Honolulu	−
Haus (house)	+	Kaiser Wilhelm (Emperor William)	Willem
Flasche (bottle, sees it)	− +	Maus (mouse)	+
Kind (child)	+	Kette (chain)	No Kette
Stuhl (chair)	−	Himmel (sky)	−
Papier (paper, shows)	+	Streichholz (match)	+ shows position
Dorf (village)	House		
Tot (dead)	−	Apfel (apple)	+
		Katze (cat)	as dog with C
Pfirsich (peach)	+		
Tinte (ink)	−	Tasse (cup)	−
Segeln (sail)	to the wind	Taube (pigeon)	−
Gott (God)	Church	Pier (pier)	+
Schulter (shoulder)	−	Kuchen (cake)	−

Examiner	Patient repeats	Examiner	Patient repeats
Kanarienvogel (canary)..	−	Vogel (bird)	+
Berlin (Berlin)	+	Artaxerxes	−
Schiff (ship)	+	Major (mayor)	−
Uhr (clock)	+		
Sofa (sofa)	there is none here		

Protocol II

Examiner	Patient repeats	Examiner	Patient repeats
Hund	+	Haus (house)	+ points to window
H	−		
Maus (mouse)	cat	Fenster (window)	+ points to it
Schiff (ship)	+		
Tisch (table)	+ (points)	Tinte (ink)	inkwell
Flasche (bottle)	funnel	Schulter (shoulder)	− shows it
Himmel (sky)	wind, storm	Gestern (yesterday).....	−
Streichholz (match)	to light	Kopf (head)	−
Segeln (sail)	−	Fisch (fish)	+
Dorf (village)	street	Canarienvogel (canary).	−
Geld (money)	−	Artaxerxes	−
Taube (pigeon)	−	Berlin (Berlin)	+
		Major (mayor)	−
		Federhalter (penholder).	points to inkwell

Sentences: (What is the time?) He is unable to repeat, but apparently understands the meaning: He says: "About noontime." (The dog is beautiful)....
He gives no reply. (I have twenty dollars) He says: "I have money." Texts of known songs he recognizes, but cannot repeat them. He *never repeats anything paraphasic.* Either he is able to repeat it correctly or remains silent. Senseless syllables he does not repeat at all. He *repeats only words he has understood.*

Reading: This is without defect; letters, words, sentences are apparently as good as he was able to read them before. He seems, in general, to understand what he reads. Sometimes he repeats, by spelling, words he does not understand. He can also read words which are presented in an abnormal manner, e.g., written upside down or with wide spaces between the letters. He is able to read those words correctly which he does not repeat if heard. He understands some by reading, but not by hearing. He asks the examiner, therefore, to write down what he wants. He recognizes the numbers. He *cannot be induced to spell words.* But it is not certain whether he cannot do it or is not willing to do it. The same applies for the task of putting together letters into words.

Writing: He refuses to write upon command. If he has written something, he does not like to show it: it is, in his opinion, so bad. He writes his name and residence correctly. In a letter to his parents, he writes a number of understandable things he wants to communicate. He leaves out words, here, but the construction of the sentences is not so bad. It may be that he was never able to write better than this. He recognizes mistakes in such a letter but is not able to correct them.

Copying: This is correct both as to printed material and written.

Writing on dictation: The same performance is noted as with repetition of heard words. What he is unable to repeat, he is unable to write; what he repeats, he is able to write; e.g., he is able to repeat the German word "hund" and writes it, but not the letter h.

The condition was essentially unchanged during observation of about four months.

The main symptoms of the case are *disturbances of speech perception and repetition*. The first defect shows the characteristics of subcortical sensory aphasia. However, there are a number of peculiarities. The patient *sometimes seems to understand, sometimes not at all*. The defect becomes particularly impressive when words which have nothing to do with the present situation, are presented. In such instances, he does not even pay any attention to what is said. Examination of his capacity to hear leaves no doubt that *we are not dealing with a hearing defect*. Further mitigating against such a defect is the fact that the patient understands a number of words quite well. That the cause is not a general lack of attention is proven by his behavior in general. In a situation where hearing of speech is not involved, he is attentive in a normal way.

It is further interesting that he frequently perceives *words better than the sounds of which the words consist*.

In respect to the greatest number of words, the patient behaves like other patients with pure speech deafness; he does not understand the words and cannot repeat them. It is remarkable that the patient is *unable to repeat a number of words which*—according to his reactions to them— *he has (see later) "understood" as to their meaning*. It was not quite certain whether the patient did not have some disturbances in the sense of dedifferentiation of inner speech; with his good repetition of a number of words, however, it was improbable that his inability to repeat others was due to a defect in this respect. We can assume that acoustic perception of a number of words must have been *sufficient to awaken the meaning but not the movements necessary for repetition*.

We have some analogous behavior in normals, in the situation of learning language. The child "understands," in a certain state of development, many words which he cannot speak and repeat. Adults are in a similar situation when they learn a foreign language. By "understanding" we mean here that hearing of a sound complex awakens some ideas which are related to it, even if it is not perceived correctly. The perception of the patient seems to be of this kind. But his behavior shows more: *the sound complex may be sufficiently precise to awaken a realm of ideas to which the idea belongs, without being precise enough to awaken the individual idea which belongs especially to the presented word*. The reactions of the patient point definitely to such a condition. When he says, instead of God, *church*, instead of village, *house*, of mouse, *cat*, etc. (see also, regarding this phenomenon, p. 66), this cannot be the effect of confusion of words similar as to their acoustic appearance. He did not confound such words. It is apparently due to the fact that the imperfect perception awoke a realm, or a sphere to which a number of words belong and not *one* special idea of this sphere.

This reaction speaks for a defect in a sphere in which the ideas or the words are composed as to their contents. We are not sure about the psychologic or anatomic "localization" of this phenomenon. Probably we should locate it in the sphere of "speech-concepts" ("Sprachvorstellungen"). Normally, in the hearing of a word, a sphere of speech concepts and ideas comes to our mind, among which one stands out as being particularly related to the heard sound. We may assume, if the perception of the word sound complex is not correct, that the perception may be sufficient to evoke this sphere, but not the special word. Therefore, the patient reacts with a word which belongs to this sphere.

This explanation would be in agreement with the fact that the patient understands words and is able to repeat them better if the acoustic stimulation is enforced by other stimulations. The patient is better able to repeat words (which previously he had not been able to repeat) *after* he has understood them. Repetition is still better when the patient has occasion to see an object to which the heard word fits. Both conditions seem to be suited to enforce the acoustic experience in the sense that the specific speech sound complexes become more precise.

There is one phenomenon which needs a further short discussion. Why did the patient *not* repeat the sound complexes as imperfectly as he perceived them, but preferred to remain silent? We mentioned a similar observation of Ziehl. In this respect it is remarkable that the patient also did not like to imitate other noises; indeed, he was particularly obstinate to any repetition of those which had any similarity to speech sounds. Apparently it was because he was aware of his defect and was ashamed to speak something which he realized as wrong, as nonsense. This phenomenon points to the significance of general psychologic factors for the development of some symptoms which I have stressed particularly (see p. 10).

Summarizing, we can say: The patient is suffering from imperfect acoustic speech perception. Why some perceptions are preserved, we are not able to say. Words are better perceived, as in most cases, than letters. Some words the patient is able to understand and repeat; others he can *understand only in so far as the sphere of ideas to which the word belongs is stimulated*, not the special word, and the patient repeats a word which belongs to the sphere but which does not correspond to the heard word. Why he repeats a particular word we cannot definitely say (see p. 66).

As little as we can say about the anatomic lesion in this case, we may assume a lesion of the extended acoustic area. Because there are symptoms which speak for some light damage of inner speech, we may further assume an affection of the region between temporal lobe and the Isle of Reil (see p. 239).   We are not able to say something definite about the nature of the disturbance of wordfinding, because finer examination is missing.   The fact that this defect greatly improved inclines me to assume that we are dealing here with a slight damage of instrumentalities and not an expression of impairment of abstract attitude (see p. 67) which did not show in any other symptoms.

CHAPTER VII

Central Aphasia

BESIDES the pure aphasias and the transcortical symptom complexes there are aphasic patients who present a *complex picture of sensory and motor disturbances*. These pictures are usually called cortical sensory or motor aphasia. The motor disturbances in cases termed sensory aphasia are considered secondary to the damage of the sensory images or of the sensory speech area—an interpretation the incorrectness of which, in principle, I have tried to show (see p. 83). Sensory disturbances appearing in motor aphasia, first described by *Dejerine and Thomas*, were the object of much discussion, without any clarification of their origin being reached. But there were in these cases in addition to the motor and sensory defects, often even in the foreground, other disturbances such as repetition, literal and verbal paraphasia, paralectic and paragraphic phenomena, incapacity of the patients to spell words and to put letters presented separately together into a word, and finally disturbance of the syntactical order of sentences. These symptoms could not be explained as effect of a sensory or motor aphasia, not even of a combination of both, not as signs of dedifferentiation of the motor or perceptual speech area.

The disturbances may not always become manifest; they may be more or less covered by substitution through motor or sensory instrumentalities (see p. 95). Some words may be spoken or written correctly because the patient uses his motor automatisms and the defect may come to the fore only if one hinders him in the use of these. The syntactical defect (see p. 98) may be covered by use of motor series (see p. 95), etc. That the symptoms are not secondary to motor or sensory defect becomes evident when *they occur without any definite motor or perceptual changes in the patient*. They are "complications" of the motor or sensory aphasia "plus symptoms" as I have called them (p. 94), which always show (although they may or may not accompany a sensory or motor aphasia)—about the same picture.

Wernicke, who has termed this symptom complex "Leitungsaphasie" (conduction aphasia), considered expression of damage of "concepts of words"; later he abandoned this theory (see p. 93). I have tried to show that it is a picture which becomes understandable as expression of dedifferentiation of inner speech and termed it *central aphasia*. The name conduction aphasia did not appear correct to me, because we are not dealing with a defect of conduction, as Wernicke had assumed as cause particularly of the disturbance of repetition and of the paraphasia, but with dedifferentiation of a complex apparatus which I believed to be justified to "localize" in the center of the speech area (see further, p. 239). The anatomic neighborhood of the motor and sensory speech centers makes it understandable that in central aphasia there are frequently real motor and sensory speech disturbances. Anomalies of spontaneous speech and understanding belong also to central aphasia, but they are of another type than those due to lesion of the motor or sensory center. I have characterized them before when I described the symptoms in dedifferentiation of inner speech (see p. 98).

Not only my interpretation but even the existence of the clinical picture is not at all generally acknowledged in the literature. I admit that one can doubt the correctness of the interpretation, but not the existence of the symptom complex. After Wernicke described this form of aphasia, other cases were published by Pick, Heilbronner, Kleist, Liepmann, Stertz, Stengel, and myself. It seldom occurs clinically in pure form, but mostly in a state of improvement of more complicated pictures of the type of so-called cortical sensory aphasia or in a progressive condition in cases which show first amnesic aphasia (observations of Heilbronner, Kleist, and myself, see p. 231).

The psychologic interpretation of the symptom complex is not at all satisfactory. Further studies are urgently needed. They will be of great clinical value because symptoms corresponding to central aphasia frequently appear as complications of other forms of aphasia and will obscure the interpretation of these as long as we do understand central aphasia only imperfectly. Analysis of central aphasia promises much clarification of the phenomenon of inner speech and will thus be of great significance for psychology and philosophy of speech.

In correspondence to the concept that in this form of aphasia we are dealing with an *impairment of the central part of language* (as far as instrumentalities are concerned), *all speech performances are more or less affected* in these forms of aphasia. At best preserved and often not modified at all are the pure motor and sensory performances. The intactness of motor actions is revealed by the fact that patients speak the letters well, a number of phrases also, and at least some of the motor series; the intactness of the acoustic speech sphere is demonstrated by the fact that the understanding of language is usually the least disturbed function, that the patients recognize their defect in speaking and that—when they were tested in this respect—they prove to be very well able to differentiate between acoustically correctly and wrongly presented words.

The different speech performances are not disturbed to the same degree. As we have said, understanding is usually preserved best, repetition and spontaneous speech are always severely damaged. There is a difference in so far as in some cases repetition is more severely damaged than spontaneous speech and vice versa. Reading and writing are always damaged, writing usually more than reading, and here again, dictation in particular. Literal paraphasia is the most outstanding defect. Verbal paraphasia also is often to be found—it might even seem *always* if one takes adequate consideration of this symptom. As far as we can see, in all cases the patients have difficulty with regard to composing letters into words and to spelling. Usually there is some difficulty in finding words. According to our previous discussion (see p. 91), a more careful investigation of each symptom is necessary before we can give a more precise description of this form of aphasia.

From what we have said, we expect to find in *damage of inner speech* in central aphasia a *symptom complex* which consists mainly of: (1) impairment of spontaneous speech and understanding, the latter less than the first; (2) literal and verbal paraphasia; (3) paralexia and particularly paragraphia; (4) disturbance of repetition; (5) disturbance of spelling and of the capacity to combine letters into words. To be noted as not infrequent complications are amnesic aphasia and signs of pure acoustic aphasia.

Case 8*

This case will be reported later (see p. 286) as one of *amnesic aphasia*. This was the outstanding symptom in the first state of this progressive condition.

Already in this state the patient showed some symptoms which we considered as expression of a defect of inner speech. These symptoms gradually increased. The amnesic aphasic symptoms persisted, but they were covered by a *paraphasic destruction of the words, which became the outstanding symptom* in naming as well as in repetition and in spontaneous speech. It was *particularly severe in repetition*. *Repetition became increasingly more disturbed*, especially for words difficult to pronounce or those unknown to the patient. Senseless combinations of syllables—if they were not difficult to pronounce—were better preserved than words hard to pronounce. Repetition of letters was correct. The first parts of the words were often well repeated, then paraphasia set in. In the rest of the repeated words, the vowels and some consonants appeared, but mostly in incorrect position.

Reading, which later became paraphasic, was still good at the same time as repetition and spontaneous speaking of the same words showed definite paraphasia. It was somewhat preserved when understanding of what was read was lost.

The *paraphasia was most outspoken in writing*, though writing of letters was good for a long time. Some words, like his name, names of certain months and other well known words, he wrote correctly for a long period. Copying was preserved best, some lines at times without errors. Later, his writing was disturbed in the form of an apractic agraphia (see p. 128).

The *capacity to spell and to combine letters into words became increasingly worse.*

---

* Published by Goldstein, (81).

As to this defect, it may be mentioned that the patient, even if he was not able to bring the letters into the right order, frequently uttered the right word.

Understanding of speech remained much better than the other speech performances till the latest period of the disease.   Understanding of sentences suffered first, then that of words.

The symptom complex corresponded now to the *picture of central aphasia* (see p. 229).

In addition, there was an *increasing defect in writing of letters*. We mentioned before (see p. 289) that he showed modifications of writing such as we find in amnesic aphasic patients and which I call amnesic-aphasic agraphia.   This defect was later covered by a severe *failure in the production of the forms of the letters*.   The patient hesitated before he began to write a letter, made wrong arcs or hooks, put them in wrong directions.   Thus, he produced very distorted letters (see p. 128).   Copying remained better than spontaneous production.

He showed abnormalities of a similar character in execution of other motor actions. All these disturbances I was inclined to consider as expression of *ideatory apraxia*.

In the end period the patient became deteriorated to such a degree that examination was scarcely possible.

Thus, we can distinguish different phases.

1. *Amnesic aphasia* (nearly alone in the first state)
2. *Symptoms of a central aphasia* (in the second state)
3. Symptoms of *ideatory apraxia* and finally *general mental deterioration*

The succession of the symptoms and the progress of the general condition led us to assume that we were dealing with a *tumor in the left hemisphere* concerning the temporal lobe and the Insula Reili.   The motor and perceptual speech area could be considered intact.

This assumption was confirmed by the autopsy, in so far as we found a *tumor* of carcinomatous character, which showed greatest extension in the white matter of the middle part of the temporal lobe, where the cortex also was affected.   There was an enlargement of the volumen of the hemisphere, apparently due to the pressure through the tumor.

The anterior end of the tumor was near the tip of the temporal lobe in the white matter of the Gyrus temporalis medialis, expanded widely in this gyrus; a peak went into the Gyrus temporalis superior, another one into the inferior gyrus.   It infiltrated the Island of Reil and the subthalamic region.   The cortex was very little affected. More posteriorly, the Gyrus temporalis superior was free, the Gyrus inferior very much affected; also more affected was the Island of Reil.   Its last spurs were in the middle and superior lobe.

There were no *lesions in the rest of the brain*.   The left ventricle was narrowed, the right one much enlarged.

We have mentioned before that the amnesic aphasia in the beginning could be considered as an effect of the pressure of the tumor, which was well suited to produce this symptom complex (see p. 290).   The tumor increasingly affected the central area in the Insula Reili and the temporal lobe, and hence the central aphasia originated; with increasing pressure, other mental functions became affected.

There is the question of whether the sequence of the appearance of the different symptoms permits the assumption that each following symptom corresponds to more severe damage of the same substrate. If this is the case, one should expect that in a case of improvement of about the same defect the symptoms would disappear in a reverse sequence. We chose, for comparison, a case published by *Heilbronner* in which the restitution was followed up step by step. The correspondences between the sequence of appearance and disappearance of definite symptoms is conspicuous if we except the amnesic aphasia which in one case appeared first but in Heilbronner's case disappeared earlier than the other symptoms (see below, regarding the explanation of this discrepancy).

Our case showed the symptoms in the following sequence:

In *Heilbronner's case*, the symptom complex consisted in the beginning of a severe defect in understanding of speech, repetition, paraphasia in all forms of speaking, reading aloud and understanding severely disturbed. There was severe paragraphia; copying was intact.

Restitution occurred:

(1) disturbances of speaking and paragraphia

(1) in understanding of speech first for words, then for sentences

(2) paraphasia in repetition, spontaneous speech and naming

(2) understanding of read material

(3) paralexia

(3) reading

(4) disturbances of understanding of read material, first sentences, then words

(4) repetition

(5) disturbances of understanding of speech

(5) writing

This correspondence allows us to assume that we are dealing with increasing or decreasing damage of the same apparatus. Such comparisons give us insight into the structure of the central speech area and allow us to understand the way of dedifferentiation (see p. 3).

Concerning the mentioned discrepancy, it is explainable by the difference of the underlying processes in the two cases. The amnesic aphasia presupposes a widespread damage of the brain cortex (see p. 290). This was present in our tumor case from the beginning; hence, the early appearance of amnesic aphasia. The symptoms of central aphasia appear step by step with the increasing localized damage. Such a diffuse effect was to be expected in Heilbronner's traumatic case only in the beginning; hence, the early disappearance of the amnesic aphasia while the other disturbances improved gradually with the increasing restitution of the localized damage.

Case 9*

A 61 year old vagrant, with nothing known of his previous history except that he was an alcoholic and asocial, and had been in jail several times, underwent a transient disturbance of speech one year before onset of the present development. In the past few years, he had had heart trouble and "asthma." *The first examination was two and one-half months before death.* Arteriosclerosis of peripheral arteries was noted, and hypertrophy of the heart. The pulse was irregular. There were essential neurologic symptoms, no agnosia, no apraxia.

Well *oriented, he behaved in a correct way, was interested* in the persons and events in the environment, gave in general the impression of a *particularly intelligent man.* He showed fine tact and behaved like a well educated man.

He had a *"full understanding"* of his defect, complained about the difficulty to speak and was depressed by his deficiencies. He "does not want to live any more." Very ready for all examinations, he did not quickly fatigue. There was no recognizable disturbance of memory in general.

The *speech condition remained about the same up to his death*, although showing a little improvement of some components.

Spontaneous speech: The patient had a *great impulse to speak.* His vocabulary was not poor but some word categories were missing, particularly *nouns.* He had, in *general, difficulty in finding the words* and his *speech consisted mainly of phrases which he spoke fluently and without paraphasia;* within these phrases, nouns also were uttered without paraphasia. He uttered frequently and repeatedly such phrases as 'Ich kann nicht sprechen" (I cannot speak), "Das weiss ich nicht" (I do not know that), "Wie heisst es gleich?" (How is it called, by the way?), "Wie sagt man doch eigentlich?" (How do you say that, by the way?). When he began to *think what to say, the paraphasia increased immediately.* The *paraphasic distortions* in his spontaneous speech consisted of: wrong position of the consonants, use of wrong consonants while number of syllables or vowels were often correct. Examples: Laufmann, Fleher, Mastha instead of Kaufmann, Fehler, Asthma. Vowels were often wrong as: Refulation, Madrese, getrifen, instead of Revolution, Matrose, getroffen. Sometimes there was a prolongation of the word: Kute instead of Kuh, wrong flexions, leaving out of a syllable: wesen instead of gewesen. Sometimes he used combinations of two words.

Verbal paraphasias, which were infrequent, showed *similarities as to the sounds,* or the words produced belonged to the *same sphere* as the demanded word. The patient frequently reiterated the same word, but *perseveration played no rôle in the* origin of the paraphasias.

Construction of sentences was severely modified: he would leave out in sentences "ich" and "es" ("I" and "it"), but utter these words on other occasions, beginning, for example, many sentences with "I." Pronouns, verbs, auxiliary verbs had wrong inflections: geleben instead of gelebt. He uttered words in correct tenses. There were not so many mistakes as to the order of words and the use of the right grammatical form. However, the *construction of the sentences was very simple*, clauses scarcely ever appearing.

Example: "Dass ich bei einem Laufmann—bei einem Kaufmann wieder...dass

---

* Published by Liepmann and Pappenheim (190).

ich koennte wieder auf de...es war zu viel...zu viel—alles zu bes...wie sagt man..."
"Ich...ja...wie ich einmal...zu Haus gekommen...bin ich einmal zu Haus gekommen—und da ist...ist ein—na wie heisst es gleich...ein...gewisser...der ist von
mir...der hat einmal gesagt zu Haus..." We note a telegram style, with lack of
nouns and verbs.

When he had difficulty in finding the words, he showed an increase of expressive
movements in the face muscles. Later the patient spoke a number of short sentences
without paraphasia, otherwise he showed in principle the same disturbances.

Speaking of series: numbers, days of the week were good. Months were not possible
or imperfect with many defects. When reciting one series he side-tracked easily
into another one.

Naming of objects: A number of names for certain objects were found, others not.
Often he began to think and found the word afterwards. He used *circumlocutions
infrequently.* The words he found were often produced with *paraphasic distortions.*
The paraphasias showed a definite relation to the right word. The paraphasic distortions were still more outstanding in naming of objects than in conversation; as
the author mentions, probably because he was forced to speak difficult words which
he avoided in spontaneous speech, the paraphasic distortions appeared particularly
in long words. The patient sometimes found words in writing which he could not
find orally.

Repetition: Severely damaged, in the sense of paraphasias. The patient usually
was aware of mistakes, and identified the right word. Short words were better than
long words; he would often repeat parts correctly, particularly the first part.

Examples:
(Goldfisch)   Gold-Goldgewlschten (sheer paraphasia)
(Elefant)   El...fant...Feudenwand, Elefande
(Eisenbahn)   Eisebaende, -Eisse- Euse- Eiss- Eiseband
Letters: He would repeat most of them correctly, but not all.
Senseless syllables: very bad repetition.
He *completed* imperfect words or senseless syllable combination *to correct words.*
He would add to numbers the word "mark," i.e., producing it as a word for money.
Numbers were mostly good, often confounding the position.
Verbal paraphasias were largely similar to presented words.
Short sentences could not be repeated, while he might repeat the words of which
they consisted.

Writing was disturbed in a *similar way as repetition.* Words *which he spoke correctly
he would usually write correctly too.* Words uttered with paraphasia he wrote in this
manner. Sometimes he did not write such words at all or only the first part. Sometimes he could write a word correctly which he spoke with paraphasia. Sometimes
when he could not find a word at all he would write it down correctly. *Dictation
was severely disturbed,* of letters more than of words; thus, e.g., he could not write *p*
but wrote Pferd (horse).

Reading: He could follow simple directions, presented in written form, as: "Where
is your nose?", "Show your third finger," etc.

He read newspapers and said he understood the contents but when he was asked to
repeat what he had read he was so paraphasic that it was impossible to decide whether
he really had understood. He found acoustically presented words out of a definite
text.

Reading aloud: Letters were correct; *words were correct, also those which he could
repeat only with paraphasia.* Reading of sentences was performed quite well, but he

would repeat words frequently. *In quick reading, paraphasic* distortions of difficult words was noted. Later, reading improved best.

There was particularly a discrepancy between reading and repetition. He would *read words correctly which he could repeat only with paraphasia.*

The *spelling* of words presented in written form was correct with few mistakes. The *spelling of words presented acoustically was impossible.*

Autopsy revealed: Right hemisphere macroscopic and microscopic normal. Left hemisphere: third convolution, Island of Reil normal, without anomalies. The same was true for anterior and posterior central convolution. *Softening*, beginning in a cross section before the Ganyl. gen. lat. *Here cortex and subcortical marklayer of Heschl's convolution was affected and the more posterior dorsal medial part of Wernicke's convolution* (only the medial part which looks to the Fossa Sylvii). Farther back, a *second lesion* began, which was confluent with the first. It was small but had *a great extent in the longitudinal direction and was located in the white matter of Gyrus supramarginalis, angularis and temporalis II.*

Case 10*

F. S., 52 years old, a bookdealer, suddenly began to suffer headaches and disturbance of speech. He could not talk, did not find words, or used wrong or distorted words; could no longer write or read. He did not understand language. Slow improvement occurred in the next months: *Understanding improved greatly;* he understood people with whom he was acquainted, but not people with whom he had never spoken. *Understanding of written material improved.* He was apparently a left-handed individual.

Examination was made some months after the beginning of the disease. Findings were about the same up to death, six years later.

Neurologic findings: Pupils were not round, and showed differences. Reaction was sluggish. Left facial paresis was noted. Apparently, the cause of the accident was syphilitic thrombosis.

General intelligence and activity was intact. The patient was interested in the examinations, showed great effort to fulfill the tasks. He was *very cautious* and hesitated to produce wrong performances; he usually spoke only if he were certain that he would do it correctly. *He seldom displayed perseveration.*

Spontaneous speech: Initiative to speak was good, but *spontaneous speech was poor.*

Repetition: Letters were usually correct, but great effort was necessary to fulfill the tasks. The mistakes consisted mostly in *literal paraphasia.* A part (particularly the first part) of words was produced correctly. Paraphasia consisted of wrong position of sounds, wrong sounds interposed. *Verbal paraphasia was seldom noted* in repetition. Particularly bad was repetition of long or unknown words and combinations of senseless syllables. Sometimes he failed with a very common and short word, while on other occasions he would repeat even a long and rare word correctly.

Naming of objects: there was more difficulty with long, unknown words than with known and short ones. Words for abstractions were disturbed in the same way as naming of concrete objects. About 50 per cent of words were found. *Literal paraphasia:* He confused sounds within the word, produced only outstanding sounds, as, e.g., sch...sch...sch, in "Heuschrecke." Sometimes he would leave out a part of a word, as, for example:

Zuckerhut (candy cone)   Zucker (sugar)

---

* Published by Kleist, 1916 (164).

Malkasten (paint box)   Mal—Mal—Mal (paint)
Zirkusdirektor (circus director)   Zirkus—Zirkusreiter (circus horseman)
Vogelhaus (bird house)   Vogel—Vogel (bird)

The words showed similarities as to sounds, as:

Blumen*toepfe*   Blumen—Blumen*knoepfe*

Verbal paraphasias were more frequent than in repetition:

Oberarm (upper arm)   Muskel, oder wie man sagt
Hüften (hips)   Gesäss (backside), also das ist das Bein dazu?
Kunstreiterin   Tänzerin

Also in naming of objects perseveration occurred infrequently. Repetition was a little better than naming. Destruction of the words was in both performances about the same. Repetition of non-language noises was bad.

Understanding of speech: On examination, hearing was intact: also sounds tested with continuous series of tones, small diminution of hearing of high pitches was observed.

Understanding of words was disturbed to a certain degree. The performance depended on the length, familiarity and concreteness of the meaning of the words. There was word deafness for foreign languages (French and English, which the patient had understood before).

Understanding of words *for objects, colors, parts of the body* was only slightly disturbed, but frequent *difficulties in understanding* of *numbers* and *abstract words* were noted.

The patient had *difficulty* in grasping the *acoustic perception of presented words:* "It is as if I do not hear and I hear in spite of that." The *acoustic perception rapidly disappeared. Memory for acoustic experience was poor* (other memory undisturbed).

The involuntary attention to spoken words was *diminished.* He was easily distracted from speech sounds. No agnosia was noted for other noises, or for music. *Understanding was very much less disturbed than repetition.* Of fifty words, only two were not understood, but eighteen could not be repeated and fifteen others only with difficulty.

Reading aloud at first was slow and with *paraphasia. Later, long, difficult words also were read without any difficulty.* He understood what he had read but was unable to repeat it.

Understanding of written material was better than understanding of heard speech. *Writing* on dictation showed the *same defect as repetition of heard words.* Sometimes words could be repeated but not written on dictation. On the other hand, he could write down parts of heard words and later complete them correctly. Copying was intact.

Naming by writing down the name was the same as naming by speaking.

Spelling was disturbed in the same way as repetition, but sometimes more than repetition.

Combining of acoustically presented letters to words was very much disturbed.

A letter the patient wrote to a brother-in-law showed no paragraphia and had good construction of sentences.

Writing, in comparison with other speech functions, was little disturbed.

Case 11*

A 40 year old woman, a chronic alcoholic, was admitted to the hospital in a state of disturbed consciousness, speaking with a low voice, scarcely understandable. *She*

---

* Published by Stengel (281).

answered some questions, e.g., "How are you?", quite well but then continued with almost unintelligible words, showing *literal and verbal paraphasia*. On demand, she would close her eyes, but often did not follow directions.

In *naming and repetition: severe paraphasia. The same was noted in reading.*

The neurologic symptoms, hemiplegia and particularly the findings in the spinal fluid, suggested the existence of a pachymeningitis hemorrhagica on alcoholic basis. Therefore, operation was deemed necessary. Exposition of the lower part of the central convolutions revealed diffuse yellow coloration of the brain. There was further found a *cyst filled with blood*, which was extirpated. *Immediately after operation*, the patient was able to move her right extremities a little better. *She took part in conversation*, showed that she recognized her speech defect, and was *often desperate about it*. She would soon become very *attentive and interested*. There was slight right side paresis, hemianopsia. *Examination of hearing:* The right side was normal, the *left side showing some impairment of hearing the low tones.*

Spontaneous speech was much improved; although fluent, it revealed *literal and verbal paraphasia, difficulty in finding words*, and defects in the grammatical structure—not the usual telegram style, but paragrammatism (wrong grammatical forms and wrong positions of the words).

If she had to *recount* something, her language was *particularly bad;* then she needed to make considerable effort to speak. Her speech even showed articulatory defects. In the spontaneous speech, the *nouns* were missing, she used few circumlocutions, many expletives.

Speaking of series was essentially undisturbed, showing only motor difficulties.

The words she could not find spontaneously, or in *naming*, or in which paraphasia showed, were *not better produced in repetition.*

Naming revealed *literal and verbal paraphasia*. Naming of abstract concepts was more disturbed than naming of concrete objects. She had a tendency to produce a relation between the task she had to fulfill and the concrete situation; e.g., asked "what the feeling is if one is alone," she would reply: "*You* are afraid."

Example of spontaneous utterances: "Mein Bruder hat in der Violine (grammatical defect) sehr gut gesprochen (verbal paraphasia)—gespielt, 14 Jahre war er dort im...jetzt kann ichs nicht sprechen was, er von mein Vater...er hat Sie ja alles gelernt (grammatical defect) dazumal, wie er Professor war dort. Mein Vater war Portier, und ich war Beamterin."

Most disturbance was noted in repetition, severe paraphasia. Even after operation, repetition showed *the most severe defects.*

The paraphasias were of the following kinds: Confusion of letters, omissions, wrong cases and tenses; *often relation of the uttered word to the sphere of the demanded word.*

She was aware of the defect and tried again and again to find the right word somehow, usually thus developing *more severe paraphasia*. The first part of the word was often correctly repeated, short words were usually correct; of compound words, she would repeat only the first part. Letters were, in most instances, correctly repeated. Senseless syllable compositions in particular were badly repeated. *Repetition of adjectives and verbs was worse than that of nouns.* Single numbers were given promptly, but not numbers consisting of two or more digits; there was confusion of the position. Sometimes she would say a wrong number, then count until she came to the right number. *She tried to proceed in the same way as in counting in repetition.* Sentences were repeated in like manner as words. Success or failure in repetition depended upon the general attitude. *In hypnosis, better performance. was noted than outside of this condition.*

Spelling of words was severely disturbed, particularly of those words she would repeat wrongly. She was unable to say, or to indicate by knocking, how many syllables or letters a word had.

Understanding: "Practically intact," she understood also a complicated command which consisted of different parts. However, she had *difficulty in understanding the language of persons who did not speak directly to her and in understanding longer stories.* She did not understand witticisms.

Reading: She read aloud slowly, with some motor difficulties, but was *little* disturbed; understanding of written material was about the same as understanding of heard speech.

Writing: This was *spontaneous,* with the same paraphasia and paragrammatisms, but fluent. *Writing on dictation was severely disturbed,* the same words showing about the same *defect in repetition and in writing on dictation.* (She would speak silently what she wrote on dictation.)

Intelligence: No general intelligence defects were noted; orientation in space and concerning her own body was intact. There was no finger agnosia, no other agnostic disturbance. Praxis was normal.

In *association experiments,* it became apparent that the patient possessed a great number of associations, and that the relation of the associations to the presented word was about like that of normals. Words which *were correctly produced in the association experiment were very often shortly afterwards repeated with paraphasia.* The words which she *could not find as associations* usually were those *she could not repeat.*

Later the patient showed paranoic symptoms. She had repeated epileptic attacks. She died after about two years of observation of a bronchopneumonia.

Postmortem: Right hemisphere normal. *Left: corresponding to the posterior two thirds of the second temporal convolution, softening extending into the Gyrus angularis. Also the lower part of the first temporal convolution affected.* Abnormal dilatation of the ventricles.

Our knowledge concerning the *anatomic lesion underlying central aphasia* is poor. It was Wernicke who first assumed that the part of the brain located between the "sensory and motor speech centers" is paramount for the construction of the "Wortbegriff" (concept of words) and who considered accordingly "conduction aphasia" as effect of a lesion in the region of the Insula Reili. There was much discussion about this and opposition to Wernicke's theory. He assumed particularly a destruction of association fibers connecting the sensory and motor speech areas as anatomic basis.

I considered the theory as, in principle, correct, but from my general point of view was not inclined to assume a disruption of a simple pathway as basis of a psychologic defect. Repetition is not at all such a simple performance as Wernicke presupposed (see p. 70). If we want to bring the disturbance of repetition into relation with some anatomic defect, we cannot assume a defect of a simple fiber connection but dysfunction of a cortical apparatus.* This is still more valid concerning the other symptoms which occur in these cases.

The anatomic findings themselves do not correspond to Wernicke's assumption. In spite of lesion of the long association fibers between temporal lobe and frontal lobe, repetition can be preserved as it was in the cases of Bleuler (16), Pick (234), von Monakov (209), Bischoff (14), et al.

While in the beginning I emphasized the significance of the Insula, later I included in the central speech area also "adjacent" areas in the temporal and parietal lobe.

Our knowledge of the relation of definite aphasic symptoms which we can bring into connection with lesions of the Insula Reili is not great. In lesions of the Insula, very different aphasic pictures are described:

Dejerine and Bastian spoke of motor speech defects, Monakow has observed mixed forms, where more or less all speech functions were affected. According to Liepmann, we observe some motor defects and paraphasia; reading and writing are affected.

The differences would be understandable if one considered that the lesions have different extension, and that more or less affection of the adjacent motor and sensory region must modify the picture.

As far as I can see, there is only one case known where the lesion was restricted to the Insula alone, the case of Voisin (83). Here a lesion in the cortex of the posterior part of the Insula had affected all speech functions, particularly repetition. The patient died five days after insult and we do not know how much of the speech functions would later have improved so that the patient would have presented a clearer picture of central aphasia. In any case, the observation stresses the significance of a lesion in the Insula for disturbances of repetition. There is no doubt that a much greater destruction of the Insula is not necessary to be followed by the characteristic picture of central aphasia. Indeed, a decision concerning how much of the Insula must be affected to produce it is not possible because of lack of material. We are on a somewhat more certain basis when we look for cases where parts of the Insula Reili and adjacent areas are more or less affected in "central aphasia." A case of Pick (234) is to the point.

In a case which I have published, I believed it is justified to bring that part of the picture which corresponds to the central aphasia into relation to a damage of the Insula Reili and the temporal lobe (see 81). The case is not particularly good evidence as the underlying affection was a tumor. But the development of the symptoms and the functional damage of the Insula made me believe that I was justified in my assumption.

For the relation of this region to the picture of central aphasia, the case which is reported on p. 279 must be considered. Here, motor speech and understanding were preserved, repetition was totally impossible. The autopsy revealed a total destruction of the insula and adjacent regions (see p. 285), and thus we believed it justifiable to bring the defect in repetition into relation with this anatomic lesion. There is one difficulty: the lack of paraphasia. One might assume that the good motor speech was due to the undamaged 3rd frontal convolution, were it not that usually, even when this convolution is intact, destruction of Wernicke's area or the Insula Reili results in paraphasia. On the other hand, were we to assume that the absence of paraphasia was due to the function of the intact speech area in the right hemisphere, we would then have to ask, why was not the right hemisphere also able to guarantee repetition and word-finding? Thus, this latter assumption is difficult to maintain, and we would prefer to explain the absence of paraphasia as due to the functioning of the motor speech area of the left hemisphere, perhaps in cooperation with the corresponding convolution in the right hemisphere. But does this assumption not contradict the concept that correct speech depends on the function of the Insula Reili and the temporal lobe? Not necessarily. Not infrequently, even in cases with lesions in these areas, some words and sentences may be spoken without paraphasia—namely, such utterances which the patient has been accustomed to make motorically, which are delivered as mere motor automatisms. How much speech can be effectuated in this way by an individual depends on his capacity for automatic motor speech. There are great individual differences. Owing to this varying capacity, a defect in other speech performances can be masked to a greater or lesser degree. The same mechanism can operate in a patient with paraphasia produced by a lesion of the Insula Reili or the temporal lobe, i.e., with central aphasia. If the patient speaks little, and if his speech is largely restricted to the same well-known words and sentences, particularly if he possesses many such—then his paraphasia might not be discovered. There is some justification for assuming that this was the case in our patient. Although he spoke fairly well, he generally did not attempt to say much and usually uttered the *same phrases and words*. Although a simple man, he spoke five languages, and it is probable that being a simple man, he had developed his motor speech automatisms especially well in all these languages. Thus, the lack of paraphasia need not be in contradiction with the assumption of central aphasia.

There is another point to be considered in relation to the lack of paraphasia. Paraphasia is an expression of a dysfunction of inner speech, not of a lack of it. If inner speech is out of function totally, then we may have no paraphasia. From the total incapacity to repeat, we can assume that inner speech in this case was severely disturbed. I have also seen in other patients with inability to repeat that the language did not show paraphasia, or at least very little.

There are, in relation to our problem, particularly two cases to be considered, the case of Stengel (281) and the case of Liepmann and Pappenheim (190). In both cases, the Insula Reili *was not affected.* In the case of Stengel, the softening concerned the posterior two thirds of the second temporal convolution and extended into the Gyrus angularis. Also the lower part of the first temporal convolution was affected. The importance of the case of Liepmann and Pappenheim induces me to discuss it in detail. We have reported before the clinical findings of the case which leave no doubt that it belongs in the group of "central aphasia." The authors see in the case a confirmation of Liepmann's assumption that the "conduction aphasia" is a type of sensory aphasia and the effect of a lesion of a part of Wernicke's center. They consider the symptom complex as an expression of the "paramount significance which the acoustic engrams of the left side have for speaking, writing and reading."

They consider the lesion of Heschl's convolution and of the region at its transition to Gyrus temporalis I so severe that the acoustic speech images must be so damaged that they could no longer have guaranteed understanding. The preserved understanding of the patient must thus be related to the function of the other intact hemisphere, while repetition and spontaneous speech of the patient was the effect of the function of the damaged left hemisphere. I think the authors are right in assuming that the right temporal lobe is able to substitute for the left one for understanding, but not for speaking, repetition and spontaneous speech (see p. 55). However, such an interpretation of their case is somewhat in contradiction to the findings in sensory aphasia where paraphasia comes to the fore particularly in spontaneous speech, not so much in repetition; in their case, repetition is particularly disturbed. The authors do not overlook this difficulty. They are further aware that the difference cannot be explained as an effect of a quantitative, more or less intensive lesion of the same area, and assume, therefore, that the lesion in conduction aphasia concerns *particular parts* of Wernicke's area. But why should we assume that the affected area is a part of Wernicke's area, *why not that the lesion of this area produces conduction aphasia because it does not belong to the region of* "*sensory aphasia*"?

If we consider this area a part of the sensory speech sphere, which cannot guarantee the acoustic performances of speech, the word "sensorisch" (perceptive) takes on a very ambiguous meaning. The authors themselves say that with this assumption "das Wort 'sensorisch' behält nicht mehr

ganz seinen ursprünglichen Sinn, indem bei der 'Leitungsaphasie' gerade
der durch den Gehörssinn vermittelte Aufnahmeakt leidlich vonstatten
geht." ("The word 'sensorial' does not maintain its original meaning,
because in conduction aphasia, acoustic word perception and acoustic
understanding is about normal.")   In spite of all this, the name "sensorial"
may seem justified, insofar as one assumes that the acoustic engrams fail
in one part of their function, namely in that which they have for expressive
speech; but it is not justified if one considers this theory of the dependence
of speaking upon acoustic engrams as incorrect (as we do) (see p. 83).
An interpretation which needs the assumption of such a *qualitative* modification of the function of the acoustic engrams has little plausibility and
appears a very much ad hoc hypothesis.   Besides that, the findings in this
case do not favor such an interpretation.   The symptom complex can be
explained in a much simpler way by assumption that the paraphasia in
spontaneous speech and repetition, the whole picture of "central aphasia,"
is the effect of the lesion of the area outside of the acoustic speech area
which one can consider as belonging to the "central speech area."   The
central aphasia of the patient is consequent to a lesion which is suited to
damage inner speech.   The preservation of understanding may be due to
the preserved function of the left acoustic speech sphere or to that of the
other side or more probably to the cooperation of the lesioned and the
preserved one.   We know that it is not necessary to have more severe
lesions of the left Heschl's convolution for essential disturbances of understanding of speech to follow (see Monakow: Die Localisation im Grosshirn
(209, p. 824).   In this respect a comparison of the anatomic findings in this
case with those in cases with pure sensory aphasia is particularly interesting,
e.g., in the cases of Henschen (case Nielson) (139) and of Poetzl (246).
In these cases, those parts of the temporal lobe, which were affected here
(middle part of second convolution and especially the lateral part of the
convolution), were preserved in the case of Liepmann and Pappenheim
(190).   That part, preserved in those cases (the medial part which goes
over in Heschl's area and the Insula) was affected in the observation of
Liepmann and Pappenheim.

This comparison seems to justify still more the assumption that in the
case of Liepmann and Pappenheim the region of word deafness in the left
hemisphere was not affected to such a degree that it could not guarantee
understanding.   But it may be that the other hemisphere played an
important role for this function.   If we come in this way to the result that
we must consider the region affected in the case as a part of the "central
speech area," it certainly is not in agreement with the original theory of
Wernicke's and others, and also of mine, which considered the Insula as

the important area.   But it is well in agreement with my later assumption that besides the Insula, the adjacent areas in temporal and parietal lobes are of significance.

The main point of my theory, the assumption of *an area outside of the acoustic speech area, is not altered at all by this case.*   It may be that differences between the clinical picture in cases of central aphasia are due to the fact that once the whole central speech area (inclusive of the Insula) is affected, in other cases only parts of it, those located in the temporal and the parietal lobe.   The latter lobe was lesioned in the cases of Liepmann and Pappenheim and Stengel.

It may be that the lesion in Liepmann and Pappenheim's case represents a particular small affection of the concerned area.   To such an assumption would correspond the fact that the functional disturbance was not very outspoken.   However definitely spontaneous speech and repetition showed distortions, there were a number of normal performances.   As to the spontaneous speech, one has to consider further that it might have been better if it had not have been disturbed by the concomitantly present amnesic aphasia, which can be explained easily by the lesion in the temporal and parietal lobes (see p. 290)   If one disregards the effect of the difficulty in finding words due to amnesic aphasia, spontaneous speech was not very severely affected, not at all very paraphasic.   As to repetition, it cannot be overlooked that words consisting of one syllable were repeated correctly and sometimes even complicated words like, for example, Madagaskar, Turteltaube.   Moreoever, repetition improved during observation.

We agree that the temporal lobes are very important for the occurrence of central aphasia and reject only the idea that this form of aphasia has something to do with the acoustic sphere.

I have discussed the case of Liepmann and Pappenheim so much in detail as a demonstration of how difficult it is to evaluate a definite anatomic lesion in relation to a clinical picture.   We are not dealing here with a simple correlation.   Besides all the factors which complicate such a procedure (see p. 45), we see how the whole endeavor is determined by theoretic assumptions, in this instance by the very dubious relationship between paraphasia and lesion of the acoustic sphere.

Indeed, I am aware that the cases mentioned cannot at all be suited to prove which part the lesion of the Insula Reili takes in the production of central aphasia.   We have seen that from observations of cases where the Insula was or was not affected we cannot learn much in this respect.   It may be mentioned that in principle it is difficult to come to a definite idea about the significance of lesions in the Insula Reili for language; there are many factors which are to be considered in an evaluation of the findings and it is not easy to evaluate some of them correctly.   The Insula Reili has a great extension, consists of various convolutions and different sub-cortical fiber systems. Among them, the tractus longitudinalis inferior suggests a particular rôle for repetition because it connects those parts of the temporal and frontal lobes which are certainly important for language. Only infrequently is the Insula affected totally or alone; other adjacent parts of the cortex are lesioned to some degree, too. There is to be added another factor which complicates the problem, namely, that particularly for the maintenance of that function which we are inclined to bring into relation to the Insula, repetition, the taking over by the other hemisphere is in no way clear (see p. 55).

CHAPTER VIII

Amnesic Aphasia

THE outstanding symptom of amnesic aphasia is the lack of nouns, adjectives, verbs and especially names for concrete objects in speech. The defect shows most strikingly in the task to name objects; the patient is unable to find the names for the most ordinary objects of everyday life. He need not present any additional disturbance of speech; at least others need not become manifest immediately (see p. 270). He repeats words without hesitating, he accepts among a number of words presented orally or written, only the one which belongs to the object; he shows no paraphasia, no disturbances in writing and reading (see exceptions, p. 252).

We have explained before that difficulty in finding words can be due to different causes. Only those cases with word finding difficulties where this defect is related to impairment of abstract attitude should be called *amnesic aphasia*. Thus, symptoms due to impairment of abstract attitude belong intrinsically to this form of aphasia.

The cases are not very frequent, at least not in pure form. If there are other symptoms present besides the difficulty in finding words, we have to find out whether they belong to the picture of amnesic aphasia intrinsically or are only concomitant symptoms due to other lesions of the brain.

Case 13*

A woman, aged 60, German, coming from a low income group, was not highly educated but evidently had considerable native intelligence and an average schooling. She had worked hard, and had brought up children. She attributed the development of her disease to a trauma, having been hit on the head; little was known about the consequences of this injury.

She gave in general the impression of a woman of her age. Physical examination showed no signs of arteriosclerosis on the peripheral arteries nor on the heart; no neurologic symptoms on reflexes, sensibility, motility, etc. She had no hallucinations or delusions.

The patient's behavior in general did not deviate particularly from that of a woman of her background. *She was friendly, vivacious, showed many expressive movements*, spoke much; in her language, certain outstanding *sterotyped sentences* were repeatedly noticed (see further). She was clean, ate by herself, dressed by herself. She never did anything abnormal, never used an object incorrectly, etc.

She was oriented as to space, but was not quite correct as to time. She knew where she was and how long she had been there, but not exactly the date and the month. She recognized the people around, nurses, the doctor, whom she called the "highest," by which word she designated his position on the ward.

---

* Published by the author, 1906 (77).

She wanted to go home, and expressed this wish again and again, but was easily quieted, and never angry.

The examination was somewhat diff cult because of the fact that she was easily distracted by any events in the environment, but after she became more acquainted with the doctor the results of examinations reported show great constancy.

Sense perceptions did not seem to be disturbed essentially. Visual acuity, visual field, and hearing were somewhat diminished, but sufficient for correct recognition of objects presented (see further, protocol).

"Intelligence" in general was certainly not much diminished, her judgment seemed to be essentially preserved as could be concluded from the way she talked about the actual situation and about things of her life. Occasional utterances gave a better insight into her way of thinking than systematic examinations, which were rendered difficult because of her distractability. That she had good judgment and understanding showed, e.g., in the good judgment she revealed regarding the position of different people: calling the physician, the mayor, the head of the state in which she lived, the rooster in a picture which showed him with the hens, "the highest."

Memory for previous events was almost intact. She knows her name, date of birth, name of the place where she lived, the name of the aunt to which it belonged, she knew the small town is a spa, etc. She remembered the main data of her life history.

Recollection for recent events was poor, better in the visual sphere than in the acoustic. However, there was a discrepancy between what she kept in mind, if she were asked to do it in experimental situation, and what she experienced in everyday life. She remembered, even after an interval of days during which she was not examined, what she had been asked in previous examinations, sometimes particulars, which one would hardly have thought she had paid attention to.

School knowledge was poor; probably she had never possessed much more. She knew in which seasons the numerous religious holidays are celebrated, and could promptly recite several prayers.

Alphabet: Difficulty in getting started; if the first letters were said, she followed: a, b, c, d, e, f, g, h, m, n, o, b, c, d, e, ...

Months: Forward correctly; backward: December, October, February, April, May, June.

Days of the week: Forward correctly, but not backward.

Series of numbers: 1–50 promptly; backward with many mistakes.

Series of "tens": 10–200 promptly; also backward correctly if one presented the first numbers.

Arithmetic: Poor, but multiplication table of 4's and 5's almost correct, 7 and 10 very incorrect; isolated multiplication very slow, but not exceptionally bad. The same was true as to additions, as $8 + 14$, $14 + 26$, which she solved correctly, but only when written down.

Performance tests were not administered. In the Heilbronner test of recognition of uncompleted pictures she showed very poor results.

No disturbance of recognition of objects and of pictures representing objects was noted. There were *never any apractic failures*. The patient pointed immediately to many objects presented to her which she is asked to identify.

Examination of language.

Spontaneous speech: She spoke animatedly, with normal emphasis and rhythm, accompanying her speech with correct *somewhat exaggerated expressive movements*. Often when she did not find a certain word, she would try to communicate what she wanted to say by *very characteristic expressive movements*. The syntactical structure of the sentences was correct, *though very simple*. The grammatical forms did not show essential deviations from the norm. *Paraphasia* was *never* observed. In her spontaneous speech, she missed definite categories of words—nouns, adjectives, verbs—which we use in order to designate concrete objects or events; this lack was striking. She expressed what she wanted to say with *circumlocutions* or by the use of words which fitted certain properties of the object, event, etc. Thus, she usually expressed all different activities with one and the same word, the German word "überfahren," which is dialect for "ausfuehren" and could be translated as "perform." She used for many objects the word "Ding"—thing (see p. 63).

The defect became still more apparent when she had to fulfill a definite speech performance, particularly if she were asked to *name objects or events*. Some examples may illustrate:

Objects shown	*Answer*
Uhr (watch)	Ein Stückle, wo man sieht, ein schöns Stückle, hätt ich nur so ein.
Wozu ist es? (what is it for?)	Es ist jetzt halb fünf (correct), schöns Stückle, Rundellele, eins, zwei, drei, vier, fünf.
Schlüssel (key)	schöns Stückle, so zu machen, wo man kann überfahren (makes movements of locking the door).
Bleistift (pencil)	so überfahren auf schöns Stückle (makes movements of writing on paper).
Messer (knife)	Stückle zum überfahren, wenn ichs nur hätt (tries to sharpen the pencil). schöns Stuckle, hatte ich nur so ein.
Handtuck (handkerchief) Was macht man damit? (What do you do with it?)	Nas putzen (makes movements of blowing her nose).
Nase (nose)	schöns Stückle, wo man kann überfahren, wo man kann Nasputzen.
Geldbeutel (purse)	Da ist Dings drin, schön Stückle, geben Sie mir ein, zehn Sous, ein Mark.
Funfpfennigmarke (five cent stamp)	Lug jetzt, man muss es auf etwas lege, man macht es drauf (tries to paste it on an envelope).
Borte (braids)	schöns Stückle, als ich 16 was ist der Höchst (after being questioned: the archduke) bei uns gewesen, da hab ich 2 solch lange Stückle bis dahin (indicates the floor) gehabt, da gab es Tanz, da hat der Höchst gesagt, ich sollt sie hochbinden, sonst wer ich drauftreten.
Gabel (fork)	Wo man kann fahre mit (puts it to the mouth), wo man kann essen mit.
Ist es ein Messer? (Is it a knife?)	Nein.
Löffel? (spoon?)	Nein.
Gabel? (fork?)	Ja, Gabel, Gabel.
Schüssel (bowl)	wo man ebbis dreinmacht, ein Runellele, man kann kochen mit (makes movement of stirring in the plate).
Ist es eine Gabel? (is it a fork?)	Ja. (doubtful).

Objects shown	*Answer*
Schüssel? (bowl?)	Ja, Schüssel, Schüssel, Schüssel.
Zum essen? (for eating?)	Ja, Schüssel, Schüssel.
Papier (paper)	So ein Stückle, wo man kann überfahre mit (makes writing movement).
Feder? (pen?)	Nein.
Papier? (paper?)	Ja, Papier, Papier.

A few objects she named correctly. For instance, bread, window. Touching did not help her when she did not find the name immediately.

Pictures shown	*Answer*
Kuh (cow)	Wo man's Ding holt, wo man tut überfahren (shows the udders and makes milking movement). Milch, wissen Sie wir hatten zehn Kühe.
Huhn (hen)	Wo man Eier bekommt, weisse Rudellele.
Ziege (goat)	Ich weiss schon wir haben 4 gehabt.
Was 4? (four what?)	Wir haben vier Geisle gehabt.
Regenschirm (umbrella)	Ich weiss schon, schöns Stückle, wenns regnet, da macht man auf, ich hab zwei Stückle daheim, drei hab ich gehabt.
Bürste (brush)	Weiss schon was, wo man kann die Stückli (shows braids) überfahren. Ich hab auch solche Stückli gehabt.
Ist es ein Eimer? (is it a pail?)	Nein.
Ist es ein Kamm? (Is it a comb?)	Nein.
Ist's ein Bürste? (is it a brush?)	Ja, Bürste, ja ein Bürste.

From the beginning, she named coins correctly, all of them, even when they were shown to her only from the side with the eagle (German currency).

Skeins shown	*Answer*	*Color named*	*She shows*
red....................	Stückli, wo man kann daruber machen (shows stockings).	red	finds corresponding nuances
		green	"
		blue	"
Ist est grün? (is it green?).................	Nein, rothlächt. (dialect)	brown	"
	Anders	yellow	"
Ist es rot? (is it red?)....	Nein.		
Blau? (blue?)..........	Nein.		
Grün? (green?)..........	Ja, grün.		
Blau (blue).............	Weiss nicht		
Ist es rot? (is it red?)...	Nicht so ganz rot.		
Schwarz? (black?)......	Nein.		
Blau? (blue?)..........	Ja, blau.		

Recognition of the objects as well as of pictures is prompt so that a detailed protocol is not necessary.

Naming from tactile sense:

Schlüssel (key)	Wo man kann überfahren, an Kasten machen.
Streichholzbüchse (match box)	Es ist ebbis drin, wo man kann überfahren mit, wo man kann Kaffee kochen, wo man kann kochen mit.
Schere (scissors)	Wo man ebbis macht, mit, wo man ebbis macht (shows her skirt, makes cutting movement under the table without looking).
Ist es ein Messer? (is it a knife?)	Nein.
Ist es eine Schere? (are these scissors?)	Ja, Schere.
Flasche (bottle)	Wo man ebbis kann drübermachen, Milch oder Wasser rein machen.
Ist es ein Löffel? (is it a spoon?)	Nein.
Ist es eine Flasche? (is it a bottle?)	Ja Flasche.
Geltbeutel (purse)	Schöns Stückli, das dar ich mitnehme (laughs), weiss schon, was drin ist, Geld is drin, Geld.
Ist es eine Flasche? (is it a bottle?)	Nein.
Ist es ein Ball? (is it a ball?)	Nein.
Ist es ein Portemonnaie? (is it a purse?)	Ja.

Coins were correctly recognized and named. She found all the mentioned objects correctly out of a number of touched objects when they were named.

Naming of acoustically perceived objects (without looking)

Examiner sneezes	Gesundheit! (+)
Wie heisst man das? (how do you call that?)	Weiss schon.
Husten (coughing?)	Nein.
Niesen (sneezing?)	Ja.
Examiner coughs.	Weiss schon was.
Niesen (sneezing?)	Nein.
Schreien (shouting?)	Nein, kein schreien.
Husten (coughing?)	Ja Huste.
Examiner shuffles with his feet.	Überfahre mit dem Stückli (shows her foot).
Klopfen? (is it knocking?)	Nein.
Scharren (is it shuffling?)	Ja scharren.
Händeklatchen (clapping of hands)	. . . So überfahre mit dem Dingli da (shows her hands).
Husten (coughing?)	Nein.
Schreien (shouting?)	Nein.

Händeklatschen (clapping of hands?)	Ja.
Jingle of money.	Weiss schon was, schöns Stückli, wo man kann nehmen dafür, Geld, 5 Mark, 10 Mark.

Recognition of objects when named, prompt.

Taste (all other senses excluded):

Vinegar on the tongue

Zucker (sugar?)	Nein.
Pfeffer (pepper?)	(Doubtful)
Salz (salt?)	Nein.
Essig (vinegar?)	Ja, Essig.
Brot (bread)	Weiss schon was, wo ich beim Bur gewesen bin, hab ich es mache müsse. Zuerst habe ich von der Kuh genommen (speaks of milk).
Fleisch? (is it meat?)	Nein, kein Fleisch.
Frucht? (is it fruit?)	Nein.
Given into her hand.	Weiss schon was, beim Bur hab ichs gehabts.
"Weckle" (dialect for roll)	Ja, Weckle, Weckle, Weckle.

Recognition from the name prompt.

Smell was so poorly developed that a more detailed examination was not possible.

There is no doubt that the patient presented the typical symptoms of amnesic aphasia:

1. *Lack of nouns, adjectives, verbs in spontaneous speech.*

2. *Lack of names for objects* with correct acceptance of the right word ("Einschnappen"), "catching on"; frequently using words in sentences which she could not find as names; circumlocutions and use of the objects showed that she recognized the objects which she could not name.

3. *Correct repetition,* no paraphasia.

4. According to our discussion about the relation of this form of disturbance of word-finding to impairment of abstract attitude we should expect that the patient would present symptoms of such impairment.

She was observed before the time the significance of the impairment of abstraction for the difficulty in finding words (see p. 61) was recognized. Therefore, she was not tested specifically in this respect. From the observation of the patient in general there can be scarcely any doubt that she was impaired in the abstract attitude. Her attitude toward the world, particularly toward the objects she was asked to name, was *concrete in the typical way.*

The patient presented some further symptoms which need explanation, because they do not seem to belong to amnesic aphasia.

1. *Disturbances in understanding:*

Understanding was in general intact insofar as one can assume from her behavior in following a simple direction and finding named objects. Whether she understood more complicated sentences cannot be said with certainty. The same holds true for the question whether her understanding was restricted to concrete words or sentences (see p. 270).

2. *Repetition:*

Repetition was correct for short and known long words, even for senseless combinations of syllables (as many as 5 or 6). Unknown words were often repeated only as to their sounds, and then sometimes with exchange of similarly sounding consonants in a way normal uneducated individuals sometimes do. The last words were usually repeated the worst. It should be mentioned that even though repetition was somewhat affected, *paraphasia was never* observed. The disturbances in repetition can find an explanation by the abnormal concreteness of the patient (see p. 71).

3. *Disturbances of Writing and Reading:*

Writing and reading in general were poor, corresponding to the low educational level of the patient, but were not disturbed as far as reading or writing of letters within words was concerned. *Spontaneous writing* showed similar omissions of words as did spontaneous speech. Writing on dictation of words did not show any pathology; also names she could not find could be written on dictation. The only deviation in writing was an at first strange way of *writing letters on dictation:*

Sounds were always correctly written. If one dictated the letters in the usual way, i.e., dictated the name of the letter, the patient wrote in the following way:

v	(spoken fau)	vau		r	(spoken er)	ruh
w	(" ve)	woe		f	(" ef)	öf
z	(" zet)	zet		r	(" er)	ehr
l	(" el)	el		b	(" be)	böh
g	(" ge)	ge		d	(" de)	döh
k	(" ka)	ka		h	(" ha)	hah
m	(" äm)	äm		e	(" e)	öh
n	(" en)	en		s	(" es)	ess
t	(" te)	te				

Vowels, where sound and letter name are equal, were always written correctly. Apparently the patient considered letters presented with their names as *words* and wrote the word she heard or a word *in which the heard letter was dominant.*

If she had to write the numbers on dictation she did not produce digits, but words corresponding to the spoken sound complex. From other observation there was no doubt that she knew what the numbers meant: 3 (drei) dreu; 4 (vier) wür; 5 (fünf) fün, 6 (sechs) sech; 7 (sieben) säbe; 8 (acht) acht; 10 (zehn) sehn.

Sometimes she might write first digits, but soon she wrote them again in the way mentioned above. The explanation of this behavior is that the sound complexes are more concrete for patients than the digits.

Copying of letters, words, numbers was normal in each respect, also copying of printed words.

Reading showed similar peculiarities as writing. The patient read words and sentences quite normally, much quicker than parts of words or letters. She was able to recognize a heard word in a number of presented written words. She understood what she read in correspondence to her education.

If one presented *parts* of words she tried to *complete them to senseful words; wrongly written words she read as correct ones,* if their distortion was not too great. If that were the case, she read letters, not words. She was able to find letters presented acoustically in a number of written presented letters. She read *letters usually as words:* b, be; c, ce; d, de; f, ef; h, ha; l (el), elf; w (we), wem; z (zet) zeit; f (ef), elf; q (ku), kuh; r (er), reih; w (we), war; z (zet), ze; r (er), rixheim (birthplace); o, dotter (German word for yolk); b, bab; te, pet; w, wet; t, gut.

She was apparently aware that the presented visual objects (the letters) belonged to known words, to "names." Because she was not able to find the names, due to the disturbances of her capacity of "naming," she would try to find a word which contained the presented letter, or build a word by addition of vowels to the consonants.

The anomalies in reading and writing point both to a defect in the capacity of *"naming."* Because in writing and reading of words naming is not necessary, she did not make mistakes here.

Thus we see that the *symptoms of the patient which at first did not seem to belong to amnesic aphasia* could be considered also as *expression of the underlying basic defect.* We shall discuss the disturbances of understanding more in detail in connection with the findings in case 15 (see p. 270).

The kind of anatomic lesion in this case is not clear. Probably we are dealing with a general damage of the brain-cortex due to arteriosclerosis. Whether there is any localized process we do not know. The lack of any pyramidal tract and other symptoms leads us to assume that such a process does not exist. Whether or which rôle the trauma the patient spoke about played in the development of the symptoms, we do not know. The patient did not show any signs of hysteria.

The next case concerns the patient observed by myself together with A. Gelb (1925), from which the *new concept of amnesic aphasia* (see p. 60) originated.

Case 14*

B. Minor, 23 years old, underwent injury by grenade shell at the parietal region of the left side. The wound healed without scar of the skull. Directly after injury, paresis and disturbance of sensation of the right arm were noted. No particularly conspicuous disturbance of speech was observed. Examination two years later: a small amount of paresis of the right arm, otherwise no neurologic symptoms; some headache and dizziness. Objectively, there was no disturbance of equilibrium. The patient was a very cooperative, friendly man, very attentive and ready to be examined. He gave the data of his prewar life sufficiently. He had the education of a child of a poor family. Apparently he was intelligent and eager to learn. He could read and write, read newspapers, books. His memory for new experiences was somewhat reduced but he could repeat 5 and 6 numbers, also backward, without difficulty. His arithmetic capacity was somewhat poor but he did not fail in simple tasks.

* Published by A. Gelb and the author, 1924 (113).

He talked *quite a lot*, apparently had no motor difficulty and showed normal sentence formation. He accompanied his speech with a *great number of expressive movements*. His spontaneous speech showed a lack of nouns, adjectives, verbs, and particularly names of concrete objects. Otherwise, his spontaneous language showed no conspicuous deviation from the norm, particularly no *literal or verbal paraphasia*. Understanding and repetition of words, sounds, short sentences was in general normal.

Examination of the different senses showed no deviation from the norm; his tone and sound perception, his visual acuity, visual field were normal.

He read letters, words, sentences normally, with good understanding. He could write spontaneously without difficulty, *his written language* showing in principle the same defects as his spontaneous speech, but his writing might contain words which he usually did not utter in speaking.

His intellectual capacity seemed to be in general preserved; he showed good judgment about the events of everyday life, good combinatory capacities, for instance, in the Heilbronner test; emotional behavior normal.

He usually *failed in the test to name concrete objects*, even the most common ones of everyday life. He showed by using the objects and by his circumlocutions that he *recognized well the objects he could not name*. A knife was called "for cutting," scissors "for cutting," a tape measure "to measure," penholder "for writing," etc. He accompanied these utterances with very *characteristic expressive pantomimic movements*.

His *difficulty in naming* concerned in the same way *abstract objects* and events; he could not characterize them—thus—e.g., the meaning of justice, hatred, communication, agreement, etc.

Among a great number of objects he always selected immediately and with certainty that corresponding to the name which was presented to him (he "caught on"). He could repeat the words without hesitation.

He also showed the defect of naming in respect to *colors*. Because the analysis of the behavior of the patient toward colors revealed his basic defect and led to the introduction of the color sorting test as essential means to detect it, we give first a detailed report of the behavior of the patient in this respect (see organization and administration of the test, p. 167).

The patient, when asked *to name this or that color* taken out from the heap of the Holmgreen colored wool skeins, only *seldom uttered the right name* and when he did so, only with great hesitation and doubt as to whether he was correct. Only infrequently did he utter a wrong name, but usually *remained silent*. He never seemed to proceed by guessing. Frequently it was to be observed that the patient used words like "cherry-red," "like an orange," "like a forget-me-not," when he was confronted with definite nuances of the concerned colors.

If a number of color names were presented for choice, he usually did not reject the wrong ones definitely and often did not choose the right one. *He did not show the characteristic "catching on,"* which he showed in the same test with objects (see p. 251).

Usually he repeated the heard color name in a way which gave one the impression that he did not *recognize the name as a known one*. He repeated the name with a low voice, again and again, and looked over the heap of colors without being successful in finding the right color. One increasingly gained the impression that the *name was to him a meaningless sound complex*. Sometimes he pointed to the right skein, but this was the effect of an indirect procedure, which we shall discuss later (see p. 167).

If the patient were asked to give the *name* of the color of *very well known objects*, as a violet, a cherry, poppy, etc., he *could not do it*. If he was effectively successful he proceeded in a roundabout way (see p. 2).

He had *very good visualization* and the heard word produced easily the *visual image of a colored* object in its natural color, but he could not name these visual colors. He could find the color out of a presented group of colored papers or skeins if the concerned object possessed a characteristic color (strawberry, letterbox [always dark blue in Germany], violet, chalk and others). If he did not find the correct color nuance he chose a *very similar* one, stressing that it was not quite correct. Never did he choose the wrong color or a nuance which differed much from the correct one. If he could not find a very similar one, he restrained from choosing any.

In our attempt to find the cause for the patient's behavior, we had first to determine whether there existed a defect in language or in color recognition.

If asked to give a *number of color names*, the patient *often produced several without difficulty* in a series such as "red, green, blue," etc. Thus we are justified in assuming that there was no difficulty in general to pronounce or to elicit color names.

In relation to *color recognition*, there was from the beginning *no doubt that the patient had a very good color perception*. His discrimination for colors became particularly evident by his capacity to distinguish between very small differences in nuances of the same color. At Nagel's anomaloscope, he behaved absolutely like a normal person, showed not the slightest indication of a congenital or acquired color insufficiency, yet he showed amazing failures in the *color sorting test* (see p. 167).

If he were asked to choose, using a given sample in a heap of many nuances of all colors (Holmgreen's set of color skeins for testing efficiency), all similar ones, regardless of brightness or darkness, he proceeded very hesitatingly and slowly; he picked out *seemingly totally wrong ones* and put them aside; sometimes he rejected a (for us) right one, after he had taken it in his hand; he apparently had the greatest difficulty with this task. He compared the sample again and again with the skeins in the heap, till he chose some which were *identical or very similar to the sample*. Thus, of course, he could choose only very few. The task of choosing identical colors he fulfilled quickly and absolutely correctly.

Apparently the patient *did not make his choices according to the basic color quality, but to the experience he had with each individual skein*. This became evident in other kinds of behavior: he might match a given very bright shade of red with a blue or green skein of great brightness, apparently determined in his choice by the identical brightness. His choice might be determined by another attribute of the given skein, by coldness, warmth, etc. But it is an amazing thing that this patient, who seemed to be choosing according to a certain attribute, was not able to follow this procedure if it were demanded of him, e.g., to choose all bright ones. He further did *not seem to be able to hold on to a certain procedure*. He would transfer the selection suddenly to another characteristic attribute. He might just have arranged the skeins as if guided by an attempt to produce a scale of brightness. He would begin with a very bright red, then add one less bright and so on to a dull red one. But if we were to ask him later to place the skeins in a succession according to their brightness he showed himself incapable of performance, even if it were demonstrated to him.

These two approaches correspond to the abstract and concrete behavior. The patient's approach was directed *not to the color categories* to which the skein belonged but to the *individual appearance of the skein*. He could accept belonging together only according to the *immediate sensory coherence*, i.e., if the presented objects were sensorically identical or very similar. According to which characteristic of the sample impressed him in the moment he proceeded, he *did not sort, but simply matched.* Never did he sort by the basic color which is not given immediately as sensory experience but experienced only in the abstract attitude. Thus it would be a wrong description to say that he chose voluntarily once according to the one characteristic, another time according to another one; the choice was forced upon him by the coherence experience which impressed him. As a matter of fact, he lacked any principle of sorting. Thus we came to the result: *the failure of the patient in sorting of colors was due to impairment of the abstract attitude* (see p. 63).

Can we understand from this defect the difficulty of the patient in *naming colors?* If normals designate a color with a definite name, they are not determined by the individual nuance in which it appears (if the nuance does not particularly come to the fore), but by the *category* to which the presented color belongs; in this—the abstract—attitude, we use the words red, blue, etc. If we want to designate the individual color nuance, we approach the problem from the concrete attitude, we choose words which correspond to the individual object, usually those which are taken from the names of objects which have the characteristic color. The patient apparently was capable only of proceeding in the second way (concrete) because of his lack of abstract attitude. Therefore, he could bring into connection with the colors only the latter kind of names, as sky-blue, strawberry-red, not the generic names which correspond to the category.

In the same way it is to be explained that the patient was unable to choose the correct color to a given name. To fulfill this task, he must be able to comprehend the word as a sign for a category, the presented colors as representatives of categories of colors. It is a totally different task if one has to show the color of an object, violet, cherry, etc. In this latter instance, one does not need the categorical attitude, one looks for a nuance which fits the object or its visual image. Therefore, the patient fulfilled this task.

What we have said as to the patient's behavior in respect to colors is valid in the same way in respect to objects.

If a normal person tries to order the different objects as presented in this test,* he can do it in different ways, according to diverse attitudes. He may arrange them by size, color, function, in terms of activity or thinking, etc. He is further able to shift from one attitude and one kind of order to another, and to effect any one arrangement on demand. The patient preferred sorting according to the possibility of using objects together in a situation which the objects awoke in him. He could bring them together also as to material, say, all wooden ones or all metal. In this case one might gather the impression that he sorted according to a chosen quality which he abstracted. But further experiments revealed that he was not able to do that intentionally on demand. As a matter of fact, he proceeded *not determined by a category*

---

* The object sorting test (see p. 172).

but was determined in his procedure by the *outstanding same experience*, sometimes by the characteristic of wood, sometimes of metal, etc.

This became particularly evident in the experiment where the patient had to bring together the bottle with a cork loosely set in its neck and a corkscrew, which we have described elsewhere (see 104, p. 306).

We are inclined to assume from these observations that the patient's attitude toward objects was also much *more concrete than that of normals* and that his *lack of capacity of naming objects* was due to this impairment of abstract attitude.

As I have stated on another occasion (see 104, p. 306), to each of these two different approaches toward the world, correspond a particular kind of language.   It is in the *abstract attitude* in which we *name objects*.

When we speak of "table," we do not mean a special given table with all the accidental properties, but we mean the category table to which this individual table belongs as representative.   The word is used as symbol for this category, the "idea" table.   In this approach toward the world, language plays a very great rôle.   In the concrete approach, this is not the case.

Our words accompany our acts and express a property of the object itself, such as color, size, etc.   This fact is shown in the particular kind of words which we use in such situations.   The words are especially adapted to the individuality of the given object.   We do not say "red," "pink," but "dark red," "strawberry red," "sky blue," "grass green," etc. Often when we have no word for naming a given object, we do so in a roundabout way.

Since the patient faces the world in the particular attitude to which speech is nonrelevant, the normal attitude from which we name objects is so alien to him that he cannot even understand how we name objects. Thus, the nominal words do not even occur to him.   When such words are mentioned to him and he does accept them, he does not understand them as names but as purely external correlates of the objects.

If he finds such an external correlate by himself, or if he is prompted in that direction, he will seemingly succeed in naming an object, but in such cases he is again only making an external correlation and not really giving a name is made evident by closer analysis.   That the words used by the patient have no categorical meaning to him is shown by the following.   Even when the patient is given the proper word, he is unable to sort the colors in an abstract way, nor can he attain the abstract approach when he repeats the words, which he will often do.   We would frequently observe that the patient, asked to name a color, told over to himself various color names: red, blue, yellow, etc.   He might even pronounce the name appropriate to the given color, but in spite of this he would remain unable to bring this correct name into connection with the color itself. In point of fact, the patient has apparently *not lost the words but his words appear to have lost to him the peculiarity requisite for use in a categorical sense for being employed as symbols.* It may indeed be thought that the words have become for the patient empty sounds, which may belong to a definite object as this object's property, but which can no longer be used as generic words and cannot serve as symbols for an idea, i.e., serve as language.

That becomes evident in the circumstance that the patient pronounces the words much as we would pronounce the words of a foreign language, which have a familiar sound but have no familiar meaning.

The change in the words which we have described, is shown with special clearness in patients with amnesic aphasia, whose speech is not exceptionally impoverished, but who have a fairly ample vocabulary, and verbal knowledge. Such patients may even attach the right words to some objects, for example, colors, but it can be demonstrated that in these cases, too, such words have not the significance of symbols. We shall (p. 259) describe such a patient in the next case.

There is one phenomenon observed in this patient which needs some further discussion. If we compare the *behavior of the patient in respect to colors and objects,* then a difference becomes apparent which, at first glance, may be in contradiction to the fact that we explain the difficulty in word-finding in both conditions by the same basic defect.

The patient is able to find the objects to the presented names, but not the colors. The difference can be understood in the following way. The relation between a word and an object is much more immediate than that between a word and a color. As we said before, in the task to find the color the abstract approach is much nearer at hand, the word does not fit one color immediately (if it fits, then the patient finds it). The word fits much more immediately one of the presented objects. Therefore, the patient never fails in this task. The difference between word finding for colors and objects comes to the fore also in the fact that the color words may appear strange to the patient, and this never seems to be so evident with the words for objects.

Conclusion: The examination of the patient shows that the difficulty in finding words is *not due to a loss of memory but is an expression of a more general mental impairment, of the impairment of the capacity to take the abstract attitude.* The case is thus a proof of our interpretation of the amnesic aphasia (see, for the interpretation and discussion of the criticism of this concept, p. 64).

Case 15*

Female, aged 48, single; secretary. Personal history noncontributory. Usual childhood diseases. Menstruation normal and regular. No pregnancies or abortions, no venereal infection. Successful and independent in her work. Has occupied for a number of years a *respected position to the great satisfaction* of her employers who commend especially her conscientiousness and industriousness.

Several weeks before onset of present condition, patient complained about weakness of left arm and leg. Three days before admission, while at work, sudden inability to speak. She was out shopping in the morning. Remembers that on her return to the apartment she went to the bathroom where apparently she lay unconscious and paralyzed for some time. Tells that she heard her girl friend ring the doorbell, but was unable to get up. Somewhat later she rose without difficulty, went to bed immediately and fell asleep. Did not react to repeated ringing of telephone. Next morning went as usual to the office; people there noticed confusion in her speech and she herself realized that she had great difficulty in taking dictation. She was sent to the hospital.

Physical examination: Well nourished, good general condition. Looks, if anything, less than her age. Slight cyanosis, especially of the lips. Local cyanosis of both lower extremities which appear cool, especially left. No edema or exanthema. Skull and spinal column normal. Everything else normal with exception of *marked dilation of heart;* arrhythmia perpetua; tachycardia. Pulse 114, pulsus parvus. Radial and axillary pulse cannot be felt in right arm for several days, only in subclavia weak pulsation. Blood pressure 115/75 mm. Hg. EKG: arrhythmia perpetua. Extremities without abnormality.

Neurologic examination: Cranial nerves: Eye movements normal, no nystagmus. Pupils normal, bilaterally equal and reacting to light and convergence. No visual field constriction. Eyeground on repeated examination without pathology. Conjunctival and corneal reflexes bilaterally sluggish. Left corner of mouth somewhat dropped, left nasolabial crease less pronounced than right. On active mouth movements, left side sluggish. No other symptoms of cranial nerves. No abnormal reflexes. No pyramidal tract symptoms. No cerebellar signs. No sensory or motor disturbance of extremities.

Laboratory findings: Blood sedation rate not accelerated, 5/19. Microscopic: leukocytosis with relative lymphocytosis. At times, arrhythmia and fluctuating spasms of blood vessels receded almost altogether. Patient had to be kept constantly under medication. Occasional typical attacks of angina pectoris.

Patient spent many months in hospital. Special investigations extended over *many months;* most important and basic experiments were between May and July 1932, at which time patient showed first pronounced improvement in physical condition. Experiments did *not seem to tire her,* she even enjoyed them very much, while otherwise she was rather suspicious about everything in the hospital. However, she became very much *attached* to *physicians,* especially Dr. G., asking often, even when quite ill whether she would not soon be examined again. This attachment remained unaltered, even after conclusion of main experiments. Often mentioned examinations in her conversation, asking, e.g., "Did I make a fool of myself when I talked to the doctor?", or "Please ask me the colors again (*cf. later*), I am sure I can do it much better now." From these occasional utterances much additional material supporting the original findings was obtained.

* Published first by my co-worker, Dr. Eva Rothmann, as doctor thesis, 1934 (260).

Further course of illness noncontributory to present discussion. At times, paranoid picture. Physical condition became rapidly worse and no further experiments could be conducted. No new cerebral symptoms. Two months after the examination, sudden death of heart failure (see autoptic findings later, p. 278).

The patient shows a peculiar *behavior in general*. She is usually quiet, speaks little, does not try to establish much contact with others. She appears always somewhat depressed; pronounced feeling of being ill. Without clear perception of what she cannot do, she often says: "Is that incorrect?" "Why can't I do that?"

At the acute onset of the illness, she immediately had the feeling that she had lost ground; she tells again and again how terrible this experience was. Apparently, she was a very ambitious, thorough and conscientious person, and even now her main motivation is "not to make a fool of herself." She willingly cooperates in all the experiments, even asks to be examined and is very cooperative and attentive. She is very sensitive to what appears to her as "being slighted" by others—though actually her environment attempts to treat her with greatest care and consideration.

At first she was on a floor which she did not like. On her request, she was transferred to another floor, to a room which, objectively, was very much better. When seen there for the first time by the physician, she was very discontented, almost crying. On insistent questioning as to the cause of her dissatisfaction, seeing that her request had been fulfilled, she finally said that she had not received a fresh gown (due to her transfer, this change had not yet been taken care of). She was extremely annoyed by this and could not be made to see the triviality of the whole thing; similarly, once when the physician did not pay enough attention to her, did not give her his hand on saying good-bye, etc.

Actually, all these situations would, certainly after reasonable explanation at least, have been understood by the patient under normal conditions without giving rise to such serious discontent, especially as she was an intelligent and adaptable individual. In contrast to this *abnormal sensitivity* under certain conditions, she was often *extremely and almost abnormally devoted* to the physicians.

In bed, patient always looked neat and orderly. Similarly, her things arranged on the bedside table were always in good order. This, according to the relatives, corresponds entirely to the patient's premorbid personality. Before her illness, as has been said, she occupied the position of a secretary and was described to us as intelligent and efficient; once when the large business where she worked was forced to dismiss most of its employees, she was retained as the only one in the office. She was a model typist and stenographer, was also able to handle the payroll, to keep books, etc.

Orientation: Patient is oriented in all respects, answers promptly routine questions. It was surprising, however, to see her *fail to understand* altogether as soon as she was asked a *question somewhat outside of the particular situation* (which, nevertheless, would have been understood without doubt by other patients and by her on other occasions). On closer observation, it could be established that such failure was not accidental, nor determined by fatigue or similar factors, but that her *understanding failed*, or at least became very difficult in *definite situations or tasks*. In such situations, the patient either did not follow a request at all, or started to execute it but seemed to be at a loss as to how to proceed. Her face became immobile, flushed, her expression one of helplessness, desperate, angry. Sometimes she would start to swear—*would come into a typical catastrophic condition*. It should be noted that she only very rarely produced an incorrect result, that much more often she did not react. It was very difficult to get information from her in such moments as to what was going on inside her mind, what it was that she could not do. Usually, one could infer this only from a few isolated words and her general behavior, perhaps by means of very specialized questions which could be answered simply by yes and no. *Such alternation between good performance and failure could be observed in all performance fields*, irrespective of whether we were dealing with arithmetic, series enumeration, spatial performances or recognition of pictures, changes which, before recognizing the basic disturbance of the patient, were quite incomprehensible to us. Thus, sometimes the patient could be examined for a very long time without fatigue or sudden failure. The findings which thus resulted are particularly used for systematic presentation in the following, though the attempt will be made to retain somewhat the order of the single experiments, her successes and failures. Altogether, there was very little change with regard to the individual performance fields over a period of many weeks.

The *variability* of her performances was especially impressive with *regard to language*. Vocabulary, verbal fluency, grammatical expression varied very much from one situation to another. No *primary defect of motor speech* was ever observed (e.g. no *unclear pronunciation*, no *paraphasia*). Nor were there any striking deviations in conversation with her about everyday topics about her work, politics, etc. Under such conditions the patient could at times lead a *conversation fluently*, without marked lack in her vocabulary. *Spontaneously*, however, *she spoke very little*, except perhaps a sentence or so when emotionally aroused. It appeared as if the stimulus of a question or concrete situation was a necessary condition to get the patient to speak.

When required to answer definite questions, i.e., in situations where a *definite task was put to her*, her speech became *halting;* often her answers consisted merely of single words and more lacking altogether in the fluency of her conversational speech. Yet, when she could fulfill the given task by means of certain verbal habits (automatisms) or knowledge of long standing, she frequently performed very well. Again, she failed completely, speaking haltingly and *very poorly* altogether, whenever it was necessary for her to *account for anything to herself*. This appeared in such simple tasks as, e.g., to enumerate the capitals of the European countries, or animal names, or the names of flowers, or parts of the body. From many conversations, it became obvious that the patient certainly *knew the things and words* which were necessary for these tasks; only when she was to enumerate them did she fail in an often surprising degree. Why this was so shall be discussed later (see p. 271).

As long as the patient gave good answers, i.e., those answers she believed to be correct, the examination proceeded swiftly and patient obviously enjoyed it. But whenever she failed, further examination in that particular performance field was severely hampered. Patient exerted a great deal of effort, became upset, her face became flushed, etc. Considering her heart condition, we had to break off the examination, especially since on continued examination she would fail even in performances which she had executed previously quite well.

Intelligence in general: Good appreciation of a given situation; good school knowledge. Memory for old material certainly good, even though it was difficult to unearth this knowledge under certain conditions. On the basis of occasional remarks of hers and dispensing the knowledge on other occasions, it became evident that her knowledge was well above average. The situations where the knowledge became apparent were of the *concrete type* while she failed if knowledge could be brought to the fore only in taking the abstract attitude.

Some examples may illustrate: Asked to name the countries in Europe and their capitals, she failed to a high degree. But during a conversation about travels, she might visualize the map of Europe and name then the various countries and their most important towns and cities, proceeding orderly from one country to the next, always with accompanying movements. When she was asked to enumerate the pieces of furniture in her bedroom at home she experienced great difficulties; her answers were rather poor. On the other hand, when during a conversation about her home she imagined herself walking around in her own bedroom she could enumerate the pieces of furniture while pointing to and demonstrating each mimically.

These examples could be multiplied (see p. 261). Poor memory with regard to enumeration apparently results from the fact that such enumeration demands that the individual *account to himself* for his knowledge. This very capacity seems to be disturbed in our patient. One can say in general: Whenever she was required to account for certain processes or procedures, she failed, while a little later in a concrete context, she performed very well and showed a recollection of a great number of things. *Under concrete conditions her memory was* excellent (see also, p. 152).

Language: We have described some characteristics of her language before (see p. 000). There is to be mentioned, further, that she showed some *difficulty in finding words for concrete objects;* however, this defect *was so little in the foreground that one would scarcely, from the failures in this respect, be induced to assume that the patient was a typical case of amnesic aphasia.* We shall see later (p. 261) that, as a matter of fact, her language was modified in the same way as in amnesic aphasia but that the defect was covered so much that it did not come to the fore in the typical impairment of finding words.

We were astonished, from the before-mentioned concept of amnesic aphasia, to find in a patient with severe impairment of abstract attitude so little disturbance of word-finding. This induced us to investigate the non-language behavior particularly carefully.

After having reported the results of these investigations we will come back to the patient's language.

Investigation with our *object sorting tests* (see p. 000) revealed the following:

The patient is presented with the following objects in random arrangement and is asked to "bring them together in an orderly fashion," "to put together what belongs together."

Object	material	color	form
1. book (Dostoevski)	linen (bound)	red	rectangular
2. travel guide	paper (unbound)	green	rectangular
3. songbook	paper	green	rectangular
4. pencil sharpener	plastic	green	rectangular
5. penholder	wood	green	oblong
6. small pencil	wood	red	oblong
7. red-blue pencil	wood	½red-½blue	oblong
8. letter opener	metal	silver	oblong
9. eraser	rubber & metal	silver	oblong
10. ashtray (small plate)	plastic	red	round
11. metal tape measure	metal	silver	round
12. top of darning block	wood	brown	round
13. spool of thread	wood, cotton	black	cylinder
14. crocheting needle	bone	white	oblong
15. fish knife	metal	silver	oblong

Object	material	color	form
16. fish fork	metal	silver	oblong
17. small scissors	metal	silver	oblong
18. glass bar (prism, used to put fork and knife on)	glass	colorless	oblong
19. skin cream (jar)	metal	blue	round

Experiment 1: Patient seems to understand the instruction without difficulty and starts in immediately. Picks up *fishknife*, saying, "That first." Asked to verbalize what she is doing, she points to the fishknife, saying, "This is the fishknife" (I. choice). She then picks up the red pencil, saying, "This is a pencil," adds red-blue pencil saying, "Another pencil," then the eraser, "Also the eraser," and finally the ashtray, "Ashtray goes also here" (II. grouping). Then takes top of darning block and measuring tape, saying, "These are the sewing things" (III. grouping). Proceeds to put pencil sharpener to group II, saying "Here is an eraser." Takes little glass bar (prism), turns it over, doesn't seem to know what to do with it, asks "What is that?" and gives the answer herself "A prism." Puts it down by itself. Picks up in this order the book, travel guide, songbook, saying "All these are books." She hesitates, however, before putting them together, saying, as she points to the travel guide: "This really does not belong because it is a travel guide, and this one, the songbook." Finally puts the three books next to each other without conviction, saying, "Perhaps each one extra." Puts scissors to group III. Takes letter opener, saying with hesitation, "This is a letter opener," puts it to group II. Picks up crocheting needle, asks whether this is crocheting needle, and adds it to group III. Picks up skin cream jar, laughs, puts it with travel guide. Being questioned about the combination, she says, "Air and sun. To put on you. Ointment. For instance when you go bathing you cover your skin, with ointment." Adds spool to group III.

Experiment 2: Retaining the order in which patient arranged the objects, experimenter asks: "How else could the objects be put together? Is there a different way?" Patient *does not seem to understand.* The question is repeated emphatically. Thereupon patient takes red-blue pencil and pencil sharpener, puts down these two objects together. Then puts together small pencil and eraser. Then fishknife and fishfork. Does not know how to go on. Examiner asks: "Why did you bring together the pencil sharpener, pencil, eraser, etc.?" Patient points to the pencil sharpener, saying, "to sharpen the pencil." Examiner: "But why did you put them together?" Patient: "Because they belong together." Examiner: "Why do they belong together?" Patient: "The pencil could also go with these (books), ...but...no..." Examiner now presents patient with group II (pencils, etc.), removing all the other objects, asking why patient had brought these together. Patient: "This could be on a desk." Examiner: "Did you think of that before when you put them together?" Patient: "No." Examiner: "What did you think when you put them together?" Patient: "Because...because they belong together." Examiner: "What do you mean?" Patient: "You can write with the pencil and with this you sharpen it and with this you erase it and with this (letter opener) you can open up." Examiner: "What are all these together?" Patient: "Office materials." Examiner: "Did you realize that when you put them together?" Patient: "No, only afterwards."

Experiment 3: Examiner presents the patient with the following group: *red* book, *red* ashtray, *red* pencil. Asks: "Could they go together this way?" Patient: "Yes, they could." Examiner: "Why?" Patient, pointing to the pencil: "If you want to

mark the book, for other people. The ashtray if you want to smoke." Examiner:
"One could say something else about this way of putting them together." Patient
does not seem to understand. Examiner now puts together the two *green* books and
the (*green*) pencil sharpener. On questioning, it becomes apparent that the patient
does not understand this grouping (as to colours). While the patient watches, Examiner picks out all the silver-colored objects. She does not understand at all
what Examiner is doing, is very unhappy about her own lack of comprehension and
asks whether she is very stupid. Examiner attempts to quiet her by reminding her
that, after all, "doctors have a way of asking funny questions," and that being unable
to answer these is no indication of being stupid. Thereupon, patient points to the
group and says: "When things are shown in a show window, it does not matter what
the things are." She apparently means that in a show window, articles which do
not necessarily belong together are arranged together.

Experiment 4: While patient looks on, Examiner now arranges all the objects
according to their *shape*, i.e., one group of *lengthy* objects, one of *rectangular* things
and one of *round* things. Patient continues to explain the grouping on the basis of
usage of the objects: "These are the books, then things you have at home, here office
things...no...I don't know..." Patient realizes that the groups cannot be understood in this way, but still has no idea about the underlying basis for the groupings.

Experiment 5: Examiner presents red book and blue jar at some distance from
each other, then hands patient the red-blue pencil in such a way that the blue end
points towards the red book and the red end towards the blue jar. Asked to put the
pencil with either object, wherever it belongs, patient at first seems to be at a loss,
hesitates, finally saying "With the book." Examiner: "Do you notice anything
special here?", turning the pencil so that now the blue end points towards the blue
jar and the red end towards the red book. Patient's face suddenly lights up and
she says: "Oh, the colors."

Experiment 6: Patient is now asked to order all the objects "in this way." Patient: "You mean by color?" On confirmation, promptly arranges the objects in
the following way:

I. Red book, red ashtray, red-blue pencil.

II. Green penholder, green pencil sharpener, green tourist guide, green songbook.

III. Blue jar next to group I, puts red-blue pencil across both groups, saying,
"This one ought to be cut in half."

IV. Puts all silver-colored objects together.

Patient picks up red pencil, holds it next to the metal objects, finally puts it with
apparent hesitation to group I. Examiner is unsuccessful in attempts to discover
the reasons for this performance.

Patient then picks up spool (black), and, after long hesitation, finally puts it down
by itself. Similarly with the glass bar, which she cannot be brought to add to any
of the groups. She is just as puzzled with regard to the eraser, attempts to put it
down by itself, too. On pressure from Examiner, to add it to one of the other groups,
patient says: "But this is gray." Examiner suggests that it might nevertheless be
added to one of the groups. Thereupon, patient finally decided to put it with group
IV (on account of the metal part), but reiterates that it does not really belong there.

Experiment 7: While patient looks on, Examiner repeats the arrangement according to shape, asking on completion: "Can they also be grouped in this way? Why
do you think?" Patient points to the group of *long* objects, saying: "All these are
things *you use at home*." Examiner points to the letter opener, patient hesitates,
does not know what to do.

Examiner combines *red* book, *red* pencil and *red* ashtray, asking whether this grouping is also correct. Patient: *"The book is for reading."*

Examiner: "Didn't you find another reason to bring these things together a little while ago?"

Patient seems to think about this for a long time, has to be encouraged repeatedly before she finally says: "Well, I already said it, according to color." It appeared, however, from her general behavior, that she had completely forgotten this principle. Examiner now presents: letter opener, penholder, red-blue pencil (all of about the same shape).

Patient: "These are *office things.*" Examiner now presents *round* jar and *round* top of darning block. Patient: *"This is a cosmetic and this is to darn."* Examiner again presents red group. Patient: "On account of the color?" Examiner again presents the long objects and the round objects in two groups next to each other. Patient: "Two kinds of tools." Examiner adds a third group of rectangular objects and hands patient the crocheting needle, asking: "Where does this fit best?" Patient looks on with a helpless expression. Examiner: "A little while ago you sorted according to color; perhaps one could do it quite differently, for instance, according to size or shape or something." Patient: "The books are rather large and this here (pencil sharpener) is not so large." After extended fixation of the objects, patient suddenly seems to "catch on," a very marked "aha-effect" can be observed. She now places the crocheting needle properly, even though only after great hesitation. Calls the round objects "oval."

Experiment 8: Objects are again presented to the patient in random arrangement. Examiner says: "If you had *to sort out all these objects into different drawers, for instance a round drawer, a long one and a large rectangular one, how would you arrange these things?"* Patient begins by arguing that there are no round drawers. Examiner suggests she might imagine a round sewing basket instead. Patient thereupon sorts in the following manner:

I. The books, hesitates, proceeds to pick up:

II. All long objects; a little later adds the red-blue pencil which had slipped away to one side. Patient asks again about the drawers, then adds scissors to this group.

III. Pencil sharpener, a jar, tape measure, eraser, top of darning block, ashtray.

Experiment 9: Examiner brings together again the red objects, asking patient whether this is correct. Patient, somewhat annoyed: *"I told you before, this is a book, an ashtray, a pencil to mark the book."* Examiner brings together the long objects. Patient: "That is a.... Perhaps one could put them by themselves." Examiner presents the travel guide and the ashtray at considerable distance from each other. Hands patient red pencil to be added wherever it belongs. Patient puts it with ashtray "on account of the color."

Experiment 10: Examiner arranges two groups:

I. A *metal* ashtray, a *metal* reflex hammer (the use of which has been explained to the patient), a *metal* pencil.

II. A *wooden* pencil and a *wooden* paperweight.

Patient again enumerates various usages of these objects but does not hit the basis of the grouping, the *material* of which they are made. Examiner then proceeds to explain to patient that the one group contains wooden things, the other metal things. Patient says: "Oh," without much conviction. Apparently she does not understand this order. Examiner attempts, without success, to push patient towards the superordinate concept, "material"; finally Examiner writes down on a piece of paper "red" and "blue," asking patient: "What are these?" Patient answers, "Colors," only after Examiner has put down a number of further color names. Now Examiner adds underneath, "metal, wood," asking: "What are these?" Finally patient understands, says, "Materials"; admits immediately: *"I would never have thought of this by myself."*

We note in this protocol a striking deviation of the patient's behavior from that of normal individuals under similar conditions. The latter will group the objects, depending on the particular task or situation, according to color, size, shape, or some functional similarity or belongingness; they can be brought without difficulty to shift from one type of grouping to another by means of verbal instructions and/or demonstration. Not so our patient *who was dominated once and for all by the same tendency: to bring the objects together in a way in which they can be used in a concrete situation,* or, in other words, as they are experienced as *part of a definite activity.*

Grouping *according to form* and *color was almost impossible for her.* Even when, as in experiment 6, she achieved an apparent sorting according to color, closer observation and analysis of her performance showed that she was not determined here by color concepts, but rather by the *immediate sensory coherence of certain colors,* and the lack of such coherence among others. The very instability of her grouping also demonstrates the *lack of a systematic grouping principle,* a superordinate concept on the basis of which the objects were to be sorted. We should not be misled here by her use of the words "sewing materials" and "office materials," etc. (see p. 65). She herself indicated explicitly that these expressions arose *after* the objects had been sorted. Similarly, when, on another occasion, we offered the verbal concepts, the patient was unable to group according to these concepts. Her performance in experiment 9 is rather characteristic. Only a short time previously, in experiment 7, she had been induced to bring the objects together according to color. Now the same grouping was again presented to her, whereupon her only response was: "This is a book, an ashtray, a pencil to mark the book."

Sorting objects according to color per se was utterly foreign to her. A once induced attitude had to be continually reinforced, otherwise it disappeared completely from one experiment to the next.

The same can be said about her performance with respect to form, size, etc. The attitude cannot be induced by simple verbal request; in such a situation the patient does not understand what is asked of her. She succeeds only if the objects are presented in such a way that a given property, e.g. color, *imposes itself particularly vividly on her.* In other words, *she seemed altogether incapable of sorting on the basis of a systematic principle or superordinate concept, nor was she able to understand any explanation of such concepts.*

Summarizing, we can say:

1. *Only one way of procedure was natural to her, namely to bring the objects together in a way in which they can be used in a concrete situation, as they are experienced as part of a definite activity.*

2. *Sorting according to special characteristics as color, form, size, the recognition of which needs "abstraction" from the predominant impression, that this is a thing which can be used in a certain situation, was impossible. If she seemed to proceed in this way, her behavior was, as a matter of fact, the effect of the overwhelming impression of certain experiences. This occurs only in special occasions and cannot be induced by words.*

3. *The patient totally lacks the ability to shift from one procedure to another.*

4. *The patient shows in the test extreme lack of abstract capacity.*

The results of the *color sorting experiments* (see p. 167) are *basically identical* with those of the experiments on sorting of objects.

If the patient is presented with a given skein, e.g., a light green, with the request to "pick out those that belong with the given skein," two ways of procedure can be observed at different times. Either the patient chooses an *identical* or almost identical skein, and this as the *only one*. Further additions arc made only after considerable encouragement to continue. Each such addition is again a *"match" to the previously selected skein*, i.e., identical or very nearly identical to that. If prevented from this individual matching, the patient cannot proceed at all.

She is *unable to make heaps* of a number of reds or blues, etc. If she selects a greater number of skeins of the same basic color, she does not bring them together in a heap, but always leaves similar ones in a separated group. This becomes particularly evident if she puts these pairs one beside the other, so that one might gather the impression that she has sorted according to a principle, the principle of *brightness*. But closer *observation of the organization of the "series" shows that this was not the case.*

The patient put to the first one a similar one, then she brought this into a certain interval from the first one, then she looked for one which would fit the second one, put this third one at an interval from the second one and looked for one fitting the third one, brought the fourth one at an interval from the third one, and so forth. That she really always selected only one became evident when one eliminated the one which she had placed last. Then she was unable to proceed. *What appeared like a brightness series was, as a matter of fact, an organization always according to two similar or nearly identical skeins in pairs.* Not before we had recognized the procedure of the patient did this fact become clear to us. That she had not proceeded in building a brightness series showed, too, by the fact that she was unable to repeat the performance on demand; she even seemed not to understand what was asked of her.

How easily one could be deceived about her behavior shows in the following: Sometimes she brought together skeins which for us did not seem to belong together at all; one might first have the impression that the patient was color blind. That that was not the case was without doubt. In objective tests (e.g. Stilling's), she behaved quite normally. She distinguished in her groupings all nuances, *even seemed to have a finer discrimination than normals.* So there must be some other reason why she, for instance, put together a light green, a dark blue and a white.

She proceeded very deliberately, considered her combinations carefully, sometimes discarded a color to substitute another one, etc., until she achieved a grouping which she considered satisfactory. On questioning as to why she put them together, she answered, e.g.: "This is the sweater, this is the skirt, and this the blouse." Asked on other occasions why she discarded a skein, she replied, "This does not fit, it is not a color for the summer." Again and again we found that if she did not pick out very similar ones, she chose colors as if *selecting them for a concrete practical situation.*

On request to put together all the light ones and the dark ones, she did not understand what she was to do; presented with two such piles, the patient immediately said: "They don't belong together." If the examiner succeeded in explaining and pointing out that those on one side were "light" when compared with those on the other side, the patient sometimes took up there, said "light," and brought together a row of light skeins and another one of dark skeins. Such procedure was, however, not easy for her, nor was she satisfied with the result. Asked why she arranged the skeins in this way, she never answered "because they belong together" or referred to the common characteristic of the skeins, but retorted in a rather tense manner: "You said to put together the light ones." Actually, she *did not group according to brightness*, as could be assumed erroneously, *but she picked out those skeins to which in her experience the word "light" belonged.*

Spontaneously, she never sorted according to brightness, just as she did not group according to hue qualities, not even when the name of the hue (green, red, etc.) was given. Thus she did not succeed any better when requested to pick out all "red ones" or "green ones." In such a case, she usually picked one or two well saturated skeins, of the color indicated, then stopped and proceeded only after considerable prodding.

The patient was *unable to group the skeins according to the basic hues*, in other words, *unable to abstract from the individual given color and to consider the skein as a representative of a definite color category.* Therefore she could not bring it together with another skein which belonged to the same category. She was determined in her procedure by the sense experience in the given moment, sometimes more impressed by the identity of the color, sometimes by identity of the brightness, sometimes by other experiences she had in looking at the colors in the moment, as, e.g., usefulness for practical purposes. We can say she was *unable to consider the colors in the abstract attitude* and could do something with them only in a concrete way.

As clear as this result was during the first observation, later the patient seemed to proceed like a normal individual. After repeated experiments, the patient suddenly surprised us by sorting the various nuances apparently on the basis of the basic hues and designated all the nuances by the words "red" or "green." Her selections were no longer limited quantitatively as they had been before, i.e., she now chose a greater number of skeins to be grouped together and the words apparently fitted the groups. The question arose as to whether a change had taken place, whether the patient had *regained* the capacity to abstract and use the words as names for the group. Closer observation showed that *this was not the case.* From her expression and comments, it became very clear that she did *not bring the skeins together under a concept* and that the words she used were not generic words. Asked whether all the skeins she selected belong together, she hesitated to affirm this, even denied it explicitly. Asked whether the words "red," "green" fit all these nuances, she said, *"they do not fit any one"* (see the same in her sorting as to brightness, p. 268). *She put the colors together because the doctors wanted it* and she had chosen the word because she wanted to please the doctor. *Her procedure was the effect of her good memory. Even now, the words "red," etc. were not used with the meaning of a concept.* They represented an external connection between a number of objects and a sound complex which she had acquired through the many examinations. They were not *"names"* but *"pseudonames"* (see p. 61). In principle, the behavior in the later observations was the same as in the beginning. She showed the same lack of abstraction and the words fitted only individual experiences. The words had no meaning but were merely individual words (see p. 62).

This observation is particularly important because here better than in any other case it could be objectively proved that the *words of the patient were changed in the way we consider characteristic for the behavior in general of patients with amnesic aphasia.* Usually the incapacity to find the words is so in the foreground and the patients are so unable to explain why they use some words which they utter, that the change of the words can only be guessed but not demonstrated.

The case provides also an explanation for another phenomenon, namely, for the *great differences between the patients with regard to the number of words still available.* At least one cause for the difference can be seen in the greater or lesser premorbid language ability of the patient. *If meaning is lost, the individual words come more into the foreground and the more individual words the patient possessed previously to his illness, the less the difficulty to find words will become apparent.*

This factor may produce also differences as to *which words may be missing,* which are uttered. A patient may possess a word as an individual word, while another one may be able to find the same word only in the abstract attitude.

There are, indeed, still other factors which are of influence. For instance, the effect which impairment of abstraction has on the automatisms, which we have discussed before (see p. 73). The isolation of the instrumentalities from the abstract attitude may, with time, produce more and more difficulties in evoking the latter. How much that occurs may depend also on the degree to which the automatisms were independent previously to the onset of the defect of abstraction, as, for example, in our patient.

Finally, severe lack of words may be due to a concomitant primary impairment of the instrumentalities themselves. This is frequently the case (see further, p. 291, the problem of primary damage of instrumentalities in amnesic aphasia).

The great intelligence of the patient and her readiness for examination made it possible to study more carefully some phenomena which the language of patients with amnesic aphasia presents more or less in each case: disturbances in understanding, spontaneous speech, repetition, reading, writing, calculation. Their presence always must raise the question as to whether they are complications or can be explained from the same "basic defect" of the patient.

There is first some *difficulty in understanding*, which we have mentioned before (see p. 253). Our patient had certainly no primary acoustic defect, no difficulty in perception of words. Understanding in everyday situations was totally intact. The patient also understood complicated sentences and side-remarks, e.g., discussions of the physicians while examining her.

On the other hand, as soon as the spoken language concerned any *extrinsic subject matter* unrelated to herself or the immediate situation, as a conversation already in progress, *the patient failed to comprehend even single words and short simple sentences.* She was able to repeat what she had heard, showing also here adequate acoustic comprehension, but did not grasp the meaning. To illustrate: the patient comprehended a very simple children's story when the examiner addressed her directly and told the story in vivid form, so that she could take part in what was going on. But she failed to understand the same story, even presented in simpler form, when it was read to her as an objective narration. *Figural speech was altogether incomprehensible to her.* She grasped the words in their literal meaning but could not be brought to understand the metaphorical character of the same words. For instance, asked: "What is a 'Backfisch'?" (German expression for adolescent girl; English verbal translation "baked fish"), she answered: "Fish can be baked..." After a good deal of concrete explanation and illustration by the examiner, she finally admitted that a young girl could be so designated. The same question is repeated two days later, and again she answers: "Fish can be fried or baked..." On insistent demand for another meaning of this very current expression, she eventually says: "You said the other day something about a fourteen year old girl." In these examples, the abnormal concreteness of the patient's language is very evident.

How concrete her understanding of words was, may be illustrated by reporting a conversation with her: To the question where she lived, she answered "in a 'bachelor apartment.' " Asked to tell what a bachelor is, she does not answer the question but reports about the location of the apartment or gives answers which show that she wants to escape reaction to the repeated question "What is a bachelor?" She said: "I have a good apartment, entrance hall, bedroom, kitchen. She answers correctly to the question whether the house is only for bachelors: "No, there are also big apartments, only in the rear live bachelors." Asked again what a bachelor is, she does not answer, is apparently in distress. Neither can she answer to the question whether a woman who has a husband and children is a bachelor. Asked again,, what is a bachelor, she says: "One goes up the staircase to their apartments."

Apparently she understood the *word bachelor only in relation to the concrete situation of her apartment*, but it did not mean anything to her outside of this situation.

The examples mentioned above, which could be easily augmented, show that *understanding of these patients can be disturbed under certain circumstances, namely, if it presupposes the abstract attitude.* Therefore, the patients often fail in understanding a conversation which one can understand only if one is able to follow changing contexts, which asks for a shift of attitude and with that the abstract attitude (see p. 6). Hence *failures in understanding* of the patient *can be considered as an expression of the "basic defect" in amnesic aphasia.* Whether this is the case in an individual patient has to be determined, indeed.

Spontaneous speech of the patient did not in general appear abnormal. The patient had a good vocabulary. There was not even the impression of a definite lack of nouns. No paraphasia occurred. It is true that the patient spoke *very little spontaneously*, and often sudden disruption of the flow of words was observable; this seemed to occur particularly when she had to think about what she was to say. Her language was especially poor when she had to *answer definite questions* to which she could not respond, *by using knowledge which immediately came to her mind.* If this were not the case, then her replies consisted mostly of single, but adequate words, or short sentences. This was most marked when she had to report about facts and events which had no relation to the present situation or to a situation of her previous life she was able to imagine. If she were brought into a definite situation which she remembered and imagined, then her language became much richer.

I should like to recall here what we have said before about her behavior in the task of enumerating animals, or names of females (see p. 261). Words came to the fore only when the task evoked in her fantasy an activity in a concrete situation. Therefore, she could not recount a story which had no bearing on her personal experiences. She had *speech only as a means to accompany concrete situations.* She failed when language was to be used as a means of giving account to oneself, of *representing something.* Thus, we can say: *Her spontaneous speech showed the same characteristics as her behavior in general.*

She could *repeat* letters, words, even difficult ones, and sentences, if they were not too long, also senseless combinations of syllables. She did not always understand what she had repeated. It seemed even that the better and quicker she repeated, the less she understood.

Reciting of series (number series, alphabet, etc.) was, on the whole, excellent. She also recited a number of songs, poems, etc. It was noticeable that she always had *difficulty in starting, and in shifting* rapidly from one series to another. When asked to count while leaving out each second number, she failed. Later, she showed apparent success in this task but close observation revealed that she spoke the alternate steps softly, hardly audible and emphasized the others: thus actually she recited the whole series. This inability to fulfill the task of reciting numbers while leaving out every second number is a phenomenon which is understandable as an affect of impairment of abstract attitude (see p. 184).

Usually she could *read* single *letters* correctly, though at times she had apparent difficulty in finding the name of the letter. Reading of words and sentences was often prompt, with good accentuation, giving the misleading impression that she always understood what she read. As a matter of fact, material which she read promptly, frequently was not understood. She almost always understood written requests, as long as she was asked to point to something or hand some object to the examiner. On the other hand, she did not seem to understand purely descriptive statements about objects and events not immediately related to her, even though she might read them fluently. She was often quite helpless when presented with simple stories from the first grade reader. She did not understand the newspaper, which is the reason that while under observation she never asked for the paper although she had followed the news with great interest previous to her illness. On the other hand, she understood *letters addressed to her very well.*

There was a further very striking aspect of her reading. She was not at all disturbed by misspelling, omission of letters, etc., and read words containing such faults even better than normals. Thus "Grten" was read promptly as Garten, "Hstuer" as Haustuer. She usually did not seem to notice these mistakes at all; however, if asked whether something were missing, she would begin to scrutinize the word, then admit an omission but could not point to it. Sometimes, she would manage to find it after spelling out the word quickly, but by no means always.

Spelling was excellent as long as she recited the letters in a *purely mechanical way* and quickly, producing series of letters, as it were. She explained her capacity in this respect as a *result of her past typing experience.* She would run into difficulty, however, as soon as this pure motor mechanism could not be utilized, e.g., when asked to leave a short time interval between the letters, or to omit certain letters. Similarly, if the examiner spelled out a word very rapidly she recognized it, but short time intervals would interfere with her recognition. The same difficulty appeared when she was to arrange orally presented single letters, or letter blocks, to make up a word, e.g., presented with W-O-C-H-E (week) she had no idea what the word was, said "Wonne" (joy), "Wahl" (choice), but immediately afterward spelled on demand the word Woche without difficulty, also wrote it down. On the other hand, when asked merely to look at the letters without trying to rearrange them, she would often recognize the word and pronounce it correctly, e.g., I $^{WN}_{RTE}$ was read immediately as Winter (winter) with the comment "Yes, I can say it...but it is terrible...", could not rearrange the letter blocks, but put down W I R T E N; immediately afterwards, asked to write winter, she would perform without mistake. She presented essentially the same behavior when she had to arrange sentences out of presented words. She had great difficulty in properly arranging words: Jäger- Hasen-den- der schiesst (Answer: Der Jäger schiesst den Hasen). She seemed to think for a long time, but could not rearrange the words, even though she pronounced the whole sentence correctly. Similarly: Wiese-die-ist-grün (Die Wiese ist grün). After several vain attempts to order the words in a sentence, she would say "Die Wiese ist grün." She could write it down correctly. The sentence was now cut up again into the single words; the patient put down: "Die Wiese grün ist." Just as she had difficulty in constructing out of the given words a sentence with grammatical correctness, we also noticed certain grammatical defects in her spontaneous speech, though far more in her writing than in her spoken language. She usually spoke in short, well constructed sentences and even when she occasionally used subclauses, questions, etc., she did not make mistakes.

The behavior in her reading can be explained by lack of abstraction and substitution of the defect by excellent motor and visual performances.

Writing: At the beginning, she had *great difficulty in writing single letters;* however, she was able to write *simple words correctly* at that time, especially on dictation. She was very sensitive to her poor performance and disliked having to write. She improved essentially as to her writing capacity. Letters written by her were characterized by general messiness and disorderly composition, which was the more striking because in the past she had been especially neat with regard to such tasks. She did not keep to the line; even single words deviated upward and downward, though this improved later. The sentence structure was, especially at first, very simple, but only rarely faulty. The content centered about herself, just as her conversation did. Considerable difficulty was experienced in reporting an objective event or something which she had read; in such cases, many words were misspelled, others omitted—altogether, just as poor as her oral reporting.

A striking fact was her frequent *misspelling of words, many omissions* and *additions of letters, reversals of sequence.* As long as she was able to perform without too much difficulty, details were executed fairly well. As soon as she had to interrupt herself, however, and *to exert a special effort, everything seemed to go wrong. Often she did not seem to know how to form a given letter* which she had just written without difficulty in another word. Confusion, particularly with regard to capital letters, was noted; often she put down capitals instead of small letters and vice versa. Frequently she wrote wrong words which she subsequently would strike out and correct. Altogether, given enough time, she did considerable correcting, until there remained only a few mistakes in her writing. For this reason, she needed much time, often several hours for a letter. She would often destroy what she wrote only to begin anew.

Later, individual letters were usually written correctly, but it was striking how often she had to stop and think how to form a letter. Occasionally she showed total failure on a letter which had been written fluently within a word just a few minutes earlier. There was great improvement in her spelling over the course of time.

Most of the anomalies of her writing can be understood as due to her "basic defect." But the defects and malformations of single letters, the defective arrangement and deviations from the line all point to another impairment, to a primary defect of writing, as we observe it in so-called *pure agraphia.* In the course of time, the mistakes due to this pure motor impairment disappeared. Whether the mistakes within the words, the difficulties in spelling, can be subsumed under the "basic defect" is difficult to say. There is a destruction of the word involved, which is of a similar type as we shall find it in dedifferentiation of inner speech in "central aphasia." I think we are dealing here with the effect of such a destruction (see p. 229).

The patient showed *changes in orientation as to space.*

The patient was oriented as to space, in the environment as well as to her own person. She could show on demand where things were in the room, the door, window, the direction of up or down, right or left. However, she had difficulty if it were necessary to account to herself about place and direction in objective space. *She had difficulty in indicating up, or down, in a presented pencil.* One might present the pencil in any direction, but she always called the sharpened end down, the other end up. She explained this by pointing to the fact that in writing, the pointed end was down. In the same way, she behaved in respect to all objects which are usually used in a definite position, for instance, with a *key, the ring was up for her.* She demonstrated that by holding the key as if she were going to put it into a keyhole.

The words "up" and "down" had meaning for her only in relation to the use of things in a concrete known situation. She could not understand that there is an up and down in objective space. If, later, she sometimes seemingly gave the correct answer, it was not difficult to disclose that she had used a roundabout way. Thus, later, *she might call the unsharpened end of a pencil down if it were presented with this end downward, because she recognized that it pointed to the floor, which is down.* Asked whether this end were really down she said, "No, that is wrong, the sharpened end is down (cf. the corresponding behavior as to colors, p. 269). The patient demonstrated the right hand correctly. The *left hand was for her the "other one."* She knew that right was the hand which one uses in activities, particularly in writing. The direction to show the right hand, meant for her, to show the hand which one uses for writing, etc. *Right and left in the outer world were determined by her right and left arm.* To indicate forward, and backward, she put her hands on the anterior or posterior surface of her body. Up and down was determined by the position of the ceiling and the floor. With closed eyes she had great difficulty in indicating up and down.

Asked to give the left hand, she usually gave the right one. If then asked to give the right one, she proceeded correctly and then also gave the left one correctly on demand. Sometimes she would take the left hand with her right one and say: "That is my left hand."

She made mistakes in the same way in pointing on demand to an individual finger of her own or of the examiner:

(Show your thumb) she stretches out both thumbs.

(Little finger) +

(Index finger of the left hand) shows thumb of the left hand.

(Index finger) again thumb.

In the beginning, she *was unable to give the names of the fingers, called them with numbers, first finger, second finger, etc.*

(Point to the doctor!) Immediately correct pointing movement with right index finger.

(Which is left hand?) +

(Which is right ear?) Points to both.

(Right ear) +

(Left hand to the right eye)   Goes with the left hand to the left eye.
(What did I ask you to do?)   Left hand to left eye.
Only *seldom did she make mistakes with the thumb and the little finger.*   If she were to show other fingers, she would proceed in an indirect way, counting silently.   She made mistakes also if she had to show other parts of the body (particularly if she were asked to show a definite part on a definite side) when one asked her to show this part with a definite hand.   She seemed to be confused when she heard such commands.

One could say she *reacted correctly if the command determined her activity immediately,* right hand—right side, etc.   *She would fail as soon as she had to give account to herself about what she was to do.*   She was successful in this instance also if she were able to use a roundabout way.   One cannot say she had an agnosia or apraxia.   Her failures were due to her difficulty if she had to do more than react immediately, if she had to take the abstract attitude which is presupposition for giving account to oneself (see p. 6).*

The patient was not able to understand what *direction and space meant, but she did not fail even in such tasks where the average person's proceeding is based on knowing directions, because she fulfilled the task with the help of visualization.*   She used all objects in the right way, showed *no signs of apraxia,* but if she were asked to show *how to use an object, she had difficulty.* She could do this if by description of the situation to which the activity belonged she was "brought into the situation."   She behaved similarly in the task to show how to beckon, threaten, swear.   If the words brought her into the concerned situation, she then performed the actions.

Recognition of objects and situations which immediately can be grasped as wholes showed no deviation from the norm.   She recognized, e.g., simple pictures.   *But presented with pictures which can be recognized only if one brings the parts they contain into a meaningful connection she failed. She grasped parts of the picture very well, particularly activities which were presented, but not the whole picture.*

This may be illustrated by the following example:

Presented with the "snowball picture" of the old Binet-Simon scale and asked to tell what was going on in the picture she said: "A broken window...the whole thing is a story...a farmer (pointing to the man)...a boy coming from school...he is hiding...(Story?) the boy...has broken the window (points to boy).   (Why?)... (patient fumbles)...because this one is hiding (pointing to the other boy)...I am sure he has done it.   (What is the farmer doing with the boy?)   I have to think about it....(Long pause; finally examiner asked: "He is pulling the boy's hair. Why do you think he does it?)....Because he thinks that the boy did it.   (Examiner: "Did you think so too?")...First I thought it was the other one.   (Examiner: "Didn't you see what the farmer was doing?")   Yes...I knew the movement he is making...("Why did you say this one did it?")...(Patient points to boy in hiding)

---

* Her behavior was very similar to that of so-called "Fingeragnosia," described by Gerstmann (76).

Because...he would get beaten if he were about...("What did he break the window with?") Oh...anything. ("What does the boy have in his hand?") A snowball. ("Now tell me the story.") He broke the window...with the snowball...then the other one came...from school...so he hides...."

The patient continued to interpret various parts of the picture, but it was quite evident that she had not recognized the essence of the story.

Even after detailed explanation by the examiner, the patient did not seem to get the point. Her description of other pictures corresponded to the above protocol. It can be said that the patient was always eager to answer something, that her response was correct as far as it concerned a part of the picture, e.g., in the above the broken window. She did not, however, recognize the action portrayed by the whole picture.

She failed because she was *not able to give account to herself about the relationship of the* parts to each other and the structure of the whole. She tried to find out what she could grasp and would apparently grasp all which represented action. If she discovered such a part, the rest of the picture was in the background, she no longer paid attention to it.

She did not look for other things because she wanted to avoid catastrophes (see p. 13); she did not feel forced to do it, because she was under the impression that her task was fulfilled; if she were eager to discover whether she might not find something else, she would search for other parts which represented actions, etc. Thus, she might grasp more and more details. It did not help her to understand the whole picture if one explained to her the meaning of the picture by words. This would demand, again, the same attitude for which she had no capacity. But she might grasp the meaning suddenly. One gathered the impression that she suddenly grasped what was going on in the situation the picture presented.

Her behavior corresponded to that in the sorting tests. *The immediate sensory experience alone enabled the correct reactions.* It may be mentioned that a similar behavior was to be observed with other cases which Lange, (177) Conrad (39) and I (124, 265) have published.

Arithmetical performances

Numbers consisting of 1 to 3 digits she read correctly, but was not able to grasp the value of the position of the digits in bigger numbers. She therefore made mistakes in reading and writing of such numbers. She read, e.g., 350,000 as three millions 500 thousands; 35,000 as three hundred fifty hundred. She would write numbers with 4 digits correctly. Numbers like 3,500,000 she would write as 350,500. Reading even of bigger numbers became better if they were presented in a way structured by free interspaces. The same was the case if one put after the number the word "Mark" (German money), so that the number represented money to her.

She *understood* the signs of counting in *concrete examples*, but was *not able to explain what these signs meant if they were presented isolated*. If she were asked to write the sign of multiplication she did not react at all, or she would write 2×3, or put it down but immediately afterwards put before and behind it a number.

As long as the patient could fulfill a task in arithmetic by using material learned previously, she was successful, but *not if the task could be solved only if one were to give account to oneself about the procedure*. Thus, it became understandable that she was unable to solve a simple subtraction but performed well those tasks with percentage calculation, the results of which she knew by heart. *The anomalies in arithmetic were thus understandable from the "basic defect" of the patient.*

Considering the fact that the disturbances of the patient concerned so many performance fields, we must ask ourselves *whether all these symptoms represent a unitary syndrome and whether we are justified in calling it amnesic aphasia.* For most of the failures we could show that they are understandable as due to impairment of abstract attitude. In this respect, they certainly belong together, and there is no reason not to consider them a unitary syndrome. The defect in word-finding appears as one symptom of the latter. Because usually the cases where this form of disturbance in word-finding is found are called amnesic aphasia, we may at least for the time being keep this name.

But there is the question of whether all patients with this type of disturbance of word-finding show this multitude of symptoms. This question is not to be answered definitely from the reports in the literature. Usually the patients are not investigated in such a way that one can say something definite about their behavior in all the mentioned respects. There is, further, the important fact that the defects may not always have come to the fore because sometimes they were more or less covered by various means; and adequate attention may not have been paid to this fact. As far as I can judge, all cases with the typical amnesic disturbance of word-finding show other symptoms of impairment of abstract attitude. If the interpretation is correct, we should find, in turn, in all cases with impairment of abstraction, a difficulty in finding words. This is actually the case. But the disturbances of word-finding may not always appear predominant. The just mentioned case is illustrative. It should further be considered that the word-finding defect is outstanding only if there is, at the same time, some damage of the instrumentalities of speech. That this assumption does not alter my interpretation of amnesic aphasia, I have explained in another place (see p. 291). We faced some symptoms in our patient which could not be understood simply as effect of the "basic defect." There was the defect in writing which we diagnosed as a slight damage of motor writing performances, probably due to a special lesion in the second frontal convolution (see p. 129).

There were further symptoms about which we can at least be doubtful as to whether they are not an *expression of a damage of inner speech,* hence the *disturbances in spelling, in combining letters to words,* in writing. A combination of amnesic aphasia with symptoms of central aphasia is frequent (see p. 231). There arises the question of whether we are dealing with an accidental combination due to similar locality of the underlying lesion, or whether there is an inner relationship between both defects.   As little as we are able to say now, the latter possibility is worth pondering in respect to the closeness of the phenomenon of inner speech to the non-speech mental processes (see p. 94).   It should, indeed (if in central aphasia, symptoms of difficulty of finding words appear), always be carefully analyzed as to whether we are dealing with real amnesic aphasia or with another type of disturbance of word-finding.   In a lesion of the instrumentalities, difficulties in finding of words may also occur as due to a heightening of the threshold of stimulability of words, which certainly should be differentiated from amnesic aphasia (see p. 64).

The autoptic findings in the brain of the patient.
The autopsy revealed a brain which showed well developed Gyri and Sulci in general.   There were *two large* and *three small softenings:*
1. *A large lesion,* which concerned the middle part of the *Island of Reil,* which had destroyed the cortex totally, affected somewhat the claustrum, but left the external capsule intact.   The most anterior and most posterior parts of the Island and the transition of the latter to the parietal and temporal convolutions seemed to be intact.
2. *A second large lesion* in the *left temporal lobe.*   Also here, the cortex particularly was affected.   The softening concerned the anterior part of the first and second convolutions, expanded backward in the first and second convolutions and affected downward the third.   The posterior part of the first and second convolutions, also the medial parts of them and the transition to the parietal lobe and to the Island of Reil were intact.
3. *A small defect,* essentially affecting the cortex, at the place where second and third frontal convolution encounter the anterior central convolution.   *Broca's region* was essentially intact, and likewise the greatest part of Frontalis II and the lowest part of the anterior central convolution.
4. There was a very small softening on the transition of the central part of the left posterior central convolution to the parietal lobe; further
5. A superficial lesion of about ⅓ inch diameter in the region where the right second frontal convolution encounters the anterior central convolution.
If we try to bring the clinical picture into relation to the autopsy findings, there should first be mentioned that there is *no reason to assume that there existed a diffuse damage of the brain.*   Neither the macroscopic picture nor the microscopic examination supposed such an assumption.   The frontal lobe, the area of Broca, Wernicke's region, the central convolutions, the occipital and parietal lobes proved to be microscopically without deviations from the norm.   The lack of such symptoms as abnormal fatigue, distractiveness, dizziness, headaches speaks also against a general damage.   The symptom complex developed out of seemingly full health, suddenly.   There were no signs of a brain damage before.
Thus, we can make essentially the *localized lesions responsible for the symptoms.*   In this respect we can say that, anatomically, the regions significant for *speech perception and motor speech were intact.*   This finds its expression in the perfection of the performances which we can bring into connection with the functioning of these regions.
The defect in *writing,* which improved later, can be brought into relation to the *small lesion we mentioned* (2, above).

For the "basic defect" the two large lesions have to be considered responsible. Both lesions concern a realm which, according to what I have said in another place (see p. 244), is important for inner speech. I have mentioned before that some of the symptoms may be considered as an expression of a dedifferentiation of inner speech; hence, the defect in spelling, in composition of letters to words, in composition of words to sentences, etc. The intactness of repetition seems to speak against central aphasia. The lack of paraphasia, indeed, we could try to explain as due to the fact that the patient covers this defect by her excellent motor performances, her excellent "knowledge of language" (see p. 25), and that her spontaneous speech was poor and did not consist of many words where paraphasia could come to the fore. Thus the disturbances of inner speech could easily be brought into connection with the lesion in the temporal lobe and the Island of Reil.

We have considered most of the symptoms as expression of impairment of abstract attitude. It is certainly not easy to bring this impairment in relation to the anatomic findings. Those parts, which usually are damaged in the presence of this defect, are not lesioned, i.e., the frontal lobes and the parietal lobe. We have thus to bring the impairment into connection with the lesion of the Island of Reil and of the temporal lobe, certainly parts of the brain which are not so significant for higher mental function. I have explained that in amnesic aphasia there is to be expected, besides some damage of the speech area, a lesion of the parts of the brain important for the non-speech performances (see p. 315). The patient shows the first kind of lesion, not the latter.

Now, to consider the whole picture as central aphasia is certainly not possible. Thus, we must confess that we are not able to explain fully the picture from the anatomic findings. We have simply to register the findings. It may be that further studies will result in a better explanation.

The next case shows the combination between amnesic aphasia and central aphasia in a more dramatic way.

Case 16*

This 56 year old white man was admitted to the Montefiore Hospital on August 25, 1935, with a history of a "stroke" eight months previously, followed by sudden onset of unconsciousness and paralysis of the right side of the body. He recovered consciousness after about one hour, seemed quite clear mentally and was able to talk coherently. Six hours later, however, he developed *difficulty in speaking*, although he seemed to understand what was said to him. There was bladder and rectal incontinence during the first week, but not thereafter. After one month the motor weakness, especially of the leg, improved and he was able to walk. The speech disability, however, persisted.

The past and family history were not important except that the patient's father had died of "apoplexy" at the age of 52.

The patient was a poorly nourished, elderly man. Heart sounds were regular, but of poor quality and there was a faint systolic murmur at the apex. Peripheral vessels were moderately thickened. Blood pressure was 130/84.

There was a right spastic hemiparesis, with the arm in extension. The leg was less involved than the arm. Deep reflexes were increased on the right, with right ankle clonus. Abdominals and cremasterics were all present, but markedly diminished on the right. Troemner, Babinski, Rossolimo, and other confirmatory signs were

---

* Published by Goldstein and Marmor, 1938 (114).

present on the right. There was a mild, right-sided hemisensory syndrome, including the face, extending to the left of the mid-line, and involving all modalities. Sensory impairment was greatest in the hand. There was also distinct hyperpathia on stroking or pinching the right half of the body. The pupils reacted somewhat sluggishly to light and accommodation. The fundi were normal. There was questionable impairment of vision in the right homonymous fields. The face showed a slight right supranuclear weakness.

The patient sat quietly in a chair most of the day, *took no part and showed no interest in the ward activities, and spoke not at all to his fellow-patients.* However, *in any situation which directly concerned him, this otherwise quiet, noncommunicative and passive individual, became animated, excited and overtalkative.* He *answered questions freely and cooperated to the best of his ability in all investigations.* He would talk incessantly to the doctors, discussing his infirmities at great length, with much facial expression and show of emotion, laughing and crying alternately.

From the history, it was noted that the patient *had been able to speak at least five languages fluently*—German, English, Yiddish, Polish, and French. At the time of our examination, he was still able to use any of these media for expression, but favored a combination of English, German, and Yiddish. His speech was best under conditions of emotional stress. At such times, he spoke fairly coherently and grammatically, utilizing a good vocabulary. Usually he uttered *short, simple sentences* which contained all types of words, although at times a subject or adverb might be missing. There was *no paraphasia.* There was a *tendency to stereotypy* and he *frequently repeated himself.* The striking thing, however, was that despite this relatively good conversational speech, he showed a *complete inability to name objects and to repeat at command either letters, words or sentences.* Although he might have just used a particular word or sentence in spontaneous speech, he was totally unable to repeat it on demand a moment later. When asked to recite the numbers from one to ten, or the letters of the alphabet, or the days of the week, he could do so only *if the first few were given to him.* Then, if asked to repeat one of the symbols, he was unable to do so unless he recited the whole series. Thus, if after counting from one to ten, he was asked to repeat the number seven, he could do so only by counting consecutively from one to seven. Often, in his *attempt to repeat* a given word, he would *utter other words,* which were *related as to their contents to the given word.* Thus, when asked to say "God," he could not do so, but would say "Himmel" (Heaven); for "children," he would say "family"; for "hospital," " Montefiore"; for "window," "glass," etc.

He could not *name even the most familiar objects,* although he was usually able to demonstrate or explain the use of an object which was shown to him, and sometimes *uttered the correct word in the course of his explanation.* When asked immediately afterward to repeat the word, however, he could never do so.

He *understood* in general quite well, obeyed simple commands, was able to point to certain parts of his body as named, could put out his tongue when asked, etc. He also seemed to understand simple conversational sentences, although he *did not comprehend even a little more complicated ones.* His understanding was always better when the spoken words fitted the particular situation which he was experiencing at the time.

The following protocol may illustrate the patient's behavior:

He was cooperative, glad to see the examiner, and quite loquacious. He preferred a mixture of German and Yiddish, sometimes interspersed with English expressions. At times, he was rather hard to understand. Paraphasia or dysarthria were not observed.   His facial expression was vivid and adequate.   ("+" indicates a correct response)

(Your name?) +

(Touch your ear.)   +

(Where, here?)   +

(Who am I?) (smiled, because question seemed so simple).   +

(Touch your eye.), repeated several times "Auge, Auge."   +

(Touch your ear.)   Idem. +

(Touch left ear with left hand.)   +

(Touch right ear with left hand.)   Perplexed, touched left ear, looked at examiner *could not succeed.*

(Touch right eye with left hand.)   Idem.   He was *not able to do test with three items,* as for instance touch with left hand first left ear then left eye.

Asked what he had to complain about "Ich kann Sie kaum es sprechen aus—Ich habe ganz viel gelernen—mein Kind sing gelernen—mein Frau ist da in Behandlung—die Kinder sind hier—ich kann bleiben.   Die Leute so schmutzig—die Finger—ich komme herein hier—sie machen so schmutzig—ich lieb nicht die Leute.   Mein Sohn verheiratet, a ganz feine Mann—ich moechte that is mein Sohn—seine Fraux—mein Tochter—sie ist in high school—English—ich moeg so gerne—I can speak French, too, parfaitement.   I was in that position there—in 100th Street—mein wife—my children, one child was home.   I got nice home—I come home—my wife—you eat something—it come 8 o'clock "Gustaf, you feel goot?"—I feel goot.   Half an hour later what happens—mein Gustaf—he's dead.   I had twenty professor—many—my children all bring—he dead—cannot sprechen—Ich habe garnicht gewissen—wass—ich weisse garnicht was (what is your son doing?).   Was von mein Sohne? was tut er? what is he doing—ja—he was there 20 years.   Er war sehr gute Mann. He has a business.   (What is the doctor doing?)   He writes.   (What with?)   Everything what you wish.—(Has your son such things—bottle of glue?)—He's a printer—yes—he's got everything, he's got a nice business—he's got such things—but he has not use for dose things.   Years ago—he used to make dem—but not now (pointed to book)—he does this things—he writes this things with a machine—a big machine—here, here and here—he's the boss—ya (what do other men do?)—I know (shakes head) (printer?)—yes—he's working over—others working for him getting $25, $40 a week.   He does every work.   He does difference work—I don't remember—I used to remember—I asked him how's business—"oh great, papa"—heute you erregnerich?—yes, it, looks like rain today—but it's cold,—the sun did not shine (does the sun shine?)—yes, no, but I can't say—I know rain, rain it is nice warmer, warmer, colder—it don't look like rain.   (Say the same words as I say):

Rain—Mein Herr.

Rain—rain, it's raining, it's raining.

Sky—I am sorry, I wish I could say every word.

God, God is always there—God—I know—I understand ("look at the sky—it's raining")—not now—not raining no more.   Gut gestern raining all night.

Holidays—kosher—yo...yontiff, I know, I understand what is yontiff, to-morrow, Sunday, Monday, Monday it will be finished, Pesach, Easter.

Writing.   He was able to print out his name in Latin capitals, *but could not write* any other words.   He could write numbers, both single and double to dictation, and was able to perform, in writing, simple arithmetic computations.

Reading.   He was able to read only his name and the heading of the *New York Times.*   However, it seemed that this was not real reading but a recognition of familiar visual pictures, since he could not read single letters or words. He could not identify a spoken word with a written word.

He apparently recognized pictures of objects although he could not name them. Similarly, he was able to recognize objects placed in his hands (with eyes closed) and could demonstrate their use, without being able to name them.

General Intelligence.—Conversations with the patient and various tests indicated that he had retained a fairly good level of general intellectual activity. His memory and judgment were apparently only moderately impaired. He had definite appreciation of the fact that his speech was changed. Sensorium was intact, and he was oriented in all directions. His reactions to concrete situations within his immediate environment were fairly good.

In contrast to this, however, he was completely *unable adequately to handle any situation which required the capacity for abstract conceptions.*

Color Sorting Test (see p. 167). The patient was asked to pick out from a heap of assorted colored yarns all those strands which are similar in color to a given sample.

(a) Medium green. He picks up a medium green. "That is a heller (brighter) green. Dies jier green, das is schoener green." He picks up a very light green. "Das heller (brighter)." He does not consider it a match and puts it aside. He picks up a dark red. Looks at the green sample, and says "No." He picks up a dark blue and a dark purple. Looks at the sample. "No, das anderes (different)." Picks up a dark green, matches it with the sample, then replaces it, apparently dissatisfied with the match. Picks up a dark purple. "No, das nicht dasselbe (not the same)." Picks up a light shade of green. "Das is greener, die mehr." Replaces it in the original heap. *Picks up a very similar green to the given sample—an almost perfect match.* "*Ja, ja, dasselbe!*" Takes other greens and attempts to match them, but returns them to the heap. Feels satisfied and joyous only when he is able to match the sample with others of almost identical shade.

(b) Goes through the same procedure with a given red.

(c) An attempt is made to demonstrate to the patient what is desired of him by putting a series of different reds in one heap, and a series of different greens in another. However, the patient was apparently *unable to grasp the principle* involved, and refused to admit correctness of the division. He showed satisfaction only when identical or near-identical shades were matched.

(d) Given a very light blue, matches with two light shades, but is dissatisfied. "No, no, auch nicht." "Beinahe, aber nicht dasselbe (almost, but not the same)." He picks other skeins of comparable brightness—very light blue, very light purple, very light grey (4 shades), very light green, very light brown, very light blue, very light yellow. However, when asked shortly afterwards to select light shades of different colors, he is unable to do so.

(e) He is shown a light blue, a dark blue, and a dark red, and is told that the light blue and dark blue match better than the dark blue and dark red. He shakes his head, saying, "No, das blue, das is ganz andere. No, das blue, everything, nicht das, nicht das."

This test reveals clearly the particular nature of the patient's intellectual deficiency. It will be noted that he seemed to be completely unable to grasp the idea of "color" as an abstract conception. He was able to think only of particular shades. Thus, he could not recognize the belongingness of light green and dark green to one and the same category, "green." To him they were different colors. When he used the words "green" or "red," it became clear that he was not using the terms in their generic sense, but was referring only to the particular shade of green or red which he had under observation at the moment. Similarly, although he, at times, would match bright shades of different colors to a given bright shade of red, he was nevertheless totally unable to grasp the *idea* of "brightness" as a concept, and could not pick out bright shades of different colors on demand.

The following tests show the same defect on other material:

Manikin Test (Pintner and Paterson, 1931): This little test, although relatively simple, involves the capacity of the patient to form a "Gestalt," i.e., to abstract a conception from a group of apparently dissociated objects. In spite of its simplicity, we see that this previously highly intelligent individual had difficulties with it. Although he finally solved it more or less correctly, he had to proceed in trial and error fashion.

First he recognizes legs and head, and then seems to recognize readily that it is a man. Puts two legs together, using words "Fuesse, shoes." Puts two arms together, and points to his own arms. Patient then puts legs to trunk, but in wrong order—he just pushes them up without looking at the form outlined. He sees error, reverses legs, and inserts correctly. Puts left arm in right socket (it being nearest), sees mistake, corrects it. Puts other arm, then head in place. Arms put close to sides—not partially abducted. Patient quite joyous upon completion. Time: 3.15 minutes.

Feature Profile Test (Pintner and Paterson, 1931): This test is somewhat more complicated than the Manikin Test in that it involves the handling of two factors by the subject—one, the grasping of the outer form of the test pieces, and the other, the grasping of lines on the test pieces which when put together properly form the eye, ear, nose, etc. The fusing of two such factors involves what we speak of as the capacity of abstract conception. As the test shows, the patient was lacking in this ability.

The patient cannot say what it is by its outline form. Uses trial and error to fit forms of profile. When he fits correctly, says, "That's right." He knows when he is right or wrong. Completes profile, then, "Oh, my God, a whole Kopf." First looks along outside of figure in order to fit earpieces. Must then be shown hole in center. Starts with trial and error inside figure—no success—then tries to put ear together outside figure. He uses the lines on the blocks—knows when he is wrong. Puts two pieces correctly, but cannot fit other two to them. He refuses to accept his own results because he knows that they are not correct. "No, sir, it's very hard, very hard." (After about six and one-half minutes work, "Shall I show you how?") Patient is asked to repeat, but no success. Illustrated once more, then asked what it might be. Patient cannot say, picks up all pieces together: "Maybe if I put it inside, I could tell you." Puts ear inside, picking up all four pieces together and thus putting them in place, smiles, points to his own ear and says "nose."

Laboratory Data: Encephalography showed marked cortical atrophy, with moderate internal hydrocephalus. In one of the anterior-posterior views there was clearly visible in the region of the left Sylvian fissure a large triangular collection of air with its base pointed outward. Gastric analysis showed free HCl of 66, total acid of 78. Stool was positive for occult blood. Gastrointestinal series indicated the presence of duodenal ulcer. Wassermann and other routine laboratory data were negative.

Course in hospital: Patient complained frequently of epigastric pain, and gastrointestinal series showed evidence of a duodenal ulcer, for which he was treated medically. On May 19, 1936, he suddenly developed signs suggestive of a ruptured duodenal ulcer. These signs subsided within twenty-four hours, and the abdomen became soft. However, the pains persisted, and on May 25, 1936, laparotomy was performed.   At operation, a small perforation was discovered in the first portion of the duodenum.   This was sealed over, and a posterior gastroenterostomy was performed.   The patient developed signs of bronchopneumonia on the third postoperative day and expired on May 29, 1936.

Diagnosis: Clinical diagnosis was: thrombosis of left middle cerebral artery, ruptured duodenal ulcer and bronchopneumonia.   Anatomic diagnosis was: thrombosis of left middle cerebral artery, duodenal ulcer with perforation and peritonitis, gastro-jejunostomy and bronchopneumonia.

For a discussion of the autopsy findings, see p. 285.

In summary, here was a man, who, after a cerebral insult, showed the following picture: Although his general intelligence was not bad, there was a *marked reduction in his spontaneity.*   His entire personality was *narrowed.* He was interested only in what was related to his person.   His contact with the outer world consisted mainly in trying to defend himself against the disturbances which arose from it.   He was friendly and cooperative in all relationships which he thought might help him, and was therefore very cooperative in all investigations.

Within certain limitations, he was able to speak words and even sentences.   He spoke *without paraphasia or dysarthria.*   He did not show any gross defect in understanding, although he did not understand more complicated things.

Compared to the relative retention of his capacity for speech and understanding, it was amazing that the patient was *unable to find the names for even the most ordinary objects,* even those names which he used in spontaneous speech.   The words, which he used had the character of "individual words" (see p. 63).   *His words had apparently lost meaning.*

Thus far, his language presents the *characteristics of amnesic aphasia.* This is in agreement with the *extreme concreteness in his spontaneous behavior* and his behavior in the tests, which leaves no doubt that he has a *severe impairment of abstraction.*

He deviates from the usual patients with amnesic aphasia, and thus also from the one previously mentioned (Case 15), by the severe *defect in repetition.*   Inasmuch as his understanding was relatively unimpaired, this inability could not be attributed to a difficulty in hearing.   Since there was no disability in motor speech, that could also be excluded as a cause.   As we have mentioned, he could not repeat at command a word which he had just used spontaneously.   Thus, we cannot but assume that we were dealing with a disturbance of *a special capacity for language repetition.*   Viewed thus, the patient shows symptoms of "central aphasia."

Autoptic findings of the brain: there was a large subarachnoid collection of fluid in the left temporal region, which escaped when the brain was removed.   The brain weighed 1200 Gm.   The vessels on the base showed moderate arteriosclerotic changes. The left hemisphere was smaller than the right and along the line of the left Sylvian fissure there was a deep excavation with *destruction of the entire superior temporal gyrus and Island of Reil and the lowermost portion of the precentral, postcentral supramarginal and angular gyri.* Broca's area and the middle and superior parietal convolutions were not involved. In a coronal section through the third ventricle the area of *softening was found to extend deeply to involve the claustrum and capsula externa,* ceasing at the border of the putamen. The temporal horn of the left lateral ventricle was slightly dilated. In sections through the substantia nigra and splerium corporis callosi, a part of the white matter of the centrum ovale was destroyed. The area of destruction extended posteriorly to the end of the angular gyrus. There was no other lesion and no special atrophy of the brain cortex.

Anatomic diagnosis: thrombosis of the left middle cerebral artery. Bronchopneumonia.

The localization of the lesion in the left hemisphere agrees with the fact that the patient was right-handed. The *defect of repetition* may be brought into connection with the *total destruction of the Island of Reil and the adjacent gyri, particularly the temporal and the parietal lobe (see p. 245), the amnesic aphasia with the defect there and in the adjacent gyri in the temporal and parietal lobes* which is suited to damage of the "non-speech mental area."

However, there are some difficulties in explaining the whole picture in relation to the anatomic findings:

First, how was it possible that the *patient heard and understood words and even sentences relatively well, if the temporal lobe of the left side was involved to such a degree by the lesion?* Not only was the so-called Wernicke region in the first temporal convolution destroyed but also the general auditory center of the left temporal lobe (the so-called Heschl's convolution). This defect forced us to assume that the patient's acoustic perception in general, and of words, must have been maintained by the corresponding part of the temporal lobe *in the right hemisphere.* However, should not the necessity of making this assumption lead us to doubt that the patient was a right-handed individual? The patient's statements, and the observation of his predominant use of the right hand made it more than probable that in essential performances he was right-handed. Furthermore, were he left-handed, it would be inconceivable that a left-sided brain lesion could produce such a severe incapacity of repetition and word-finding. Since these incapacities must be related to the left-sided lesion, it leaves no doubt as to the dominance of the left hemisphere for the concerned speech functions. Thus, we have no choice but to assume that in our patient, in spite of the dominance of the left hemisphere, the integrity of the *right hemisphere was able to guarantee understanding of speech, at least to a certain degree.*

This would not contradict other experiences. We know from other cases that a gross defect in the capacity for understanding speech usually occurs only if, in addition to a lesion in the left temporal lobe, the pathways which connect the right temporal lobe with the left hemisphere are also damaged (see p. 55).

However, there is still another difficulty. Usually in cases of destruction of the "Wernicke center," and, according to Goldstein, of the Insula Reili also, we find paraphasia. But our patient had no paraphasia: We tried to explain this when we discussed central aphasia, and I should like here to refer to this discussion which brought us to the conclusion that the *lack of paraphasia could be understood by the special condition of the case* (see p. 241).

To summarize our hypothesis, we may say: We believe that the lack of the capacity for repetition and word-finding was caused by the lesion of the left Island of Reil and adjacent convolutions in the temporal and parietal lobes of the left hemisphere, corresponding to the patient's right-handedness; his capacity for understanding speech was probably guaranteed by the right hemisphere; his capacity for speaking without paraphasia, by the 3rd frontal convolution of the left hemisphere, perhaps in connection with the corresponding convolution of the right hemisphere.

The next case shows, *in the beginning, the picture of amnesic aphasia*. With increasing damage of the brain due to a growing brain tumor, other defects appeared, such as of inner speech and of the non-speech realm of thinking and acting.

Case 17*

This 54 year old man showed no anomalies till a few weeks before admission; a slight fainting spell was the beginning of his disease. Since that time, he complained of headache on the left temporal region and fatigue. He could not speak as well as before. Particularly, he could *not find the words for concrete objects*.

At the first examination he was oriented in all respects, quiet, spoke quite well, but showed a lack of some words in spontaneous speech.

Physical examination showed no anomalies. On the left side, the temporal region was sensitive to tapping and pinprick; slight right facial paresis. No disturbances of the sense organs and of the reflexes were noted.

In general, the patient did not show any mental deviation. His judgment seemed to be good, he realized, with anger, his failures. His speech was lively, intonation was good. There was *no paraphasia*. He often searched for words, then hesitated and spoke like a stutterer.

(What age?)	54
(When born?)	January 1st (+)
(Where?)	In . . . (Suddenly he gives the correct name of the city.)
(Shortly afterwards: Where born?)	Das habe ich wieder verschmissen . . . (That I have again misplaced)

* Published by Goldstein (81).

(Where do you live?)	+
(Date today)	+
(Month?)	June, July, August, September . . . July +
(Backward)	December, January, no . . . Friday, December, November, October, November . . .
(Year?)	+
(How long sick?)	There I am already four . . . four . . . four . . . (stuttering) weeks, and this is last day, 8 days ago it started (points to his left temple).
(How many children?)	5 +
(Names)	Lise, Mina, Berta, Marie, Hans. +
(Were you in military service?)	Yes, Ostpreussische Fussartillerie. (Gives correctly the year, the name of his sergeant.)
(Afterwards?)	Coachman
(Where?)	Here in K. +
(Series of numbers)	1 to 20
(Backward)	20 . . . 19, 18, 17, 16, 15, 14 . . . 13, 12, 11, 9 . . . 87654321
(Tens)	. . .
(Backward)	with defects
(ABC)	a, b, c, d, e, f, z . . . (he says: I could never do that)
(Festivals)	New Year, Easter, Whitsuntide.
(When Christmas?)	. . .
(In winter?)	Yes, there is my birthday.
(When is Christmas?)	In the last month.
(What is the festival in December?)	W . . . We have said . . .
(Is it Whitsuntide?)	No.
(Easter?)	No.
(Christmas?)	Yes.

Naming of objects:

1. Seen objects: The patient names a number of objects correctly, as chair, heat, house, bed, table, duck, (how he proceeds in finding the word was not investigated).

(Roll of wax)	das is Seif (soap—Zungseif, wie sie da man—
(What is its use?)	zum anstecken (to light).
(Wachs?)	*Ja*, Wachs.
(Tintenwischer) (pen wiper)	Das ist auch zu diesem einzustecken, die Feder einzustecken.
(Glas?)	No.
(Tintenwischer?)	*Ja*, Tintenwischer.
(Telephon)	Das ist vom Dinge da (holds his hand to the mouth, as if he wanted to talk into a telephone) Das so Dings da man durchsprechen kann.
(Telegraph oder Telephon?)	Telephon.
(Watte) (cotton wool)	Das ist von diesem—Watte—(puts his finger in the ears).
(Bleistift) (pencil)	Das ist von so einem . . . (makes writing movements with the hand). Das ist zum aus, zum schreiben,

	schreiber, ich kann nicht darauf kommen, zum nehmen zum schreiben (takes it in hand and writes).
(Messer?) (knife)	No, kein Messer.
(Federhalter?)	
(penholder)	Ist es auch nicht, aber so etwas.
(Bleistift?) (pencil)	*Ja*, Bleistift (pencil).
(Kleiderbugel) (hanger)	Wenn ich ein Jackett aufhangen habe (takes it in his hand, makes movements of hanging dresses) wenn man die Kleider reingemacht hat, dann hängt man sie auf, ich kann nicht darauf kommen—aufhängen.

In the same way, he behaved in naming drawn objects and if the object were presented to another sense. He recognizes the object, does not find the word but *identifies the correct word*. Names the patient does not find, he cannot write down. There is no difference between the word-finding behavior in concrete object and abstract ideas.

Intelligence in general, judgment, insight into the defect seemed to be intact.

Repetition: Also repeats correctly long and complicated words, even words he does not know, as Ararat, Xerxes: xerxet. He repeats all letters.

Spelling:

(Feder)—(Messer) M-e-s-e-r; (Haus) H-o-s-a

(Ohr) O-r-r-; (Stuhl) Sch-t-u-l; (Feder) F-d-r;

(Bleistift) B-l-s; (Tinte) T-n-m-t; (Hand) H-a-t;

(Papier) P-i-i-r; (Auge) A-u-g-e; (Nase) N-a-s-e;

(Finger) Fe-e-r-m-; (Buch) B-o-r.

In the task involving *words to compose of letters*, he is very poor.

	Reads	Composes
(V-a-t-e-r)	+	V-t-a-e-r (reads Vater)
(T-e-i-z)	+	Z-t-e-i
(Zeit)		
(M-z-g-a)	—	G-z-n-a
(Zange)		G-n-a-z
		G-a-n-ze
		(reads Zange)
(O-hOr) Which is correct?	+	
(H-o-r)		
(G-a-u-e- Which is correct?	+	first he puts:
(A-u-g-e)		g-a-u-e
		then a-u-g-e
(F-ed-er)		
(R-e-d-f-e) Which is correct?	+	r-e-d-f-e
		Feder

He shows great difficulty in giving the number of letters, even if the word consists of only four letters.

Understanding of language: He follows directions, shows the parts of the body, the objects in the room, fulfills more complicated tasks, as going into the other room, taking a bottle of water there, filling a glass with water and putting down the full glass, etc.

He is able to describe properties of objects (often with circumlocutions), can express which object or idea is meant if one describes it. His judgment in respect to the things which belong to his life did not seem to be disturbed. Special examinations of his capacity of abstraction, of building of concepts, etc., were not performed. Thus, a definite conclusion as to a defect in this respect is not possible. His difficulty in understanding what one means with spelling, and in reciting series backward, and some answers which reveal particular concreteness may be interpreted as expression of a defect in this respect.

He has no apractic phenomena. Drawing is abnormally bad, he apparently has difficulty in recalling forms. His capacity of combination, as it is necessary for fulfilling the Heilbronner test, was apparently not disturbed.

Reading: Letters and numbers and a great number of words and short sentences are usually given promptly and with understanding. He also reads unknown words in a spelling way. From a number of presented written words, he indicates acoustically presented ones promptly.

Writing: He was previously a skilful writer.

Spontaneous writing: very paraphasic, the individual letters in general are given correctly.

Often it happened that he apparently did not know *how to write a letter;* he would start in a wrong way, write a false letter, finally producing or not producing the correct form. He always recognizes if he has written a letter in a false way.

On dictation, he writes words partially correctly, partially with *paraphasic* defects. He writes single numbers and those consisting of two digits promptly; in numbers with three places, he often omits some number.

He writes letters on *dictation* as follows: (a) +; (b) mbe; (c) ze; (d) de; (e) eh; (g) g; (h) ha; (i) ihm (him); (l) +; (m) mein (my); (n) nn; (p) pe; (r) er; (s) se; (u) +; (v) fau; (w) wau; (x) xil; (b) ab; (s) es.

Copying of letters, words and numbers was prompt.

In this state of the disease, the patient showed as outstanding symptom the *difficulty in finding words* for objects which he recognized very well and could always find among a number of objects which corresponded to a presented word. He showed characteristic circumlocutions which revealed that he recognized the objects. His motor speech and understanding of speech did not show defects; repetition also was normal. Thus, he showed the *typical picture of amnesic aphasia.*

His behavior revealed that he was not disturbed grossly in general as to the mental functions. Whether his capacity of abstraction was disturbed we cannot say from the protocols.

Some deviations in writing correspond to the defect in writing we have described in the previous case with amnesic aphasia (see p. 252) and can be considered as expressions of the latter.

Besides the symptoms typical for amnesic aphasia, the patient showed some other disturbances: (1) in writing; (2) in spelling and combining letters into words; some paragraphia; (3) some stuttering in the beginning of words.

Concerning the defect in writing letters on dictation which the patient presents, it corresponds to the phenomena we have mentioned in the first case of amnesic aphasia (see p. 252), and can find the same explanation (amnesic-aphasic disturbance of writing) (see p. 253). However, this is not so certain with regard to the difficulty to elicit the forms of letters spontaneously. We could consider this as due to a defect in abstraction. The voluntary production of letters in imagination certainly needs abstract attitude. Nevertheless, in consideration of the symptoms which appeared later, the defects in the production of forms of letters of ideatoric-apractic type, the mentioned difficulty to write the letters correctly, may more probably be considered as the first expression of a damage of that kind due to the damage of the parietal region by the tumor.

The case can teach us nothing definite concerning the pathology underlying amnesic aphasia, for we are dealing with a *tumor* (see autopsy findings, p. 232). But from the symptomatology and the postmortem, we can assume that at the time the patient presented amnesic aphasia as a nearly isolated symptom, the motor and sensory areas were almost intact and the tumor did not damage the region of "inner speech" (see p. 244) severely. The patient did not show paraphasia in speaking or disturbance of repetition. The effect of the tumor could be considered as *a slight damage of the "speech area" and the "non-speech mental area"* of the brain. Later, with increase of damage of inner speech area, more and more inner speech proved affected and other symptoms of speech disturbances, as well as of thinking, came to the fore. We consider this state in the discussion of "central aphasia" (see p. 232).

The Anatomic Basis of Amnesic Aphasia

The anatomic basis of amnesic aphasia is not at all clear. There are different reasons for this. The cases are rare, and the number of post-mortems in typical cases is small. Abstract attitude is a very high mental function and is thus probably related to complex anatomic structures which may be damaged early even in fine lesions. This may explain why we find it disturbed in diffuse lesions of the brain cortex which may not produce any other gross symptoms. Such is the case in arteriosclerosis, general paresis, Pick's disease, diffuse injuries of the brain, etc. If amnesic aphasia occurs in a localized affection, the latter usually concerns the *temporo-parietal region;* but it must be of a particular kind, it must not damage this region too much, otherwise disturbances of instrumentalities of speech and of the mental phenomena are so predominant that amnesic aphasia does not come clearly to the fore. A fine damage in this region which is suited to produce *a fine diffuse damage of the cortical function,* can take place particularly in tumor or abscess in this region—the two conditions in which particularly amnesic aphasia appears. I stressed such an origin of this symptom complex years ago. Impairment of abstraction appears in lesion of various parts of the brain, in lesions of the frontal and parietal lobe, and in both cases we observe the defect in naming. However, it seems that the clearest development of this symptom complex *occurs if the lesion is located in the temporo-parietal region; this would mean if the speech area were affected to a certain degree too.* One may argue that with this statement I give up my theory of the origin of amnesic aphasia as due to impairment of abstract attitude. Not at all. *Impairment of abstract attitude remains,* to my experience, *the prerequisite without which the defect in "naming" never occurs. A lesion of the "speech area" alone is never followed by the amnesic-aphasic defect in word-finding.*

Some damage of the instrumentalities seems to play a rôle, particularly for the development of the *extreme* defects of naming. Difficulties of innervation of instrumentalities can aggravate the basic defect. The intactness of the instrumentalities, on the other hand, supports "pseudo-naming" (see p. 61). Some defect of them may hinder the development of the latter and hence a particularly severe picture of disturbance of word-finding may result.

CHAPTER IX

Pictures of Speech Disturbances Due to Impairment of the Non-Language Mental Performances

THERE are to be observed clinical pictures which—as much as they may differ in their special symptomatology—have in common one phenomenon: The speech instrumentalities themselves can be assumed to be intact, to a greater or lesser degree, while the patient is not able to use them or cannot understand correctly what the words mean when he hears them. There is one group of these patients where the intactness of repetition in contrast to the defects in understanding and spontaneous speaking is particularly apparent. This was called, after Wernicke, transcortical aphasia. The name, transcortical aphasia, originated from a definite theoretic interpretation which is no longer acceptable, and is certainly not a fortunate one. However, I would consider it useful to maintain this name till we have a better understanding of the underlying functional disturbance, because we are accustomed to bring a definite symptom complex in relation to it.

A. THE TRANSCORTICAL APHASIAS

The problem of these forms of speech disturbances is not only very complex but is much confused by the various theoretic interpretations which have often hindered investigations.

I consider it my task to characterize as clearly as possible, using the literature and my own experiences, the various forms observed and to see how we can understand them from a common point of view.

Originally, transcortical motor and transcortical sensory aphasia were distinguished, and it was assumed that these forms occur if the pathways are interrupted between that part of the brain which is important for non-language mental functions and the motor or sensory speech center (Lichtheim, 185). If, in the motor form, sensory disturbances were present, an attempt was made to explain them by the dependence of motor speech on sensory speech—according to the theory we have mentioned before (see p. 83). From this point of view, it was denied that a real transcortical motor aphasia exists, and assumed that the motor disturbances, too, are due to a lesion of the "transcortical sensory" pathway (e.g., Lewandowsky, 181). Cases where the sensory functions are intact or very little disturbed induced the assumption of another possiblity for appearance of the transcortical motor symptom complex. It was considered to be the effect of a partial defect of the motor speech area itself, which disturbed particularly the voluntary, intentional speech, but left the motor functions themselves intact to such a degree that repetition was possible (see p. 82). Other authors tried to explain this form of aphasia as due to higher mental defects themselves (particularly Pierre Marie, Moutier).

The literature contains a similar diversity of interpretation of the picture of transcortical sensory aphasia. The assumption of a defect of a "transcortical" sensory pathway did not find much approval, though it was also assumed by some, e.g., Lewandowsky. Bastian (6) considered it the effect of a partial functional defect of the sensory speech center, a sensory aphasia in improvement. This idea was widely accepted. Heilbronner, who agreed with this interpretation in general, declared that restitution of function after sensory aphasia must be, in these cases, of a particular kind. Otherwise, it would not be understandable that a similar anatomic condition is followed sometimes by another symptom complex, for instance, subcortical sensory aphasia.

Still another interpretation was that these preserved performances were the effect of a function of the other hemisphere (Bastian, Liepmann, Pick; in the most definite way, Niessl v. Mayendorf, 216).

Finally also, for this form of transcortical aphasia, diffuse mental damage was assumed (Monakow, 209, Mingazzini, 204).

Grossly, one can distinguish clinically three groups of pictures of transcortical aphasias: (1) Those cases in which the defect of spontaneous speech is predominant; (2) those in which sensory defects are predominant; (3) a group, where disturbances of speaking and understanding are present.

Common to all is *preservation of repetition* and other signs of normal functioning of instrumentalities.

On another occasion (86), I have given a detailed description of these forms of aphasia. Here I shall repeat the essential results, somewhat modified by my newer general concept.

(1) *The Transcortical Motor Symptom Complexes*

1. The first way this symptom complex can originate is a *partial damage of the motor speech area*, a heightening of the threshold of the motor speech performances. We have mentioned this type when we discussed motor aphasia (see p. 82). It is distinguished from other forms of transcortical motor symptom complexes by the *lack of any other speech disturbances or mental defects* on the one hand, on the other hand, by *more or less defects in the motor act of speaking*. The patient's speech may be abrupt and accompanied by perforced movements of the face. The difference between

spontaneous speech and repetition may not be so outspoken as in other forms. Speaking in series, particularly their fluent recital and the use of those grammatical forms which are of motor origin (see p. 81), is disturbed, the patients showing more or less motor agrammatism (see p. 81). Naming of objects is better than spontaneous speech. In contrast to amnesic aphasia, spontaneous finding of words is even more disturbed than in the object naming test, in which the patients with amnesic aphasia show such a great deficiency. The reason is plausible. In amnesic aphasia, where the difficulty to find the word is due to impairment of abstract attitude (see p. 246), sensory stimulation (presentation of objects, etc.) cannot help; this may be of great help when we are dealing with a heightening of the motor threshold. The same concerns reading aloud. This is sometimes even better than repetition (Bonhoeffer, Case I; see the report of the case, p. 206). Writing must not show any deviation.

The symptom complex is mostly of a *transient character*. If we are dealing with an increasing defect, the patient will later show total motor aphasia; in decreasing damage he will also regain his spontaneous speech, etc. We find this defect, therefore, particularly after injury, where often the initial shock produces a slight damage of the motor speech area, and after disappearance of the shock, normal speech comes back. I observed this frequently after gunshot wounds (see also the cases of Lichtheim, 184, Bonhoeffer, 18, and Posthammer, 250).

2. In a second type of transcortical motor aphasia, we find besides the motor speech defect an *impairment of the impulse to speak at all*, and we are inclined to consider this impairment as essential cause. If the lack of intention to speak is of a very high degree, then we find also some disturbances of repetition. Repetition, too, presupposes certain impulses on the part of the patient (if it is not echolalic; see p. 303). However, repetition may still be possible, but not spontaneous speech. These patients usually also show a lack of speech in reaction to questions and to other stimulations. They are also impaired in their emotional speech reactions. But the patient, in general absolutely mute, may occasionally be capable in emotional situations of uttering correct sentences (Case of Noethe, 219). Indeed, his reaction in all these respects is better than spontaneous speech which may be totally lacking (cases of Rothmann, 261, Quensel, 252, personal observation 86). It is characteristic for these cases that the motor act itself is well preserved.

If we assume that the speech defect is a consequence of the defect in impulse,* an expression of an akinesis produced by an organic lesion, it

---

* It should not be overlooked that the phenomenon of impulse is not at all clear. We use a term which needs very much concretization. Particularly, the relation to the "mental disturbances," with which we shall deal soon, should be clarified.

may be surprising that the akinesis shows in speech and not in other activities of the patients. We could assume that this is due to a selective effect on different performances. I think such an assumption would not be too far-fetched.

Anatomically, we can bring this symptom complex into relation with a *lesion in the frontal lobe.* There is no doubt that in lesions of the lobe itself we find a lack of intention to speak. However, the patients show lack of intention in all performances (see case of Hartmann, 126); or other mental symptoms, characteristic for this localization of the lesion (see Goldstein, 106). This must not be so in the cases we have in mind. I am not fully satisfied with the mentioned interpretation of the defect of spontaneous speech. A closer review of the cases, also from the anatomic point of view, brought me to the conviction, that in these cases there exists *besides* the impairment of intention (anatomically designated as *a lack of the influence of the frontal lobe*) a *certain damage of the motor speech area* itself, and that this combination produces the picture differing from both the transcortical motor aphasia produced by a partial defect of the motor speech area alone, and the cases where the frontal lobe itself is severely damaged.

A lesion located in the region between the frontal lobe and motor speech area, which may not damage severely both areas themselves, may be followed by this symptom complex. This would explain, too, why sometimes more general akinesis, sometimes more real motor speech defects are present.

The case of Noethe showed for a certain time general akinesis. In one of my cases, some symptoms of direct damage of the motor acts, e.g., also in repetition, and in Rothmann's case, certain defects in reciting series, pointed to some defect of the motor speech area.

Assuming that we are dealing with a *combination between a slight damage of intention and a slight defect of the motor activities,* the behavior of the patients in the different speech performances becomes understandable, because this combination will damage the different performances in a different way corresponding to the different degree intention or motor activity have to be intact to execute them.

Most affected is spontaneous speech, often totally lacking; less affected is reactive speech following sensory stimulation by presentation of objects, etc. Naming of objects and reading may be possible to a certain degree, at times when other spontaneous speech is totally lacking. (When this difference is not present, then we are probably dealing with a combination with amnesic aphasia or with other causes, which produce a more severe damage of motor speech; Case Rothmann, 261). Writing is sometimes better preserved, particularly in naming objects, than spontaneous speech.

It may be disturbed particularly when the lesion extends in the neighborhood of the posterior part of FII., an area which is so important for the motor performances of writing (see p. 129).

Speaking of series may be lacking, if the patient has to produce the series spontaneously because beginning needs a special impulse. But it can be well preserved if one presents the first members of a series and brings the patient into the motor rhythm—at least much better than in the cases of the first mentioned form of transcortical motor aphasia (see Cases of Heilbronner, 135, Forster, 86, my case, 86).

Sometimes, in these cases, the spontaneous use of the muscles which are used in speaking is also disturbed more or less for non-speaking activities. A patient of mine showed a lack of spontaneous mimic; his face was rigid. He could not perform the movements of the mouth on demand or only slowly and with difficulty, e.g., in showing how to purse up his lips, how to blow a paper, while he was able to do all this in imitation or in response to an adequate stimulus (for instance, blowing a real paper). Similar symptoms were shown by the patient of Noethe.

The *anatomy* of these cases is not clear. The most important case in this respect is Rothmann's observation (261): a small lesion in the white matter in the posterior part of the 3rd frontal convolution so located that it has apparently particularly severed the fibers originating from the frontal convolution without affecting severely the cortex of the frontal lobe and of Broca's area. Furthermore, there should be cited the anatomic findings of Quensel and Noethe.

With the assumption of a damage of "intention," we come near to the disturbances of voluntary motor speech due to damage of the processes of the non-speech mental processes (see p. 309).

3. There is one question which must further be touched upon. Can the picture of transcortical motor aphasia be the effect of *taking over the function of repetition by the other hemisphere?* This was assumed first by Bastian (6), and later emphasized particularly by Niessl von Meyendorf (217). We have discussed in general how difficult it is to decide whether any speech function is taken over by the "other" hemisphere and how careful we should be with such an assumption (see p. 51).

In most of the cases, the left speech area was not so damaged that one was forced to assume that repetition could not have been affected by its function. Even in cases where there seems to be no other way to understand the preserved repetition, as in the cases of Farge, Bonhoeffer, which Niessl von Mayendorf uses as example for his theory, there remains the question of why was the path over the other hemisphere not used for spontaneous speech too? The intact motor speech area in the minor hemisphere should make this possible. The explanation I have given (see p. 51) seems to me more adequate to the observable facts.

(2) *The Transcortical Sensory Symptom Complexes*

We have stressed that the way from sensory speech perception to understanding goes through various steps. The observed symptom complexes are the effect of a stoppage of function at one or the other step. But a survey shows that symptom complexes are not understandable simply as effect of purely quantitative diminution of function. Each step represents more or less a qualitatively different function, and the functions are not simply added; new complexes originate. For example, repetition is not always the same, it is at one step automatic, at another, voluntary, i.e., performed with or without higher mental influences. Correct repetition, on the other hand, secondarily influences understanding of perception as well as meaning; the patient may become aware of the meaning only after repeating. The rôle which the awakening of concepts of words in repetition plays for understanding is not fully realized. All these possibilities have to be taken into consideration if one wants to judge correctly understanding and repetition in an individual case of that type.

As to the possibilities through which the transcortical sensory symptom complexes may originate, we begin with the often discussed problem: Can this form of aphasia be the *effect of a partial lesion of the sensory speech area?*

If one considers the effect of function of this area as perceptive speech experience, perception of acoustic phenomena as *speech*, it is scarcely understandable that impairment of this function should produce a picture which is characterized by lack of understanding combined with preserved repetition. Imperfect perception of sounds usually has a greater effect on repetition than on understanding; we may be unable to repeat words of a foreign language but may understand their meaning. We can observe the same thing in children in a definite stage of learning language. (This is not in contradiction to the fact that the child may repeat words which he does not "understand.") Also for grown-ups, perception of characteristics of the sound complex may be sufficient for understanding, not for repetition, particularly if we consider how much resistance many people, especially those of limited education, have when they must do things which seem to them not quite correct (see p. 72).

We have mentioned before (see p. 91) that damaged speech perception may not be sufficient to evoke the correct idea but may incite some understanding, the "sphere" of "ideas" to which this sound complex belongs; but this does not enable the person to repeat the presented words. Thus, again, we see imitation more disturbed than understanding.

Those authors, indeed, who bring transcortical sensory aphasia into relation to sensory aphasia do not mean the pure word deafness but Wernicke's aphasia, which they consider as due to a lesion of the sensory speech area, of the acoustic speech images. This, however, as I have tried to show, is an effect of a lesion of the sensory speech area and the adjacent part of the Insula Reili—functionally considered the effect of impairment of speech sounds combined with those of "speech concepts" (see p. 93). If that is the case, this defect should disturb repetition still more because the speech concepts are significant for repetition (see p. 103). As a matter of fact, I was inclined in the mentioned case of partial word deafness (see p. 103) to make responsible for the disturbances of repetition a concomitant damage of the word concepts

If I thus reject the theory that transcortical sensory aphasia is a less severe form of sensory aphasia, I do not at all deny that this symptom complex can occur clinically in a state of restitution of Wernicke's aphasia. But this does not prove that between it and sensory aphasia there is only a quantitative difference as to the underlying damage. Anatomically, there is no possibility to come to any decision concerning this point. The lesions are, in both symptom complexes, located in the temporal lobe. Lesions very similarly located may produce word deafness or Wernicke's aphasia, or transcortical sensory aphasia (see p. 227); without this, we would be able to say why one or the other symptom complex occurs, which would seem to indicate how little anatomy can help us here.

From the functional point of view, the clinical relation between transcortical sensory aphasia and Wernicke's aphasia can be explained in the following way: As long as the perceptive function is grossly disturbed, repetition and understanding are both disturbed; whether there exists besides the damage of the perceptual sphere a defect of the relation between perception and understanding (the non-language mental processes) cannot be decided because it cannot become apparent in special symptoms. Only in improvement of the perceptive symptoms can it become evident whether such another defect is present (if it did not improve, too), namely, in the more severe defect of understanding than repetition. Thus, we are confronted with the picture of transcortical sensory aphasia which in the beginning was hidden behind the severe perceptual defect. This interpretation is, in principle, different from the assumption that transcortical sensory aphasia is simply a state (or quantitatively smaller degree) of Wernicke's aphasia. If one considers more carefully what the authors really meant when they emphasized this clinical occurrence of transcortical sensory aphasia in cases of Wernicke's sensory aphasia, one sees that behind the simple description of its origin the given explanations are not so far from that given by me; thus, as to the preceding, if Heilbronner denies that transcortical sensory aphasia is simply a smaller degree of Wernicke's aphasia, and if Bonhoeffer writes that not simply the extension of the lesion in the left temporal lobe is of significance (whether the one or the other symptom complex appears), but that the transcortical picture occurs if a *definite substratum* is affected, if some association fibers are destroyed (namely those which connect the temporal lobe with other parts of the brain) and others which guarantee repetition are preserved. Pick means about the same in saying that if in temporal lobe lesions the damage of the acoustic speech center decreases, perception of words may again become possible; but understanding remains impaired because the "pathways from A–B" are lesioned.

The interpretation of transcortical sensory symptom complexes by lesion of special pathways between the peripheral areas and the "Begriffs-feld" (area of concepts) produced no difficulty for the authors who assumed such separate direct pathways. This is different for my general concept which denies isolated connections between the motor and sensory speech area and the rest of the brain, and considers instrumentalities and non-language mental performances—both motor and sensory—equally related with each other by a unitary performance which we call the concepts of words (see p. 93). Anatomically, the stimulation of the area important for the non-language mental performances goes over the central speech area. From our concept, we would expect that always not only understanding but also spontaneous speech will be affected if the relation between concepts and the non-language mental performances are severed. As a matter of fact, that is usually the case. It is often not fully realized because in these cases the motor defects are usually explained as *secondary effect of the sensory* defect according to the theory that all speaking goes the way over sensory speech. We shall see that the motor defect is to be considered as the effect of the same damage as the sensory defect, not as the consequence of the latter (see p. 301).

There exist, indeed, some observations in which the transcortical sensory defect is so in the foreground that another explanation seems necessary. I have pointed to the possibility that this picture may be the effect of a *combination* of a *slight damage of acoustic speech perceptions and a slight damage of the relation between the instrumentalities and the non-language mental performances.*

This slight damage may not impair acoustic speech perception to such a degree that it can no longer elicit repetition, but sufficiently to disturb understanding, if the *process of understanding itself is somewhat diminished, too.* On the other hand, a certain alteration of the relation between instrumentalities and non-language mental performances may impair understanding, *if the basis—the acoustic speech perception—is not quite normal*, but may not be severe enough to damage spontaneous speech, particularly if the motor instrumentalities are intact. We meet here a phenomenon to which enough attention is not paid, namely, that the *combination of two defects may produce definite symptoms, while each defect alone may not have any—at least visible-disturbing effect.* Thus, no symptoms may appear as long as one or the other of the slightly affected functions may be alone in action, but may appear if combined function of both is required for a performance.

If we so assume, at least for some cases of transcortical sensory aphasia, some damage of the sensory speech area, this is not in contradiction to our denial that they represent a state of lesser damage of the latter as has been assumed (see p. 298). Without the concomitant damage of the relation between instrumentalities and non-language mental performances, such a lesion of the sensory speech area never has this effect.

The main characteristics of these cases are: *Understanding is severely damaged*, much more than spontaneous speech. The patients speak much, they usually show some reduction of words, particularly lack of nouns, probably due to a concomitantly existing amnesic aphasia. If one subtracts this latter defect, the language appears correct, meaningful, the syntactical and grammatical structure quite well organized. Some paraphasia may be present, probably as effect of a slight damage of the central speech area. The following utterance of a patient of Bischoff can be considered as characteristic of the spontaneous utterances of these patients: "Ich bin schön heute nicht viel, ich müss jetzt hingehen zu meinen Kindern und will auch dort zu leben, ja das ich benützen so, dass ich benützen soll und dann ging ich ganz weg von hier; ist mehr Qual hier und dort, ist es bald zu Ende. Ich bin schön sehr lange—schön sehr lange verbraucht, ich schön alles und so danke ich gar so brauche—und dann werde ich tot sein." This example shows that the spontaneous speech is much less distorted than in those cases with transcortical sensory symptoms where the latter are an expression of a more general mental defect (see further, p. 309).

Speaking of series is good, the patients being able to start series voluntarily.

Reading aloud is intact; understanding usually impaired. Spontaneous writing corresponds to spontaneous speech and is usually somewhat more disturbed than the latter; writing on dictation can be intact.

Often there exists a diminution of acoustic attention and of memory for speech, which points to some damage of the acoustic speech area. The character of repetition leads us to assume that the relations between instrumentalities and non-speech performances are not strongly severed.

The patient we have in mind does not show at all echolalic repetition (see p. 303).

Our interpretation of these cases is in agreement with the appearance of this symptom complex in improvement of a severe total sensory aphasia or as the first state of a condition which later shows this form of aphasia (as in a case of Pick) and with the anatomic findings: lesions in the temporal lobe which do not directly affect the word deafness area but damage it to a certain degree and destroy more or less the posterior part of the left hemisphere (Case Bonhoeffer, 19), or a diffuse atrophy particularly affecting the temporal lobe (Pick's case, 233), or atrophy of the temporal lobes in both hemispheres (Case Bischoff, 15).

(3) Mixed Transcortical Aphasias

In a number of cases of transcortical aphasia, there are disturbances of spontaneous speech as well as of understanding. The symptom complexes are the effect of impairment of the "relationship" between the instrumentalities and the non-language mental performances, or of the mental performances themselves. Often, both factors are involved, the one more, the other less. Corresponding to the complexity of this "relationship" and the structure of the non-language mental performances (see p. 315), the clinical pictures belonging to this group of aphasia are very complex. The origin of each observable defect is not at all always clear. The picture becomes particularly complicated when as often occurs, the instrumentalities are damaged, too, more or less the motor or the sensory part— or the concepts of words. The differences between the degree of alteration of the spontaneous speech and understanding become understandable only if one takes all involved factors into consideration.

If we consider first those cases with speech defect particularly due to the damage of the "relationship", we meet different pictures as to the form in which repetition presents itself. Repetition appears more or less without understanding and more or less without intention, i.e., compulsive. As long as some understanding or intention to repeat is present, some "relation" can be assumed to be preserved; if repetition shows the character of echolalia, then the "isolation" of the speech area can be considered nearly complete.

Echolalia is particularly developed if both factors are impaired. A defect of intention alone does not produce echolalia as long as understanding is only slightly damaged, and vice versa. If understanding is disturbed, but not totally impossible, the patient may repeat without understanding, which is particularly surprising if he repeats even sentences correctly. He need not speak in an outspoken echolalic way. One has the impression that he grasps at least that he is supposed to repeat and does it somewhat voluntarily. Indeed, some understanding does not always hinder echolalic repetition (Stransky, 290).

Anatomically, the first of the defects important for origin of echolalia is related to lesions in the temporal lobes and the bridges between them and the posterior part of the brain, particularly the parietal lobe; the second, the lack of impulse, to lesions in the frontal lobes or the bridges between these and the speech area. Sometimes one can observe how, with increase of the anatomic damage, the parrot-like character of repetition becomes more apparent (as in a case of Monakow, 208), and with decrease, echolalia makes place for a more voluntary repetition (as in a case of Bonhoeffer).

The spontaneous speech is not at all lacking in such cases (if there is not a severe disturbance of impulse). Sometimes the patients even speak a great deal, although in a disconnected way. The motor performances themselves are not, or not much, disturbed, but the language of the patients lacks some categories of words, particularly nouns and syntactic forms. It consists mostly of the same phrases, as "What shall I do?" or "Let us do," "That is bad," "It is all right," etc.

I give, in the following, some spontaneous utterances of such a patient in the original (German) language, which makes the characteristics more apparent than an English translation:

"Jo, jo, Sie seien sehr orndlich, that ich bei Ihnen, das alle Tage machen genug und genug ih ha jo garnischt gemacht and soto es jo glugs, dass ich gewiss das sollte machen. Gott sei gedankt grod ock wieder do nei" (points to his arm).

Or another utterance of a patient of Quensel: "Ich bin doch hier unten, na wenn ich gewesen bin ich weess nicht, we das, nu wenn ich, ob das nun doch, noch, ja. Was Sie her, wenn ich, och ich weess nicht, we das hier war ja," etc.

The spontaneous speech in these cases differs from that in motor aphasia by the fact that it contains "small words," which are missing particularly in motor aphasia (see p. 81). While the motor execution is better preserved, syntax is disturbed (which in motor aphasia is particularly maintained). It differs from that in transcortical motor aphasia by the fact that the patients speak much more; from that in transcortical sensory aphasia (see p. 297) by the much greater destruction of the utterances. Common to both is predominance of the small words and lack of nouns. The predominance of the small words may seem to be in contradiction to our assumption that these words are particularly related to the higher mental processes. But this is not the case. This relationship concerns only the use of the words in isolation. Under this condition, the patient cannot produce them. He can utter them within definite phrases where they appear as parts of motor automatisms without being aware. In addition, these words do not mean something definite; they merely represent learned motor series which may be produced quite correctly if the patient is urged. This is revealed in the appearance of grammatical forms in the remnants of patients' speech.

(4) *Echolalia*

Case 18*

A 64 year old bookdealer, after cerebral insult, showed *total loss of speech* and paresis of the right arm, symptoms which disappeared within two weeks. One month afterwards, a *second insult* occurred: loss of speech, general confusion. Some improvement but picture not much changed up to the exitus, due to pulmonary infarct.

General condition good. The patient seems not to be confused or demented. He recognizes objects. There is unfortunately no detailed protocol about the mental condition of the patient.

Spontaneous speech: Reduced to the words "ja," "jawohl," "nun ja."

Understanding: Patient apparently does not understand what one speaks to him.

Repetition: Words and short sentences like "I am hungry" are *repeated correctly,* in an echolalic way, apparently *without understanding*.

Naming of objects: Only a few correct; usually not able to find the name.

Writing: patient writes spontaneously correct words, in a sequence that gives no meaning.

Writing on dictation: Correct.

Copying: Not examined.

Reading: Reads the newspaper aloud, apparently without understanding anything.

Postmortem: Arteriosclerosis of the basal arteries. The gyri of the whole cortex are abnormally small, the surface at different places shows very fine tubercles.

There is a yellow softening which is located on the bridge between gyrus parietalis inferior and the posterior part of gyrus supramarginalis, and temporalis I which affects the lower part of the inferior gyrus parietal and the middle gyrus parietalis from gyrus supramarginalis to the posterior end of fova sylvi in an extension of 27 mm. It is extended further in the sulcus of I and II temporal convolution so far that it has here an extension of 65 mm. The softening concerns the cortex more than the white matter. In the second temporal convolution itself there is a superficial softening.

Not affected is temporal convolution I, cortex and white matter, but near the Insula the cortex shows atrophy. The gyri frontales in both hemispheres are small. Further, there is in middle third of the corpus striatum a small softening which is extended from nucleus caudatus and lentiformis to the Claustrum.

The right hemisphere is totally intact.

This large lesion is well suited to *damage particularly the bridges between the speech area and the other parts of the left hemisphere,* especially to the parietal lobe, which is certainly very important for the non-language mental processes. The preservation of temporal convolution I, insula Reili and Broca region has *guaranteed repetition*. The severity of the

* Published by Heubner, 1889.

defect in the bridge between speech area and the area of the non-language mental performances combined with *some defect* in the *frontal lobes* can be considered as the *cause of the echolalic character of repetition*. The fact that the patient was not severely deteriorated, leads us to assume that that part of the brain responsible for the non-speech processes was not severely affected.

There is no reason to assume that repetition was here the effect of the function of the right hemisphere. It was present immediately after the severe lesion; the parts of the brain in the left hemisphere which one brings in relation to the instrumentalities were in a condition certainly suited to function in an almost normal way.

While in the preceding case of echolalia (case 18) the non-language mental performances were not severely disturbed, in the following case the echolalia goes parallel to severe general mental defects.

Case 19*

A man, 65 years old, had shown mental changes since some months before he had undergone apoplectic insult with loss of speech and right hemiplegia. Since that time, he had been confused, excited, mentally deteriorated.

Examination reveals no neurological symptoms.

Disoriented, restless. *Impairment of intention* in general to a high degree. Patient is willing to follow what one asks from him as far as he can do it; sleeps very much during the day. Often he does not recognize seen objects. Catalepsic and catatonic symptoms. He has a great inclination to *echopraxie* and *echolalia*, repeats all which is said in his presence, apparently usually without any understanding. He also usually repeats in an echolalic way when he has understood what was said. He repeats parrot-like according to the presented rhythm, etc.

Understanding of speech is certainly very poor preserved only for some words and short sentences. Thus, he follows directions as "Give me your hand," "Grasp my hand," "Shut your eyes," "Get up." He answers correctly the question how many "kreutzer" are in one "krone" (Austrian money).

A more detailed protocol is missing.

Spontaneous speech: Little inclination to speak at all; speech consists of few words, lacks particularly "concrete" words, nouns, etc. Little paraphasia.

Naming of objects: A few correct, others not.

Motor act of speech: Well preserved as far as examined or reported; series of 1–20 correct.

Reading: Paralexia without any understanding. Also, if he reads correctly, he does not understand.

Writing: In the beginning, own name spontaneously, address on dictation correct. Later only own name on dictation, finally totally impossible.

Copying: Impossible.

Stransky has considered the case as transcortical sensory aphasia. I think that is not justified. Spontaneous speech is disturbed at least to the

* Published by Stransky, 1903 (290).

same degree as understanding, or possibly even more.   On the other hand, the symptoms seem to him the effect of "a general mental weakness," which finds its expression also in other mental symptoms, particularly in echopraxia.   The report is unfortunately so incomplete that it is scarcely possible to say anything definite about the kind of mental defect.   The patient understood some sentences and produced some performances, e.g., he knew how many "kreuzer" were in one "krone," so that one can not assume a very severe defect.   It seems to me that we are dealing with an isolation of the more automatic actions and this may be due to defect of the voluntary ones.   Thus, the echolalia and apraxia would be explainable.   The lack of inclination to speak at all, the lack of spontaneity in general may have played a great rôle in the development of the picture. I think the atrophy of the frontal lobes may be particularly responsible for this.

Case 20*

A 61 year old widow had suffered disease with fever and delirium a year and a half previously.   After she recovered, she had "lost her memory," but could speak as usual, though sometimes somewhat confusedly, till about seven months before examination.

Examination reveals:

Spontaneous speech very much reduced, speaks very little usually very short sentences without special contents.   Occasionally, particularly in affect, she utters a short reasonable sentence.   (Nothing more reported.)

Understanding: Preserved for single words, otherwise *severely disturbed*.   Even of simple sentences, she understands only a part.

Naming of objects: She names some objects correctly.

Speaking of series: Series of numbers, of days of the week *correct*.

Repetition: Up to 4 words, completely correct.   Automatic echolalia, often repeats the same words several times.   Sometimes understanding of words after repetition.

Spontaneous writing: Strong paragraphia.   Writing on dictation possible with paragraphia.   She copies in imitating the letters.

Reading: Correct, but *does not understand what she reads*.

Behavior   changeable.

The patient's *intelligence* is no doubt *strongly reduced*.   Most of the time she is apathetic; sometimes she shows apractic reactions.

Autopsy revealed *atrophy of the brain, particularly developed in the frontal lobe*.   No localized lesion was noted.

Pick considers the case as transcortical sensory aphasia.   There seems to be no doubt that spontaneous speech was very severely damaged, too.

The *best performance was repetition* and it showed an *automatic echolalic* character.   Only one-half year after onset of the disease, the patient died in a condition of progressive mental deterioration.

* Published by Pick (230).

We can assume from the clinical findings that the motor and perceptive part of language certainly was not damaged severely, and that the symptom complex was the effect of a destruction of the relations between the speech apparatus and the apparatus for the non-speech mental processes. This corresponds to the anatomic findings. The echolalia may be partially due to the *outspoken atrophy of the frontal lobes.*

Case 21*

A 74 year old woman of low grade education, four years before examination showed "mental anomalies": she progressively lost her memory and became inactive. She spoke little and gave answers which people around her did not understand. She came into the hospital with the diagnosis of dementia senilis.

Neurologic symptoms: Tremor of the hands, of the tongue, pupillary reaction sluggish, no particular paralysis of the extremities, but all movements slow and uncertain. Incontinence.

Asked for her name, she says: "Ich heisse Pahl." ("My name is Pahl"—correct)

When were you born?	"1847 sind wir geboren." (We were born in 1847)
How old are you?	"Ich bin 79." (I am 79.)
Which year is it?	"Welches Jahr? Da sind wir ja geboren bei dem Kinderkrankenhaus." (Which year? That's when we were born near the children's hospital.)
Which month?	"Ich habe welchen Monat gekriegt." (I got which month.)
Are you married?	"Ja." (Yes)
What is your husband?	"Der war jarnischt weiter." (He wasn't anything special.)
Show your tongue?	"Ja, meine Zunge zeig ich." (Yes I'll show my tongue—*but does not do it*)
Where are you here?	"Wo sind Sie hier? Im Krankenhaus." (Where are you here? In the hospital)
What is the name of the hospital?	"Wie das heisst." (What is its name.)
What is the name of the hospital in which you are?	"Ach in dem Sie sind." (Oh, in which you are)
Since when have you been here?	"Seit wann sind Sie hier, ja." (Since when have you been here, yes.)

The patient showed outspoken echolalia, she repeated the questions or a part of them in a questioning way.

Two months later she no longer gave any correct answers, repeated the questions totally automatically, and no longer in the questioning way. She said spontaneously one and the same sentence quite correctly: "Gott erhalte den Vater im Krankenhaus." (God keep alive our father in the hospital.) This remark was related to the fact that her husband was in a hospital. She did not speak anything else spontaneously.

She seemed to understand offending questions, at least she protested against them. She did not name any objects and used the objects in a wrong way.

---

* Published by Liepmann (188).

Reading and writing could not be tested.

The automatic echolalia persisted till her death some weeks later.

Autopsy revealed: severe atrophy of the brain, particularly on the left side. Brain weight, 1,040 grams. On the tip of the left temporal lobe, a large atrophic depression filled with fluid. First and second temporal convolution extremely small. Broca's area on the left side smaller than on the right. Severe general arteriosclerosis of the brain vessels.

Liepmann considered the picture as transcortical sensory aphasia and as cause the atrophy of the left temporal lobe. But he assumed that the high degree of the disturbance speaks for a damage of other parts of the left hemisphere.

I think we can assume that we have a severe diffuse damage of the whole brain, which left intact to a certain degree the speech apparatus and thus made possible the occurrence of echolalia.

In the cases just mentioned, the examination could not be or was not performed carefully enough to warrant saying anything definite about the condition as to the "intelligence," as to the non-language mental functions of the patients. Speech—understanding and spontaneous utterances—was so grossly disturbed that from this, a conclusion as to the non-speech mental condition was impossible. The phenomenon of echolalia spoke for a definite isolation of the almost intact instrumentalities from the non-speech mental capacities; it could not be determined to what degree the latter may have been preserved.

Case 22*

A businessman, 50 years old, had, for several months, suffered a lack of memory and could no longer attend to his business. Three months previously, "kidney attack." He did not recognize anybody for three days, did not answer any question, often repeated the questions or said yes. Improvement followed. In the last two weeks, condition deteriorated; dizziness, disorientation, exaltation. The physician's diagnosis was "uremic condition."

In the first examination, the patient is excited, drowsy, does not show any interest. Physical examination shows hypertrophy and dilation of the heart, noises in the aorta. Pulse 100, urine shows albumin. Clinical diagnosis: chronic nephritis.

The neurologic system shows *exaggerated tendon reflexes, tremor of the hands, otherwise no neurologic symptoms*.

Patient reacts to pin prick and to questions. His attention is rather good, he looks at the investigator when addressed by the latter. He gives his name correctly. Asked for the date, he says: "The same." (Month?) "The same as usual." (When did you come here?) "This time." (Where from?) "I don't know." (Why are you here?) "Different things, what shall I say? different objects." (Are you sick?) "Yes, yes." (What is wrong?) "I don't know which objects." (He cries.)

When the orderly enters, he says: "He, too, has taken many of my things."

During further examination, it was outstanding that the patient either *did not*

---

* Published by the author, 1915 (86).

answer in an adequate way, but gave similar answers as mentioned before, or *repeated the questions echolalically, apparently mostly without understanding the words.*

He almost never speaks spontaneously.   If he is *addressed, he may speak a good deal,* but always similar sentences as mentioned before.   *Very rarely were paraphasic distortions* of words observed.   On simple demand, he never utters any of the *speech series,* but if one presents the first members of the days of the week or of the series of numbers, then—particularly if one insistes energetically that he should continue—*he does so quite correctly,* but apparently *without any understanding* of the words.

He does not name any object, says only: "Different things," or: "Do you know perhaps?"   On the other hand, he *selects* a number of everyday objects *correctly on presentation of the word.*   But failures occur in this test, too, apparently because the patient did not understand the word he repeated correctly.

Repetition: patient repeats correctly letters, sounds, words, also absolutely unknown and difficult words as "Bakairi," "Artilleriebrigade," sentences like "Die Wiese ist gruen" (The meadow is green), "Heute haben wir Donnerstag" (Today it is Thursday) and similar ones.   *He repeats without articulatory failures, without paraphasia, mostly in a typical echolalic way.*   One has the impression that he does not understand any of the words he repeats without failure.

Understanding: As we said before, some words are identified with concrete objects, but certainly he *does not understand a great number of words.*   He follows only very simple directions.   That we are not dealing with apractic symptoms becomes evident when the patient performs the same simple activities normally if one demands him by gestures to do this.   It could not be determined whether he did not have apractic disturbances, too, particularly because the patient very easily entered a condition of unconsciousness.   For this reason, the examination in general was limited.   The patient died shortly afterward in a condition of uremic coma.

The *autopsy* showed the following: The brain was very large, the convolutions appeared larger and flatter than normally.   *The left hemisphere appeared to be much larger than the right,* and the convolutions still more abnormal in the before-mentioned way.   *Particularly the region of the central convolutions, the part of the frontal lobes located before them, the gyri supermarginalis and angularis were elevated above the level of the rest of the brain.*   The convolutions were here extremely large and the sulci almost leveled.

There was *no localized* lesion to be seen.   On a transversal cutting, the whole left hemisphere appeared larger than the right and particularly the before-mentioned regions.   The enlargements of the hemisphere are due essentially to an *enlargement of the white matter.*   In several places, there were small hemorrhages, but not in the region of Borca, in the temporal lobe and in the Insula.   The microscopic investigation showed a great number of microscopic encephalitic foci.

In spite of the incomplete examination of the patient, we can say that he presents the picture of a *mixed transcortical aphasia.*   Spontaneous speech is restricted to a few repeatedly returning words and phrases.   If he is addressed and starts speaking, then he may even speak considerably in the form of logorrhoe.   Understanding is severely disturbed.   In contrast to this, his repetition is well preserved, even for complicated, certainly unknown words and sentences.

We cannot prove, indeed, whether or how much the non-speech mental processes of the patient were preserved and how much of the disturbance of spontaneous speech and understanding may be due to a defect in this sphere.   The extreme difference between the defect of spontaneous speech and understanding on the one hand, and the perfect preservation of repetition on the other, makes us assume that the origin of the picture is a *damage of the relations between speech and the non-speech mental processes.* The occurrence of a definite echolalia and logorrhoe which are symptoms of isolation of the field of speech from the rest of the personality (see p. 301) make this assumption still more probable.   The enlargement of the brain may have been well suited to damage the more complicated performances, spontaneous speech and understanding, but left undisturbed the more automatic function of repetition in the form of echolalia.   The particular affection of the gyri supermarginalis, angularis, frontalis, and the better preservation of the so-called speech apparatus may have been of importance for the development of the picture.

B. Other Types of Speech Disturbance Due to Impairment of the Non-language Mental Performances

There are a number of other cases which have some similarity with the mentioned cases of transcortical aphasia but differ from them by the fact that the impairment of the non-language mental performances are more in the foreground and the speech defects are secondary to the latter.

The pictures differ as to the individual symptoms and usually are published under different names.   In our discussion of the disturbances of the non-language mental processes we come to a distinction between impairment of abstraction and damage of the "unitary function in thinking" (see p. 117).   We were aware that these types of disturbances are closely related to each other.   There will be times when they are considered under a common denominator.   But we maintained the distinction because for the time being such a consideration is not possible and could at least not be brought to a fruitful result in the frame of our present investigation; hence, it could not be made useful for the practical purpose of description of cases.

We saw further that there may be a possibility to consider the defect not only from a psychologic point of view but also from a functional physiologic one, and to consider the symptoms as effect of the dedifferentiation of the "basic function" of the brain matter (see p. 118).   We shall apply this point of view as far as possible also in the characterization of the clinical pictures.

There are first to be mentioned those cases which are similar to amnesic aphasic patients, and the explanation that we are dealing here with the effects of impairment of abstraction is near at hand.   But such cases differ from amnesic aphasia in that the disturbance of finding words is not so apparent, and that other disturbances of language and of the non-language performances are much more dominant than in amnesic aphasias (in the latter, they are present but not so pronounced). The patients speak less spontaneously than amnesic-aphasics. They also have difficulty in finding the little words. We shall discuss later how these differences are to be understood. A case in point is the following:

Case 23*

A young man of twenty-six received a shotgun injury in the left internal carotid artery. The bullet went out at the base of the skull without apparently injuring actual brain matter. The patient was comatose for some eight hours. On awakening, he was unable to speak except for the words "yes" and "no." He seemed to understand, although with difficulty. He recognized his parents.

Physical examination was, except for the local injury, essentially negative. X-rays showed no evidence of the bullet. Clinical diagnosis was: "*Occlusion of left carotid artery with cerebral infarction.*"

From his previous history, he seemed to have learned well, was over average, particularly *had good language ability*, but was socially badly adjusted. He had been in reformatory and jail. While in the reformatory, he apparently read extensively. His knowledge of Shakespeare certainly surpassed the norm for his socio-economic or educational group. He read at least some of both Voltaire and Rosseau (probably in translation) with some understanding of what it was all about, as was evidenced on questioning. But more than that, he managed to acquire a not inconsiderable amount of Greek, probably from one of the other inmates, possibly a native of Greece. He could read and write a number of the Greek letters, and knew some vocabulary.

Even after his accident, the patient was still interested in reading, although on questioning he admitted that he could not understand what he was reading.

Throughout all the examinations, the patient was always very friendly and cooperative. He almost never fatigued. When asked how he was, he always said "fine" or "pretty good." The patient was investigated intensively over a period of eight months following the injury and observed further for four years.

His *memory seemed to be good*. He remembered previous examinations after days and weeks. His sense discrimination was normal, but in all tests which needed comparison he showed failures. He did not seem to understand what more or less meant, bigger or smaller. He had some tactile agnosia at the right hand. He differentiated qualitative differences but could not recognize the meaning of the objects. Left hand was normal.

Arithmetic: the patient could neither add or subtract, or multiply in the usual way. He *counted* within the number series the required number of steps. He thus managed to succeed in very simple addition problems. He did not seem to understand what first, second, third, meant, e.g., in a row of coins presented. He could handle money in simple practical problems, but only those coins he had to use daily. He did not know the value of the coins outside of a practical situation. His knowledge of what the hands of a watch meant corresponded to definite events, as, for instance, "lunchtime," but he had *no idea of what time meant*.

As *to space*, the patient found his way in the hospital, in town, but was not able to

---

* Observed with my student, Marianne Simmel, who is to describe the case more in detail in another publication.

tell how. He did not understand what direction meant. He had lost completely the concepts of right or left as referring to spatial position and orientation.

In the color and object sorting test, the patient displayed the characteristics of impairment of abstraction (see p. 168). He was not able to sort according to categories; he was determined in his procedure by immediate sense impressions and use in a definite concrete situation. He could not shift from one attitude to another. In the stick test, he was always successful (probably due to his excellent visual imagery).

1. *Spontaneous speech:* The patient *spoke very little spontaneously.* If he did, he would usually speak only nouns and verbs. These words meant sentences of concrete content. The utterances were frequently accompanied by vivid gestures. Thus, he said "chair," in pointing to the door as if asking, "Shall I get one?" when a chair was missing. Sometimes unable to find a word he would write down the first letter of the word, occasionally in his hand. The *pronunciation* of the few words he uttered was *very clear.*

2. *Reactive speech was better.* The patient found adequate words in some situations, or to questions. Also here he never used sentences, but the "one-word sentence," or occasionally a noun and verb or adjective together, but never the article. Instead of "a little," "maybe" and similar expressions he used "yes-no" in all more or less appropriate situations (he used adequately and without difficulty both "yes" and "no," though there was a time when he occasionally confused the two). He began to utter with increasing frequency such phrases as "pretty good," "I know," "I see," "I don't know," "I don't understand," "I'm lost" (when he failed), "I don't mind," "Good-bye." This was the more striking as the patient never used sentences, or even parts thereof in any other connection.

3. *Speaking of series:* He was *never able to start* a series. He failed also when he was asked to repeat the series the examiner presented. Only when the examiner started and the patient joined in could he continue without the examiner. He could speak the series if he were allowed to speak in a definite rhythm, but not if between the numbers (for example) a little interval was to be interpolated. He could not count backwards.

4. *Repetition:* From the beginning it was noticed that the patient could *repeat a great number of words* even if he did not speak them spontaneously or on demand or was not able to read them aloud. Even such long and complicated words as "Thanksgiving" or "staircase" he repeated fluently *without hesitation and paraphasia.* He never succeeded in repeating even a short sentence, although he might be able to repeat most of the words in it separately. He almost always *failed to repeat the "little words"* such as *in, on, of, the,* etc., which he never used and which he *could not read.* Perhaps the most striking instances are the following, where the patient succeeded or failed to repeat words of identical, or almost identical sound but different meaning (see p. 72). Presented with the word *for* he would neither repeat nor read it; presented with *four* or *4,* he would invariably repeat it and usually read it. If *for* and *four* or *4* were presented simultaneously or in quick succession, he invariably failed with *for* and succeeded with *four* and *4,* even when it was pointed out to him that all these sound alike. Similar experiments with identical results were made using *in* and *inn; of* and *off; to, too, two* and *2.* Of a sentence or short phrase, he might repeat one word of it which was known to him, or the last word pronounced by the examiner. He would repeat, however, the motor phrases that he used spontaneously, such as, "I don't mind," but had the greatest difficulty in repeating "don't" by itself. Later it became possible to get the patient to *imitate the sound of*

otherwise "unknown" words after repeated presentation. This *imitation*, however, was very *different in character— from the more genuine repetition*. When he repeated words known to him, he seemed to perceive the word as such in most instances, and in repeating used his characteristic tone of voice and accentuation. No uncertainty or hesitation was ever observed in such cases. On the other hand, when *imitating* the sounds of a word that he did not know, *his performance was slow, hesitating and uncertain:* his face had a characteristic "blank" expression and he produced sound-imitations in an echolalia-like fashion rather than repeating the words. This became especially noticeable when the examiner mispronounced a word or parts thereof, e.g., the *th*-sound. The patient in such cases would repeat the examiner's mistake, the tone of voice, etc.

Numbers of one or two digits he soon repeated well, but he failed with more digits.

He repeated a few of the *letters* but in *echolalia-like fashion*. The same was true as to *sounds*.

5. *Naming of objects:* In the beginning the patient *was unable to name any object or picture*. There was never any question as to his recognition of the objects. He always agreed to the correct name emphatically when suggested by the examiner, while he rejected incorrect names. At times the possibility of *handling the object would help him in finding its name*, and later, being allowed *to write the beginning of the word seemed to initiate it and facilitate his word-finding. Some months later* he found a great number of words for objects though sometimes even well-known names were missing.

When he found names, he *never* showed *literal paraphasia, but outspoken verbal paraphasia*. For example, he said smoke, cigar, for pipe; paint for paintbrush; eat for toaster; table for lamp. He failed particularly in names for the parts of the body; if he gave a correct answer he was not sure whether it was correct. This held true also concerning the names of clothing: tie, vest, etc.

6. *Understanding of speech:* For the superficial view the patient's success and failure in understanding presented quite a confusing picture. At one time one might feel that he was closely following a conversation between others, then again he seemed to fail completely when directly addressed. From the beginning he had been able to understand simple commands, as, "sit down," "show your nose," etc. At the same time he *failed whenever such a request contained more than one concrete item, e.g.,* "stand up and close your eyes," "open your eyes and show your tongue," etc. The patient seemed at a total loss as to what was being asked of him. The same had been observed if a request usually understood by him were *addressed to him while in the midst of some other activity.*

Whether the patient succeeded or failed to understand words or sentences which he could understand under optimum conditions, seemed to be primarily a question of the unity of a given action and the maintenance of a once-induced attitude. His understanding was altogether *independent of the length of a given word*, or the number of syllables contained therein. He might *grasp words out of a context, while remaining completely oblivious to the latter: or he might grasp the meaning of a context without clear understanding of the words.*

7. *Reading:* From the beginning the patient seemed to "recognize" a number of words even if he could not read them aloud. He often indicated that he understood a word but could not "find" it. At first he used in such instances a great many expressive movements, gestures, etc., but as he improved he substituted for words he could not find those which in a given situation had some connection with the word presented (*verbal paralexia*). Thus he would say "paint" for *draw*, "marry" for *wed*,

"time" for *era*, "loan," "money" or "safe" on different occasions when *security* was presented; "New York" for *Penn. Station*, "hot" for *oven*, etc. Sometimes he would add something to the word as when presented with *pen* he read "pencil." He might read "room" for *door*, but on another occasion, "door" for *room*. Occasionally, he would "misread" a word, such as "live" for *liver*, "flower" for *flow*, "button" for *but*, etc. Those words which he read (correctly or incorrectly) he *read immediately* upon presentation and without hesitation. *No literal paraphasia was ever noted.* He read without any mistakes in pronunciation and articulation, even such long words as *Thanksgiving* and *Massachusetts*.

Occasionally, the patient, after having failed to read the word on demand, would indicate by gestures that he "knows" it, then pick up a pencil and begin to copy it and suddenly pronounce the word fluently and correctly. During later months he was observed several times tracing a word which he could not find—or part of it—with his finger rapidly on the table which sometimes helped him, although not invariably, to find the word.

Whenever the patient was able to read a word or to arrive at a more or less correct result by some of the above-mentioned round-about ways, there was never *any question as to his understanding* of the word. He *never*, as far as could be determined, *was able to read a word which he did not understand*, while at the same time he seemed to recognize a number of words and understand them without being able to read them correctly.

He could *not read sentences*, and he was never able to bring words he could read together into a sentence.

In *reading mutilated words*, the patient's performance, in the case of words otherwise known to him, was equal *if not better* than the performance of normal individuals. *Hsptl* was immediately read as "hospital," *starcase* and *stircase* as "staircase," *gradn* as "garden." When presented with a number of mutilated forms of the same word with the correct spelling interspersed among them, he would immediately pick the correct form, point to it and read it aloud. Similarly, on tachistoscopic reading, his performance—on words known to him—at least equaled that of normals. He succeeded in reading out loud words presented only 1/100 or 1/50 second. If mutilated words were presented tachistoscopically he could read these as if not mutilated. On the other hand, he failed tachistoscopically on those words which he could not read ordinarily either.

To be exact, the patient *did not read at all* in the way in which normals do. *He recognized instantly a great number of words*, mostly nouns and verbs, but also a few adjectives, especially color names. If he did *not recognize a word instantly, no matter how much time he was given, he could not read it*. For this reason, his performance on tachistoscopic reading was at least normal, if not better on those words he knew; 1/100 sec. was almost always sufficient for such recognition. *Reading as a process starting from left to right was something completely alien to him*.

8. *Writing: Poorest* of all was the patient's *writing on dictation:* his *spontaneous writing* (e.g., if he wanted to find a word) *was somewhat better*. But the procedure in the two activities was essentially the same. Usually he *began with the first* letter or two, then *placed the last letter* and *finally attempted to fill the middle*, usually failing in the latter. He almost never wrote whole words spontaneously, since, having written the first letter or two and perhaps some such outstanding letter combination as a *ll* or *mm*, he usually found the word. The function of this writing seemed to be the initiation of the word that could not be initiated otherwise. Copying and reproduction from memory (if successful) were for the patient apparently tasks completely dif-

ferent from writing as described above. *Copying seemed to be the task in which the patient improved most rapidly during the early weeks.* He soon copied *words and even sentences*, irrespective of whether or not he understood them. No matter what he copied—well-known words, or unknown ones, senseless letter combinations, numbers or forms—he almost never made any mistakes. There seemed to be absolutely no difference for him whether he copied senseless letter combinations or a meaningful well-known (to him) word. If interrupted and asked what such a word was, he invariably became startled, and seemed to have no idea at all; frequently, he could be brought to the point where he suddenly "recognized" the well-known word, in which case the examiner had some difficulty in getting the patient back to copying. Again and again it was observed that the patient *did not copy words, but individual letters.*

His reproductions from memory showed a mixture of the processes involved in writing and in copying. Either he was able to utilize his very good visual imagery, in which case his reproductions had the same characteristics as those of his copying, or, failing this, he perceived some of the outstanding characteristics of the material presented and subsequently proceeded in a way similar to his spontaneous writing or writing on dictation, thus almost always producing correct parts, but never a totally correct reproduction. There was considerable evidence from tachistoscopic experiments that the patient reproduced very much better on material not known to him, and that to him, "meaningful" material might lead to much less successful reproduction.

If one considers only the language of the patient, the picture resembles the transcortical motor aphasia of the second type: the severe lack of spontaneous speech with well preserved repetition and good quality of the motor acts of speech themselves fit this picture well. However, there are some peculiarities of the preserved speech performances and particularly of the non-speech mental behavior which must induce us to assume at least besides the transcortical motor aphasia further anomalies. The acoustic sphere in general, and in particular as far as speech is concerned, could be considered intact; the lack of any paraphasia and well preserved repetition allows us to assume that inner speech is not disturbed. Recognition, praxis, judgment, thinking, attention, interest, knowledge in general did not show gross abnormalities. And yet *all these performances and all other ones which one may test, were modified in a characteristic way.* If we consider first understanding, which seemed to be preserved at best, it became evident that the patient understands well as long as understanding means reacting immediately to a word or sentence with a definite performance which is directly related to the linguistic demand. But when the patient is confronted with a task which demands reaction to two things which are not intrinsically connected with each other, i.e., *do not present immediately a unit for the patient, he fails.* He may fulfill each part of the task well but not both in a connection which is necessary to fulfill the task. He does not even understand what this means. He is *unable to shift voluntarily* from one subject matter to another. Therefore, he may understand quite well words and sentences in a definite situation to which, for him, they belong (in the present or in the recollection of a past situation), but not outside of such a situation, etc.   This is a defect which can be understood as expression of the damage of the basic function of the brain cortex (see p. 118).   Indeed, one can also describe it as effect of impairment of abstraction.   From this aspect, the case becomes similar to cases of central motor aphasia, to amnesic aphasia, to a patient of Boumann and Grünbaum (see p. 76), to some cases of transcortical motor aphasia, to patients suffering from that form of visual agnosia which Gelb and I have published (112a).   Cases like those of Gerstman's "fingeragnosia" may belong here too, also the case of Pick's disease which Katz and I have published (113).

I should like to refer further to the similarity with such cases as I have published with Haufmann and Rickers-Osiankina (124) and with Scheerer and Rothmann (265).

In all these cases, we are inclined to assume a lesion in the so-called "central part of the brain cortex" (see p. 46).   The differences in the symptomatology are due to a different localization of the lesion within this region, and to the fact that besides this region, other special fields are more or less affected, or the defect of the basic function concerns more or less the one or the other special performance field (visual, motor, language, etc.)   Thus, the effect shows itself in somewhat different symptoms, particularly as far as language is concerned.

Where the lesion is located in the mentioned case, we are not able definitely to say.   There is no doubt that the brain damage is the consequence of the injury of the carotid artery and in such cases the damage of the brain is related to the middle cerebral artery.   From the clinical picture, we may assume that the speech area is not directly affected.   The lesion may concern particularly the region between temporal and parietal lobe or may have damaged to a certain degree the whole "central area" of the brain cortex.

The patient presents a great number of symptomatologically interesting findings.   They will be discussed in a more extensive publication by Marianne Simmel.   I should like to stress at this point only some few which are particularly important with respect to some of the problems with which we are here concerned.

The patient showed the defect of word-finding in the *typical amnesic aphasic* way in the beginning in a very severe degree.   *Later, he improved in* this respect, but remained unchanged as to impairment of abstract attitude.   His improvement may be due to the use of roundabout ways (see p. 2).   Indeed, we cannot prove it so definitely as it was possible in the woman patient mentioned before (see p. 268).   This patient was much more disturbed in general, his language was by far not so good as that of the latter.   Thus, we could not get as much information from him as in the other case.   A roundabout way at his disposal was his *extraordinary capacity of visual memory and imagery*.   His visual memory made it possible for him to "read" a great number of words by simple recognition of the visual form (see p. 313).   The attempt to find a word for an object may have evoked in association to the seen object the visual image of the written word, which produced by association the motor word which he could not find as "name" because of his defect of the abstract attitude (see p. 61).   Sometimes he first made certain writing movements.   This procedure could indeed help him only in "finding the word" to presented objects, not in voluntary spontaneous speech; for the latter, abstract attitude is more necessary.   As a matter of fact, in this respect he did not improve—a difference from the usual amnesic aphasia patients.   The difference came to the fore particularly in his behavior as to the *"little" words* (see p. 68).   He *could not find them at all in speaking, reading and writing*.   He could not repeat them as he could not repeat any word he did not understand.   Urged, he might "repeat" the word by "imitation" of the sounds (see p. 312).   Another deviation from amnesic aphasic patients was that *he could not spell and combine letters into words* nor read by reading syllable after syllable, even if after looking at the written word he produced a word as a whole.

From these mentioned and other symptoms one could characterize the defect as *impairment of abstraction and abnormal concreteness or as impairment of the "basic function."*   The patient would have been much more disturbed if he had not been able to *cover up his defect by visual and motor associations* which passively came to the fore when he could not proceed normally (see p. 28).   This was rendered possible by his premorbid good visualization and motor skill in speech.

The differences between this patient and the usual amnesic aphasia case may be understandable from the assumption that in the latter, besides impairment of abstraction, the speech instrumentalities are somewhat affected, but not in this case (see p. 314); on the other hand, the basic function of the brain is damaged here to a higher degree than in the usual amnesic aphasia.

The next case is a characteristic example of the effect of impairment of the unifying process in thinking (see p. 114) on language.

Case 24*

This patient, a 22 year old woman, had suffered cerebral paralysis in infancy. Since that time, epileptic seizures of Jacksonian type had occurred.   Therefore, an

---

* Published by A. Pelz.   See, for a number of interesting symptoms, the original paper (223).

operation was performed. Upon operation, the brain showed a dark red spot in the central convolution. No tumor or cyst was found. *Eight days after operation, fever and difficulties in speaking were noted.* A second operation was performed which revealed a softening of the cortex in a diameter of about 2 inches. After operation, prolapsus cerebri occurred.

In the beginning, there was left flaccid hemiparesis, disturbance of sensation for touch, pressure and movements in the left side of the body, left hemianopsia. The hemiparesis and hemianopsia disappeared after a certain time, there was a slow improvement of the aphasic symptoms.

At the time of the examination the symptom complex was as follows: The patient lay normally in bed without movement and showed little interest in what was going on. From time to time she would ask for water. *If the doctor addressed her*, she was usually somewhat afraid and would utter sentences like the following: Herr Doktor, ich freue mich, ich freue mich (Doctor, I am glad, I am glad). Kopf nicht weh (Head does not hurt). Kann nicht hoeren (Cannot hear). Mama kommen!? Kommt Mama? (Mamma to come!? Is Mamma coming?). Operieren nicht! (Don't operate!) Heute frisch verbunden! (Today new dressing!) Kann nicht gesund werden. (Cannot get well.) Kann nicht essen. (Cannot eat.) Den linken Fuss—tut weh. ` (Left foot—hurts.) Kann nicht fuehlen meinen Fuss. (Cannot feel my foot.) Der Kopf tut weh. (My head hurts). Verband zu fest. (Bandage too tight.) Ich will nach Hause gehn—fahren. (I want to go—ride home). Ich muss davon doch sterben (I must die of it anyway). Suddenly in the midst of the examination: Die Judsche schreit immer so des Nachts. (The Jewish woman always cries loud during the night) (another patient). Ich—ich—gesund werden, nicht gesund werden. Ich will nach Hause. (I—I—get well, not get well. I want to go home.) (Very excited and almost crying) Bis nach Pfingsten!—Ich—Ich nicht liegen—meine Schwester, ich zu Hause bleiben (Until after Whitsuntide!—I—I not lie—my sister, I stay at home). Ich sterben (*crying bitterly:* I to die). Operiert will ich nicht werden (I don't want to be operated). Ich hier allein (I here alone). Linkes Bein tut weh (Left leg hurts). Meine Schwester ist nicht mehr gekommen. (My sister does not come anymore.) Werden Sie morgen kommen, Herr Doktor? (Will you come tomorrow, Doctor?) Ist sie jetzt schon zu Hause, meine Schwester? (Is she now already home, my sister?) Ich allein—allein—bleiben hier? (I alone, alone—stay here?) Ich kann nicht gehn! (I cannot walk.) Ich sterben. (I die.) Der Hals tut weh. Der Kopf tut weh. (My throat hurts. My head hurts.) Kann ich nicht schon bald gehn? (May I not soon go?) (*After bandaging*) Mein Kopf ist schlecht? (My head is bad?) Ich moechte zu Pfingsten aufstehen. (I want to get up at Whitsuntide.) Kann nicht sprechen. (Cannot speak.) Ist mein Kopf besser? (Is my head better?) Mein Kopf—ist doch nicht—mein Kopf ist doch nicht—(*with great effort*) schlechter, Herr Doktor? (My head—is not I hope—my head is not I hope—worse, Doctor?).

Speaking of series: She spoke the days of the week when helped with the first; also, after she had been given the first months, she could recite them all. She could recite them backwards also, almost without mistakes, but very slowly. She counted numbers promptly and correctly, even being able to give them backwards, beginning with 10. When giving the alphabet, she succeeded with the first letters after being prompted several times, but would soon say, "No, no." She knew how to recite the first line of a well known children's song, but made mistakes in the second line; she would then say, "No."

Naming of objects: She named some of the presented objects correctly, others not, but identified objects correctly when the word was presented.   She could point correctly to objects and pictures.

Repetition: She repeated letters and words correctly, even difficult and unknown words, as "Elektrizitaet" (electricity) and "Urodoabulus," also such very long ones as "Schornsteinfegermeistersgattin" (wife of a chimney sweeper).   "Sommerfahrplanbuch" (summer table), "Sanskritliteratur" (Sanskrit literature).   She could repeat simple sentences well, as, "Die Wiese ist gruen" (The meadow is green), "Die Wunde ist gut" (The wound is good), but made slight mistakes in more complicated ones.

Understanding of speech: The results were subject to change.   Questioned as to her name, her birthday, year of birth, names of sisters, father, birthplace, etc., *she answered correctly*.   She followed simple directions as: Show your tongue, Give me your hand, and similar ones.   Sometimes there was a failure due to dyspraxia.   She did not understand longer sentences and particularly if they were presented in a more complicated structure.   She understood simple statements best; she had difficulties as soon as there were subordinate clauses.   The patient showed *great difficulty in the sentence completion test*.   The sentences were very well known verses, proverbs, etc.   Normal individuals of about the same educational level fulfilled this task quickly; they uttered the whole sentence usually after having found the first words even though the other cards were not arranged yet.   The patient showed *definite failures* which we will discuss in the interpretation of the whole symptom complex (see p. 322).

The author who has published this observation mentions that one did *not at all gather the impression that the patient was deteriorated in her intelligence in general*.   Her condition seemed more severe due to the *lack of spontaneity*.   A number of occasional utterances showed that she had a good judgment as to her condition, that she was eager to help in the examination and understood situations even when she did not say anything.   Thus, for instance, when she saw that a boy wrote Hebrew, that is, from the right to the left, she said spontaneously, "Backward."

Reading: All letters, with exception of v, x, y, were read correctly in handwriting and in print.   Sometimes she had some difficulty in reading printed Latin capitals. She read correctly numbers with two and three digits, those with three and four digits only slowly and with mistakes.   She read words, even those totally unknown, quite correctly if they did not consist of more than two or three syllables.   Confronted with longer words, she read the syllables separately, or she *spelled*, and that *always correctly*.   Combining letters into a word was very difficult for her and was imperfect.   There was no paraphasia in reading.   Only very seldom was a letter misplaced.   It was not very easy to come to a judgment as to whether she understood what she was reading.   One had the impression that she did not understand when she was to react with an action to a written command.   She repeated the read words correctly.   Only after many attempts was one by demonstrations successful in making her understand what she should do, and then she readily *followed the written instructions*.   Thus, the *impression was that her understanding of reading was about the same as her understanding of spoken words*.

Spontaneous writing: She wrote a *few words quite correctly*.   Her attempt to write a letter was very poor.   *Copying* of all written and printed letters in Gothic and Latin signs was performed promptly and correctly.

The patient was able on command to make drawings of a great number of everyday objects in an apparently normal way.   She failed in some objects, as a face, but could copy them.

Her *memory* was changeable.   If she had the task of repeating six numbers, which were always correctly repeated when presented in isolation, she would generally repeat the first or the last two.

The patient died after a short time, and the anatomic findings were as follows: Necrotic softening in the right hemisphere; detailed description could not be obtained.   Because the aphasic picture occurred after the operation we can bring it into connection with this softening.

It is not mentioned whether the patient was left-handed, but the appearance of the described picture in a lesion in the right hemisphere makes it probable.

This patient shows *disturbances of spontaneous speech and understanding*. That they are *not due to motor or peripheral defects* is evident.   The patient pronounced well, showed no paraphasia, reciting of series (if she found the first figure or if it were presented to her) was mostly intact, and, finally, *repetition was correct*, also for complicated words and for sentences (although only for short ones).   Her behavior in reaction to language leaves no doubt that the perceptual sphere is intact.

The promptness of her procedure in repetition shows that *inner speech probably is normal*, too.

There is no other possibility than to assume that the disturbances in spontaneous speech and understanding are due to a defect in the *non-speech mental processes*.   Her behavior in general allows us to exclude an intellectual or emotional deterioration in general.   She has some insight into her defect, follows the examination with interest; her memory is certainly not severely diminished.   The author mentions particularly that he did not have the impression that her "intelligence" in general was diminished. Hence, we must see whether there is any special abnormality in the mental processes which may explain her speech behavior.

The patient recognizes objects with all the various senses quite normally, she has no agnostic symptoms, she reads well, words and sentences, written and printed.   She understands what she reads.   She shows some dyspractic phenomena, particularly in writing, but certainly does not have a severe apraxia.

She was not examined with abstraction tests and from the reported results of the different examinations nothing definite could be said on how good her abstract capacity was.   In her utterances there is some lack of nouns which comes to the fore particularly because she has otherwise no definite lack of any word category.   In a case with so good a preservation of instrumentalities, an assumption of some impairment of abstract capacity as origin of this lack may be justified.   To this, it would correspond further that her utterances refer nearly exclusively *to very concrete situations, particularly those which concern herself*.   This may lead us to assume *abnormal concreteness*.

The most outstanding symptom of her speech is the *simplicity of the structure of the sentences*. The sequence of the words in the sentences is almost correct but only the simplest constructions are used. There was never a subordinate clause to be observed.

Her impairment in constructing sentences showed still more when she was confronted with the sentence completion test. The patient, after some demonstration, *understood well* what she was supposed to do. She also did *quite well* as long as *sentences were presented which she knew very well*, particularly those she was accustomed to utter as series: prayers, known proverbs, etc., e.g., "Vater unser, der du bist im Himmel." (The Lord's Prayer in German.) Sometimes she had difficulty, but after she had read one word characteristic of the sentence, she could say the sentence and arrange the words correctly. This procedure shows how great a part the *motor speech series played in her success* (see p. 95).

It was particularly astonishing that the patient, after succeeding with such sentences, showed the greatest difficulty, even *incapacity, to arrange words into simple sentences for which she did not possess such motor series*, but where she *had to proceed by thinking*. For example, if presented with the words: Eltern (parents), lieben (love), die (the), sollen (ought to), Kinder (children), die (the), the patient brings the words "parents" and "children" together. Then: parents—love—children—ought to—the, or: children—love—parents; or: love—parents—children—ought to. *She is unhappy that she is not able to fulfill the task.* Der Jäger schiesst den Hasen auf dem Felde (the hunter shoots the hare in the field): she reads: "hare—shoots," and arranges: "shoots—the—hunter—in—hare," then suddenly speaks the sentence correctly and arranges the words.

Sometimes if the correct result were shown to her she would proceed correctly the next time. But not at all always, or even if successful, only after several attempts, e.g.: the hunter...(then she takes different cards, puts them down) shoots...(says no, tries different position, then she arranges correctly).

Another sentence: Ich bin operiert worden, weil ich Krämpfe hatte (I was operated on because I had convulsions). She arranges: "I—convulsions—had—because—I—convulsions—had"; then: "because—operated,—because—I—operated." In the end she does not succeed.

Wenn ich gesund bin, fahre ich nach Hause (When I am well, I go home): "when—I—I become well, home—"then she arranges the cards correctly.

We see from these experiments: (1) The patient arranges *correctly if some characteristic words awake a motorically well known sentence.* (2) She brings together *words which are in simple relation to each other:* e.g., parents and children; I, convulsions, had. (3) *She shows failure when the order* into which she has to bring the cards *presupposes thinking and finding out something about the meaningful relation of the ideas to each other.*

This is exactly the defect which clarifies the structure of her spontaneous speech and the lack of understanding: in spontaneous speech, the simplicity of the structure and the combination of such ideas which belong (for her) closely together, the preference of ideas which have to deal with her very personal affairs. Some of the results of the experiments show even poorer capacity than the spontaneous speech. The reason may be that these experiments presuppose more activity in general than spontaneous speech which originates in a situation. But the experimental results are not at all always worse than the spontaneous utterances. Contrariwise, some are very good, and these good results reveal a factor which is important for understanding the patient's speech. *From the superficial view,* these well performed sentences *appear to be complicated structures of sentences.* But, as a matter of fact, *they are not built* by the patient in the moment. They represent *learned motor series* which she produces as motor activities, stimulated by the presented material. Hence, her defect is hidden behind the use of learned automatized performances which can be executed without complex thinking.

This certainly modifies the patient's spontaneous speech. It would appear much more disturbed if the patient were not able to use such learned motor performances, and would become more apparent if we were able to eliminate them as we do in the experiments.

It seems to be in some contrast to this statement that in her spontaneous speech some words, which we are inclined to consider as motor automatisms, are missing. There is a lack of verbs, the verbs are often used in infinitive form, not in the correct one. In this respect, there is some similarity with the spontaneous speech of patients with motor aphasia. But there is an essential difference: the patient utters many of the "small" words, which we miss in motor aphasia (in motor agrammatism, see p. 81). The motor speech, in general so well preserved in our patient, does not make it probable that the mentioned anomalies of her spontaneous speech are due to a motor deficiency. It is more plausible to consider them as expression of the defect in the *process of the mental organization.* It is interesting that the preference for infinitive forms goes along with the frequency of the use of "I," an experience of the egocentrism of the patient's attitude toward the world, both corresponding apparently to a simplification and concretization due to dedifferentiation of thinking.

We can thus say that the patient's mental processes are sufficiently preserved to guarantee simple procedure as recognition of objects, combining ideas to concrete units, but not to organize material to higher units, as, for instance, to well constructed sentences. *This defect expresses itself in the defects of the spontaneous speech but is somewhat hidden under the substitute of motor-speech automatisms.*

In so far as this part of the picture is concerned, we could speak of transcortical aphasia (because repetition is so well preserved), due to a *dedifferentiation of the non-speech mental processes.*

But this dedifferentiation is not simply a type of impairment of abstract attitude. Although this attitude was indeed somewhat impaired, really outstanding was a defect which could be described as impairment of the *unifying process in thinking in general* (see p. 118).* In addition, one could speak of an effect of disturbance of the *simultaneous function.*

I think it scarcely needs further explanation that the characterized defect makes understandable the patient's disturbance in understanding speech, too. The spontaneous speech appears more disturbed than understanding because the defect influences spontaneous speech more than understanding.

What we ask from the patient as far as understanding is concerned is very simple: understanding of words or very simple sentences. It is not even necessary that one understand a sentence in all its complication to fulfill a task correctly. If we want to express our thoughts in speech, the process does need more activity in general, and a more precise organization of the thoughts is necessary. If this is disturbed, we shall hesitate to speak at all. Therefore, our patient spoke even her simple sentences usually only in reaction to our questions or if she was driven by emotions. There is another factor which may reduce spontaneous speech. If the patient recognizes the defect, as our patient does, she will be reluctant to speak at all.

Repetition, which is well preserved in this case, *does not show echolalic character.* This is understandable because understanding and intention are not disturbed totally (see p. 301).

The case is a characteristic example for those forms of aphasia *where the instrumentalities are intact, the relations between them and the non-speech mental processes are not severely disturbed, but there exists a dedifferentiation of the latter in the sense that the simple performances are possible but not the more complicated functions which produce the higher order of thinking. This defect is mirrored in definite symptoms of spontaneous speech and understanding.*

Case 25 (112a)

Finally, I should like to cite some examples of the above-mentioned patient of Gelb and myself with visual agnosia due to lack of *simultaneous*

* See particularly, Pelz (223), p. 147.

function (see p. 121). We have given before a short report of the symptoms of the patient which show—besides the severe visual agnosia of the patient —a great similarity with the last reviewed picture. Here we are particularly interested in the fact that the patient's language had lost meaning and showed all the characteristics of the language of an individual who is impaired in abstract attitude. He could not begin to speak by himself, did not understand and could not use language in a metaphoric way, etc.; even if he gave correct answers, they represented use of speech instrumentalities without real insight into what the words meant. He was able with his great knowledge of language to settle a considerable number of situations. His language was induced by the outer world, particularly by the speaking of others; in concrete situations it might not deviate much from that of a normal individual. Indeed, it was somewhat stereotyped but it was not lacking in any category of words, of grammatical and syntactical structure, although the latter was very simple. He was able to cover, by this language, his severe defect to a high degree, particularly his severe visual defect—indeed, possibly supported by the excellent utilization of kinaesthetic experiences (see p. 121). Two examples may illustrate: He was presented with a red book on a table and asked what it was. He could not recognize it by vision, only that it was "something red." Then he "traced" it in his planless way (see p. 121) and from the thus acquired kinaesthetic experiences he came to the recognition that it was a square. He said, "It is a square." Then: "Here something white"..."a red square, on the small side white; it is lying on a table. Red square, white, thick, on the table, that may be a book." Or another example: A picture hanging in a frame on the wall: he traced, and said, "A square...A square on the wall ..squares on the wall, pictures, windows, frames, doors, mirrors, calendar." Then he saw it was black. He said, "It is not a window, not a mirror, it may be a picture." He solved his task by speech associations which he utilized in an exquisite manner. Some of these associations he built during his disease, so that when he described a complicated pathway about which he had no knowledge based on visualization with a sequence of words, he said: "First ten steps straight ahead, then to the right, then there is a corner, around the corner, to the left, twenty steps, and so forth."

How good his language was in a concrete situation may be illustrated by the following example: He was interested very much in the business by which he made his living. Asked how business was, he said: "Ah, our business is excellent this year. We could hire new workers. We are not able to handle all that we have. The foreman handles too much at the same time. If I would be the businessman, I would order some at a time. I would make sure of all things during the slack time. The kind of things which are now delivered would never be delivered. If the work has to be done so quickly, naturally there are mistakes."

If the answer to a question demanded thinking first, he was at a loss. He would repeat words of the question, and while talking, more and more words would come to the fore which revealed a considerable knowledge. For example, asked "What is a frog?" he said: "Frog?...a frog?...what is a frog?...frog, quack, quack, it jumps." (What does it eat?) "That I do not know. It is in swamps, in water, on the brink." (What is its color?) "Frog...frog...tree frog, ah, color, tree-green. The tree frog is green, so!" The patient apparently begins with an action, which brings him into a definite situation: he repeats the words of the task. Then suddenly snaps in as association to frog the word "quack, quack." This association has nothing to do with the question; it is a *speech association*. Then other such associations appear which finally bring the answer to the question as to color.

He is asked on another occasion: "By what are the waves caused?" He answers, apparently as association to the word waves: "There whispers the wind, the wind." Asked what that means, he says: "There murmur the waves, there whispers the wind." This is a line out of a very well known German poem. He babbles this line again with totally expressionless features. Apparently, he does not understand the meaning of the words. Asked what the words mean, he says: "That must be a poem. I do not know how that came. How shall I explain it? What shall I say? Waves!" His behavior is more correctly described as "it spoke out of him rather than he spoke." He had to answer and he answered with words which came passively into his mind.

For this patient whose relations with the world by vision were very severely reduced, his visual recognition and imagery were totally missing, the instrumentalities of language became of greatest significance to remain in contact with the outer world, and he used the instrument of language in an excellent way. He represents an extraordinary example to demonstrate how much an individual can achieve (under favorable conditions) by a language, the "meaning" of which he does not experience but whose fitting in definite situations he knows and which is impressed on him passively and gives him the only possibility to fulfill a task he is set for.

Those who wish to study the significance of the instrumentalities of knowledge of language will find a rich material in the original description of this case. Indeed, they will at the same time realize how restricted such language without meaning is, and how unfit it is to do justice to the demands of the most essential tasks of the human being. It lacks all spontaneity and creativeness, i.e., the characteristics of man's behavior.

CHAPTER X

Treatment

A. GENERAL REMARKS

TREATMENT of aphasic disturbances was not and is not very popular among neurologists. Usually the attitude was one of pessimism as to whether one can help these patients by systematic training, and it was said: Either the condition improves spontaneously or it remains essentially unchanged in spite of all attempts at retraining.

This pessimistic attitude was at least to a certain degree understandable as long as one had to deal with patients with apoplectic insults where, indeed, due to their general condition, retraining is difficult and frequently not very successful, if also not so unpromising as often is assumed.

However, there is another group of patients where retraining gives much better results, and is very important. These are the men with injuries of the brain, particularly those with aphasia due to gunshot wounds. These cases also, who during and after the first world war came to observation in large number, were not considered by the neurologists at large as good objects for special treatment. At the end of World War I, advocation of establishment of special hospitals for treatment of soldiers with brain injuries and especially with aphasic symptoms did not meet with enthusiasm from the neurologists. Even after results had to be acknowledged, the treatment did not become a generally accepted method. One of the main reasons for this was that treatment is successful only if it is based on very careful examination of each individual case, a much more careful examination than usually was performed in studying of cases of aphasia (see the publications of Isserlin, Poppelreuter, Goldstein, et al.). The usual interpretation of the symptoms was not favorable for retraining, in contrast to the newer application of a more functional point of view. Finally, retraining can be expected to be successful only if it is performed with great effort, skill and spending of much time. If all these presuppositions are not fulfilled, disappointments must take place and the procedure comes into discredit—to the harm of these most generally neglected patients.

Those physicians who saw the problem and acted upon it accordingly, have reached good results (see Isserlin, Goldstein, Reichmann and in this country particularly Granich [during this war]).

There is no question that as a consequence of restitution of the damaged substratum, some disturbances are alleviated spontaneously—for instance, often the initial motor aphasia. This occurs particularly as result of operative procedures, elimination of a tumor, of loose splinters, abscesses, etc.

We can assume that in those cases the substratum recovered so that it functions now in the premorbid way. However, there are cases where, in spite of a defect of the brain remaining—even possibly increased by operation—improvement takes place, e.g., by extirpation of a scar in the cortex. Here we can assume, as I have explained before (see p. 9), that improvement is the effect of elimination of the disturbing effect of a scar, etc., i.e., by operation. The preserved part of the apparatus begins to function again in the previous way, thus guaranteeing the performances, at least to a certain degree.

Only in these two conditions, can one speak of *restitution*. From my experience, I cannot agree with the assumption that performances related to a definite substratum after destruction of the latter may return by taking over by a substratum which was not related to this function before (see particularly p. 51 and p. 53). Improvement by restitution takes place not only during the first weeks or months after the incident but sometimes many months later, particularly in cases of injury. Indeed, we never know definitely whether and how much spontaneous recovery will occur. But even if we can expect it, exercises are of help. Spontaneous recovery often develops slowly and before it occurs the patient may develop defensive and protective mechanisms, mannerisms, emotional reactions, wrong ways of compensation for the defect, building up of roundabout ways, etc. (see p. 192), which—useful for a certain time—later may become a severe hindrance, if real recovery sets in. Indeed, development of such intermediary reactions cannot be avoided, and sometimes should even be encouraged to help the patient go through the intermediary period. But the physician can help the patient by controlling the development of these "unnatural" reactions and by preventing him from sticking to them if they are no longer necessary.

Another reason that training is necessary is that frequently special methods have to be applied which the patient cannot find himself, because they must be based on psychologic and biologic knowledge concerning the nature of the defect; they are particularly useful because their application brings the patient the impression that he is not as disturbed as he thought (see p. 152), and thus often help to accelerate even the spontaneous recovery.

Even if spontaneous recovery is effective, there often comes a time when further improvement needs special effort on the part of the patient which he may not be able to effect alone. A motoric aphasic may be able to speak, but not fluently, and only with great effort and early fatigue, but the situation in which he lives makes it desirable for him to acquire better language. Here special training may bring the desired effect.

There are patients who, even after a long time, show no recovery and live in a situation in which it can scarcely be expected. If here some of the lost performances return, we are probably not dealing with restitution but substitution. Here the previous performances do not return, the defect is only compensated more or less by other performances, developed by using roundabout ways. We are sometimes deceived about this when we take only the effect into consideration (see p. 2). The patient may, himself, develop such compensation, but the physician can help him develop the right ones, guided by his knowledge of the means for substitutions which the investigation will reveal. These substitutes are determined by the tendency of the organism to come into the best possible condition—in spite of the remaining defect. This purpose is achieved if the performances fulfill the practical demands. This is the point of view from which alone they should be considered. The performances differ as to the variations of the personal structure, the special defect and the situation in which the patient has to live (cf. to this my explanation of the differences in two cases of visual agnosia, 90). The effect may be achieved by performances in a performance field different from the affected one or by amelioration of the defect performance itself through performances in another field. The first, e.g., is the case in severe visual agnosia where the patient learns to "read" by evaluation of kinaesthetic experiences, gained by planless tracing (see p. 121); the second, for example, if another agnostic patient makes the visual experience clearer by tracing movements and thus his reading is based on improved visual experiences (see p. 123).

In general, one can say that adaptation to an irreparable defect can occur in two ways (see 108a). The organism can yield to the defect; it restricts its performances to the preserved reduced ones, but the normal functioning of the organism is in principle unchanged. It is the more natural procedure, seems more automatic, demands less voluntary activity on the part of the individual, and hence secures more security than the second way in which the organism may react to a defect. Here the organism gives up the old procedure; because its maintenance would give too little effect, it tries to compensate by other performances. This represents a more volitional kind of behavior, leads more readily to fluctuation, involves less constancy and less security and admits a greater possibility for catastrophic situations. Some performances may be better than if the organism had stuck to the old procedure. In a mild form of visual disturbance of reading, the patient will try to use the reduced visual experiences. The patient with severe defect will give up this procedure and "read" only on the basis of kinaesthetic experiences; he may, in this respect, as far as recognition of the context of the written material is concerned, achieve better results, but the whole procedure is more difficult, more voluntary and more insecure.

These two ways of adjustment to a defect have to be considered if we want to understand spontaneous "recovery" and if we want to plan the training in the best way. Each performance has to be considered in respect to its significance for the best way of self realization of the organism in the given situation.

The various forms of aphasia are accessible to treatment in different degrees, the disturbances of the receptive side of language less than those of the motor side. Fortunately, the sensory defects show in general better spontaneous restitution because the apparatus underlying the sensory functions mostly comprise corresponding parts in both hemispheres (see p. 53). This is revealed in the severe defect in the beginning where the part of the apparatus in the minor side is disturbed in its function by the shock due to the damage in the major side, and in the recovery after disappearance of the shock.

B. Training of Patients with Motor Speech Defects

In dysarthria, our task is to help the patient to improve the distorted pronunciation. Exercises of the innervation of the concerned muscles are the means. I should like to refer, for this procedure, to the book of Froeschels and Jellineck, and to the management which Granich, who worked particularly with brain-injured soldiers, recommended and which he describes as follows (see 117, p. 48):

1. Repeating sounds after the instructor, in the attempt to perfect the sound, with running comments from the instructor by way of approval and criticism, and suggestions as to how to hold or move the mouth parts.

2. Imitation of the mouth movements of the instructor, who tilts his head back and opens his jaws wide to demonstrate the movements.

3. Directing the patient's attention in general to the appearance of the mouth parts during speech and having him visualize his own mouth movements as he tries to speak. This is best done when the patient and the instructor sit side by side in front of a large mirror.

4. For severe cases, by molding the mouth parts for the patient with a tongue depressor or fingers.

5. Having the patient feel with his fingers the mouth movements of the instructor and then his own.

6. Attempting the sound as part of a familiar short word; bringing in singing for recovery also, if it helps.

7. Placing a strip of damp paper on the tongue to increase sensation during speech.

8. Associating the movement for a given sound with some familiar non-speech act; for example, p with a type of spitting, k with clearing the throat, etc.

"P" can also be learned by making the movement of blowing out a candle, or by producing the movement of puffing smoke, as in smoking (see fig. 10). Or the patient may learn the "ng" by performing the act of swallowing, etc., or other sounds by imitation of animal sounds which are similar to human sounds; for instance, by learning the "U" by producing the "moo" of a cow, etc. This procedure can be very helpful in some cases. However, we should never forget that the sounds acquired by this method are not equal to the sounds we use in speech, and further that the sounds which one produces separately are not the same as those used in *words*. In real language, we do not speak by combining sounds into words. Thus, other kinds of training have to be added (see the following).

One might be inclined to object to this "unnatural" procedure from the point of view that it contradicts normal speaking in so far as we normally are unaware of the motor activities in speaking. Froment and Monod have, on this basis, rejected such a procedure. Froeschls was correct in stressing the point that therapeutic procedures cannot be rejected simply because other than physiologic means are used. There is an essential difference between the training of normals and the training of patients with motor aphasia. Certainly, in normals, one can and should proceed along physiologic paths and of course in pathologic cases one should also do the same thing as much as possible. But we are forced to adopt another method, at least in the beginning, if we are not successful with the "natural" procedure. Of course, later, the patient should learn to give up the conscious way of producing sounds, and he will, when he is able to speak in the natural way. In correct application of the exercises of the motor act, not only is there no danger involved, but also, by necessity, in many cases it is the only method of procedure which is successful (see the effect of this training in the cases reported before, p. 192 and p. 196).

In cases where the patient is *able to repeat sounds heard,* we shall start with repetition. The patient has to repeat sounds and words again and again, and hence also to learn to speak them spontaneously after a time. But even in these cases, the correct pronunciation will not be entirely acquired in this way alone; here, too, direct motor exercises are necessary to achieve it. Certainly, if the patient is able to speak sounds, words, so clearly that he is able to make himself understood, and only his pronunciation is incorrect, we should not torture him in this period of training with phonetic exercises. It is much more important for him to be able to use his speech for comprehensible communication than to speak correctly. There is no better means for improving motor speech than to use

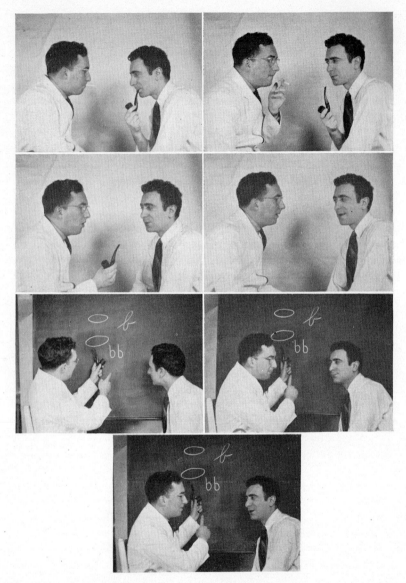

FIG. 10.   One example of retraining in speech movements.   Learning to produce the sound *b* by relation to the lip movement in emitting pipe smoke.

it for conversation and to gain the experience to be able to use his language for communication with his fellow men.   Nothing will increase the patient's hope for improvement as much as this experience and make him more ready for disagreeable exercises.   He will give up the language of signs and gestures which all patients with severe motor defects use in the beginning and which impedes progress in regaining speech.   Therefore, it is the uppermost aim of all training in this field to reach *as soon as possible a condition which renders communication possible*, and we should continue with the exercises of sounds only until this state is reached.   Better pronunciation may be regained by speaking or may be improved later by exercises.   Because the goal is to gain a language which is suited to express definite thoughts, training with words which have meaning for the patient, or meaningful sentences, as soon as possible is preferable.   This does not mean that the patient should learn to build correct sentences. But he should learn to use words as sentences, as the child does when first beginning to speak.   The patient often shows himself this tendency for the one-word sentence.   It is for this reason that it is unnecessary for the patient to learn in the beginning all the small words.   It is also not necessary that he decline verbs correctly.   He may use the verb in the infinitive, which is a simpler form.   In general, it may be stressed that one should never ask the patient to do anything which he is not able to do, or only with extreme effort.   Nothing will more diminish the effect of our exercises.

Learning of senseless combinations of syllables has been recommended on the basis that the patient might thus become capable of speaking new words, consisting of combinations of the syllables learned.   Such an assumption is not correct.   These words derived from senseless syllables do not exist either in our consciousness or in our motor action.   We do not speak combinations of syllables, but words, or better, sentences.   Certainly, in order to pronounce words which contain difficult combinations of letters, we must be able to pronounce the latter.   However, this alone will not help the pronunciation of words, and pronunciation will be learned within the word better than separately.   For some patients, it is without doubt much easier to pronounce these combinations within a word than in isolation.

As soon as possible the patient should name objects and accompany by words activities which he has to deal with in everyday life, even under conditions in which the normal does not do it.   Because he has no impairment in the capacity of naming, itself (see p. 61), he will not have difficulty in doing this, even if he pronounces the word wrongly.   He should be urged to speak as much as possible.

If we are dealing with a purely motor defect, it will be astonishing how quickly the patient regains language sufficiently for conversation after he has overcome the initial difficulty.   In this respect, there is a great difference between those patients with peripheral motor aphasia and the patients with central motor aphasia who are impaired also in the abstract attitude. The abstract attitude is an important means of learning in this "abstract" way. This is demonstrated also in the fact that training is the more successful the more intelligent the individual is.

We have pointed before (see p. 36) to the hierarchic organization of the sounds. All which we have said there has to be considered in training, particularly the rule that the production of one sound presupposes the existence of another one (see p. 38). This corresponds to the experiences with our patients. We often find that when we start with one sound, the patient is unable to learn it. But it is very easy to teach him the pronunciation of the sound concerned after he has learned other sounds. The application of this rule, which according to Jacobson, is valid here, may save time and effort. Indeed, one must never forget that it does not represent the only factor of importance but that other factors previously mentioned are also to be considered, and finally, that the selection which pathology sometimes makes may not always be in accordance with the normal stratification. If in practice we observe that a patient is not able to produce a definite sound, we should not force him, but should go over to another sound (see p. 192).

There is one type of patient who is able to speak series and familiar expressions fluently, but the pronunciation of the sounds, and, as consequence, the pronunciation of some single words, is defective. Here the pronunciation of the words by frequent speaking in any form, repetition, reading, spontaneous speech, in series, must be trained. The patients realize this themselves and recite the series to themselves, the series of numbers, days, months, etc., until they come to the desired word, which they then repeat much better than they would have been able to if uttered separately. Sometimes they can only say a word within a song. While in *singing* they may make no mistakes in pronunciation, they may have the greatest difficulty in pronouncing one of these words individually. Later, the word has to be freed from its relation to the rhythmic context.

One will use all these aids, sometimes recognized by the patients themselves, for retraining. If the *patient is able to speak* words within a series, then one *will insist that he recite the series slowly*, word by word, repeating first the series and then the single words separately. Sometimes it is useful for the patient to learn to say the word in rhythmic accentuation.

After the patient has learned to speak most of the words, prompt automatic fluency may be lacking. Spontaneous speech may be disturbed particularly because some automatisms are missing which are necessary for fluent speaking, as, for example, the grammatical forms—suffixes, prefixes, articles, the forms of conjugation, etc. (see p. 194). The patient may have to ponder each form. Therefore, his talking is slow and heavy.

The patient may try to acquire the automatisms by rote learning in the same way as children do. However, this procedure usually brings little success particularly if the abstract attitude is impaired. In the beginning one must proceed in an indirect way. The patient may use various mnemotechnic means or he may learn with the help of grammatical rules. As soon as possible, he should use what he has learned in meaningful sentences. He should complete the grammatical forms in compositions, according to the sentence completion test, etc. Speaking in correct forms will be acquired only if the patient memorizes the various forms again and again, only if the motor automatisms are rebuilt.

C. Training in Disturbances of Reading

We have described before (p. 122) how a patient with visual alexia may learn to read by systematic development of tracing movements. In cases where difficulty of spelling and composing letters into words is the basis of the reading difficulty, one may try to teach spelling, etc., but, on the other hand, the patient may learn words as wholes, particularly those which are of practical significance to him.

We have mentioned another difficulty in reading, when the patient recognizes visually the letters as known objects and is able to pronounce the sounds but has lost the capacity to connect both phenomena. It is usually not possible to rebuild this relation directly. Two indirect methods are useful in this respect: in one, visual association between the form of a letter and the form of a known object is established; the name of the object helps to find the sound belonging to the letter, e.g., the association of the form of an a and an apple, makes him find the sound a. In the other, motor association between the picture of the letter and a definite movement is formed (see p. 336).

These procedures in retraining reading capacity might be considered similar to those used in teaching children. However, there is an important difference which must not be overlooked. In teaching children, the roundabout method of relating objects to letters is employed only for a short time and only for additional aid. The child soon forgets this, recalling it only when reading difficult letters. Very soon, a direct relation between the printed and written letter and the sound is established. For the patient, the roundabout method may be the only possible procedure. He may be unable to learn the other way. This difference is of theoretic and practical importance. The child is induced to forget the roundabout method, as it interferes with fluent reading. He is perfectly able to do so. The patient, however, must keep these associations, at least for a long time, till he may gain, to a certain degree, direct associations.

The roundabout method of using motor associations consists of building

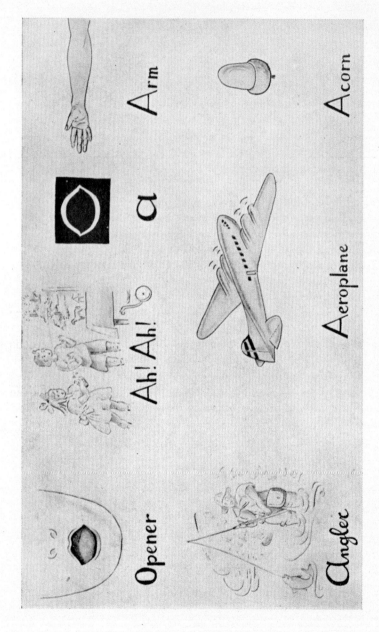

Fig. 11. The two sets of drawings reproduced here, suggesting associations of the form and sound of the letter *a*, are examples of charts usable for retraining in speech, reading and writing, by means of form-sound-movement relationship (see p. 336).

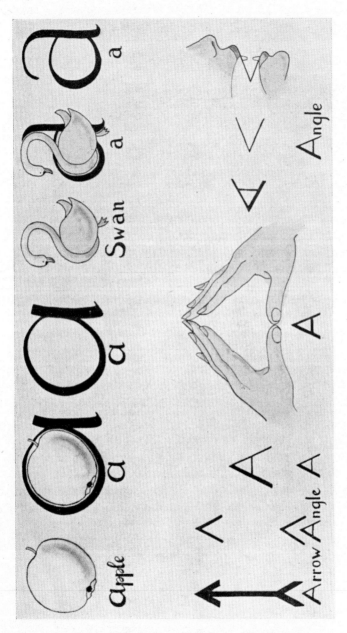

Fig. 11.—*Concluded*

an association between a seen letter and a particular movement. That in itself is suited to evoke the making of the sound. For instance, in learning to read *o*, the patient has to imitate with his mouth the form of the seen letter, and makes a blowing movement. Thus he produces the sound of *o*. With time, upon seeing *o*, he produces directly the sound of *o*. For training the patient to read the capital *A*, the similarity between the appearance of *A* on its side, ⊲, and the shape of the mouth which belongs to the making of the broad A sound, is pointed out to the patient. In this way, various motor associations can be used in learning to read.

As to the theory of treatment in general, this example shows that the methods of training patients and children have some similarity, but that a simple carrying over of the methods used in child training would be wrong and disappointing. This refers not only to retraining in reading, but is valid generally. I stress this point because it is often overlooked, and the disappointment which naturally follows may cause all attempts to retrain patients to be discredited.

Slowly memorizing the alphabet is another means of facilitating learning to read letters. This procedure originated when it was found that a patient may fail to find the correct name of a letter he sees, but may be able to select the correct name from a series of spoken letters. Hence, he may be able to find the correct letter by speaking the series slowly or silently. We therefore instructed such patients to learn the alphabet, preferably in groups of five letters (*a-b-c-d-e, f-g-h-i-j*). The vowels may be learned as a special series, *a-e-i-o-u*. Each group is represented by the five fingers of the hand, each finger representing one letter. First, the patient listens to the teacher reciting the letters, counting them off on his fingers. He then repeats this procedure. It is also helpful for the patient to learn the alphabet by writing, if he is able to write.

Usually, these patients recognize the identity of the letters of various kinds of alphabets (small letters, capitals, written, or printed letters). However, if the patient does have difficulty in this respect, simple exercises may be introduced by which the patient learns to associate the visual images of the corresponding letters of the various alphabets. This is best accomplished by sorting exercises. The patient must select, for instance, from the various kinds of alphabets, all letters related to the small *i*. A modification of this is for the patient to write down the letters of various alphabets which he associates with the visual image of the small *i*.

If the patient is able to read some letters, he starts his training by reading syllables of short words. He must combine the sounds of the single letters. Singing is helpful here.

Reading in these roundabout ways is very arduous. Therefore, we try to facilitate things by learning to read words as wholes. For this purpose, we direct the patient's attention to the similarities and differences in the visual forms of the words.

We write down, one under the other, ten words that have a similar visual appearance, such as "Hans," "hand," "hunt," "hurt." We present three words at a time. The patient must learn to recognize the similarities and to distinguish the differences in the three words. He may learn the words which belong to such groups as series. Later, he has to match a word he sees with a word he hears. Then he has to read aloud the words as wholes; here he may first recite the series of words, and then pick out the correct word in the written series.

The words selected for the patient to learn as wholes should be words which are easy to recognize visually and which are used frequently in reading.

D. Training in Disturbances of Writing

In cases when the difficulty in writing is an expression of impairment of spontaneity (see p. 127) retraining consists of improvement of spontaneity in general. For special training, the patient is instructed to copy letters and other forms, such as circles, again and again. Later, he must take dictation. If speech is intact, dictation of words in meaningful sentences should begin as soon as possible.

In other cases, the patient has forgotten the actions corresponding to the formation of letters (pure agraphia or apractic agraphia), or at least has difficulty in remembering them (see p. 129), or may remember some parts which he may be able to begin correctly, but soon does not know how to continue with the form of the letter or he may mix up single parts of the letter, etc. If the patient is able to copy the letter, even in an imperfect way, he may learn to improve his writing by copying movements. Then he may accompany his writing with uttering the sound or the name of the letter. If this is not possible, the condition has to be improved in other ways. If the patient has good visualization and the visual images can be further improved, it is advisable to make the patient aware of the visual images and let him copy the images. However, this will help only to a limited degree. It is a very imperfect method. It is rare that somebody can evoke so clear an image of a letter that he can use it as a model for writing. The following use of visualization may be more helpful. The patient learns that the form of a given letter is the same as the form of an object. Then, if asked to write, he may remember the form of the object and copy its visual image (see fig. 11). For instance, he may make an *F* by copying the visual image of a flag. This visual image need not be very definite in order to be used in the formation of the letter.

In patients with poor visual imagery, this method is naturally not applicable. Here, only retraining of the motor automatisms represented by letters can help. The procedure is as follows:

1. The teacher guides the patient's hand according to the form of the letter, repeating this several times, and letting the patient repeat the tracing again and again. The teacher gradually refrains from guiding, so that the patient acts with increasing independence. This helps to execute the movement with increased speed.

2. Tracing on a pane of glass under which the patterns of the letters are placed so that the patient can see and copy them, has proved especially successful.

3. The teacher may write the letter in the air in front of the patient's eyes, so that he is able to imitate the movement directly.

4. The patient may learn some letters by association of the movement of forming the letter with other movements.

It is useful to train the individual in forming not only letters, but also other simple shapes, such as circles, lines, and so on.

These exercises may bring improvement in a short time even in patients who have been unable to write for months or years. One of our patients, who had all the difficulty above described, and who could produce very few letters successfully, was able to write some words and short sentences spontaneously two months after beginning the treatment. It is noticeable that concomitantly with improvement of writing, the general behavior of the patient, who lacked all spontaneity, was improved. Since improvement took place step by step in relation to the exercises, there can be no doubt that it was due to these.

If, as in secondary agraphia (see p. 131), the capacity for forming letters is not impaired, but the patients are disturbed in writing capacity as a consequence of defects in their language function we have to proceed differently according to the underlying speech defect.

In defects in writing as sequelae of motor aphasia, writing may improve if speech is improved. If this is not the case, one may try to improve writing by copying and using visual images (see p. 28). If the agraphia is "pure agraphia" (see p. 129), the patient has to be retrained in the way we mentioned before.

There is another group of patients who are able to form letters, copy letters, speak sounds, and name letters, but who have lost the capacity to relate language and letters. The letters have become meaningless objects to them. An incapacity to read parallels this defect (see p. 133).

If the patient is able to write several letters or several words as wholes from dictation (as is often the case), we use these letters or words he has retained as a starting point. The teacher divides the word into sounds, and points out the relation between the sound and the corresponding letters. The patient tries to repeat the sounds. Thus, he may learn to write some letters from dictation and become able to use these letters in writing other combinations in other words. At the same time he may learn to read some letters and words. His attention may be drawn to the visual images of the letters, thus impressing and reinforcing them in his mind, providing, of course, that his visualization is good. The patient may then be able to write the letters on demand by copying this visual image.

Another procedure is as follows: The patient must copy a letter which is presented beside an object. The name of the object begins with the letter. The patient, at the same time, must say the name of the object and isolate the first letter. The association between the object and the letter can be strengthened by using an object which has a shape similar to the letter, e.g., an apple with *a*. This relation between a letter and the name of an object can also be strengthened by acoustic associations. The patient learns "a-apple," "t-trumpet," etc.

We proceed by the following steps:

1. The patient is shown the picture of the object and the letter. He has to name the object, separate the first letter of the word, point to the letter, and repeat the sound of it. He is then confronted with the picture of an object alone. He must select from a group of presented letters that letter which relates to the object, and then name the object and the letter. He must copy the letter. Then he must write the letter without a model.

2. The teacher speaks the name of the object. The patient has to select the corresponding letter from a number of letters, and copy it and then write it without the model.

3. The teacher utters the sound. The patient speaks the name of the object, and then selects the letter, copies it, and writes it without the model.

4. The teacher expresses the sound. The patient selects the letter without giving the name of the object, copies it, and writes it without the model.

5. The teacher expresses the sound and the patient writes the letter.

After some weeks of training, the patient is able to write the letter from dictation, proceeding in the roundabout way: hearing the sound of the letter, recalling the name of the object, reproducing the visual image of the object and the visual image of the letter, and copying this image. With time, this long procedure is shortened by the gradual omission of one or several of the steps, until finally, upon hearing the sound, the patient writes the letter directly.

This training can be facilitated by building up an acoustico-motor-visual response. The patient learns to express each sound by a motor act, an expressive movement. The speaking of *o* is experienced by forming an *o* with the mouth, and the patient imitates this form, at times by using a mirror.   Thus, he learns to connect the sound with a definite movement, corresponding to the form of the letter (see fig. 11).

Whether a patient will require this and other helpful methods for retraining, or whether the first method described will be sufficient, depends upon his individuality.

After learning to write the letters from dictation, the patient will be able to write words by dividing them into letters or sounds.   The capacity to divide words is usually intact in patients of this type.   Of course, separate training must be given if this capacity is disturbed.

By writing words letter by letter, the patient learns to write words as wholes.   Generally this is not very difficult, as he is not suffering from a defect in writing itself.   If he is unable to divide the words into sounds or letters, and has had little success with writing words as wholes, he must be taught to divide the words into sounds.

The exercises are to begin with phonetic reading.   The patient must experience the sounds and recognize that the spoken words can be built of combinations of sounds.   However, this alone is not sufficient for teaching him to separate sounds as is required in writing words.   The following exercises are often more successful.

The teacher carefully articulates short, simple words, separating the sounds; for example, "hand, h-a-n-d."   The patient must repeat this, pronouncing the word with pauses between the sounds.   This last step is the most difficult, but it can be facilitated by making the individual familiar with the sound in another way.   He learns the alphabet, as before said; then he has to realize the relation between the names of the letters and their sounds.   After he has grasped this, the teacher expresses the sound, the patient the letter; then the teacher the letter, and the patient the sound.

Another method is to present the patient with letters written on a piece of paper, and require him to cancel out those letters which do not belong to the specific sound he is working on.   Here, too, isolation of letters and sounds facilitates learning.   The patient must read words, letter by letter, sound by sound, and write words in the same way, with the teacher guiding his hand.

Of course such exercises in phonetic writing only develop spelling that corresponds directly to the articulate sounds.   After he has learned to write in this way, the patient must learn orthographically correct writing by spelling exercises.

In the beginning it is only natural for the patient to make many mistakes. The following are the main errors.   He may have difficulty in separating vowels and omit them.   He may mix up vowels or similar consonants such as d, t. He may not be able to separate the sounds correctly, combining parts of two sounds and making them one, etc.

With patience and determination, it will be possible to help the majority of these patients to such an extent that they will be able to write from dictation, and even spontaneously, well enough for practical purposes.

Central aphasia and sensory aphasia are almost invariably followed by some disturbances in writing ability which correspond to the defect of inner speech (see p. 229). The letters are written normally. The defect consists of mistakes in spelling, omission of letters, errors in grammar and syntax. Improvement of the underlying speech defect is difficult. We have to try to consolidate the "ideas of words" (see p. 93). We try to acquaint the patient with words and show him that variations in pronunciation need not change the meaning of the word. The patient is given the task of repeating the correct and incorrect pronunciation of a word, while remembering that it is the same word, unchanged in meaning. He must separate the letters and syllables of a word, combine them, and realize what is significant for the meaning and what is not, by comparing them with other words which are similar in sound. The words are then broken up into parts which he can speak correctly. He must repeat these, combine them, giving them the proper pronunciation, until he is able to pronounce the whole word, etc.

Exercises of repetition of different kind of words and sentences, reading and writing are essential. Besides this, building of motor and visual automatisms and those in writing are recommended, indeed especially for such performances which are of particular practical significance.

E. Treatment of Disturbances of Word-finding

As we explained before (see p. 59) this symptom can be the expression of different functional defects. We have to determine the cause in the individual case, because retraining differs accordingly.

The difficulty in word-finding can be impairment of memory, particularly in the sphere of language. These patients need not show any defect of general intelligence, particularly not impairment of abstraction (see p. 67). We are dealing with a loss of learned material, and these patients can be helped by application of the usual methods of learning.

In the group where the difficulty in word-finding, in particular in naming objects, is one symptom of the so-called amnesic aphasia, which basic defect is impairment of abstract attitude (see p. 60), we have to proceed in a totally different way.

If the damage of the brain underlying amnesic aphasia restitutes itself to a certain degree the patient may regain, more or less, his abstract attitude and the capacity to find words, also in the form of naming. This may occur after extirpation of a tumor, abscess or even spontaneously if the effect of a hemorrhage which in the beginning had damaged the brain cortex diffusely later is restricted to a more circumscribed area. Under such conditions, real improvement, not only effectual "pseudo-improvement," e.g., pseudo-naming, may occur.

If the damage of the brain matter is persistent, only "pseudo-improvement" can be achieved, i.e., building of "associations" between objects and words. To build these associations directly by rote learning is usually disappointing to the patient and the physician (see p. 63). Finding the words can take place only in an indirect, roundabout way which the patient sometimes finds himself but in which training can help him very much.

The simplest methods which the patients often apply themselves are the following: the patient asks the name of an object, writes it down, beside a simple picture of the object and trains himself by reading the word again and again while looking at the picture. The teacher may show the picture, present the name and later ask him to give the name to the picture. This procedure is strenuous and somebody who is impaired in abstract attitude will not be very successful with it due to the difficulty in rote learning (see p. 8). It may be more successful if the patient learns together words belonging to a group of objects which are in a natural concrete relationship for him. For example, he knows that a shirt, trousers, coat, waistcoat, necktie do belong together. He learns these words as a series. If he has to give a name for an object, he recites the group to which it belongs and thus achieves his result by speaking the word which fits the object. He stops when he recognizes the word wanted. This procedure is facilitated if the patient has acquired some words. These words can then be used as basis for further associations. Sometimes it helps if the patient learns the words of a series in a definite rhythm, one which is familiar to him. If he possesses such series from a previous time, certainly they should be used for finding the demanded word, as, for instance, the days of the week, series of the months, of numbers, etc. They should be intentionally repeated, otherwise they may be easily forgotten (see p. 8).

Better ways of improvement are those which use the capacity of the patient to find the word in a concrete situation to which it belongs. The patient will bring himself, or we bring him, into such a concrete situation where the demanded word may come to the fore. This will happen if the object he wants to name elicits another object which is for the patient more concrete and therefore more closely related to a word. This word may allow him to find the demanded word. One example, taken from Granich's book (117, p. 55) is the following. As the patient sits in the dining hall with his coffee before him, at a loss as to how he can ask for cream, he may remember the object, ice cream, and then may ask for "cream."

If he is asked to give the name of a person, he may remember a situation in which he was meeting him and addressing him by name, and thus may recall the name.   He may not recall the name of a street, but he remembers that the street has the same name as the first name of a friend.   This recollection brings the name to his mind in connection with other characteristics of his friend.   Or he may recite a little verse which he knows is related to an object and contains the word he cannot find.   While repeating the verse he recognizes the word and repeats it (see 108, p. 157).

There is a further possibility of improving word-finding by use of images, particularly visualization.

The patient may visualize the written word and read it.   Or he may visualize with the presented object another object, the name of which he knows and which by association may bring the demanded word to the fore (see 108, p. 157).

Another method is to let the patient learn meaningful sentences which contain required words.   A patient unable to find the words hunter, hare, shoot, learned in a deposited rhythm, "The hunter shoots the hare."   Later he could find all these words with the help of this sentence.   The sentences learned in this way should depict concrete situations.

The form of the sentence completion test can be used as material for exercises.   First sentences are used which are familiar to the patient and easily understood.   Words the patient has difficulty in finding are omitted. The sentences are modified; words he has learned are brought into new connections and new words are introduced.

However, all these ways are not real word-finding.   The most conclusive evidence of this is that, immediately afterward, on being asked again the name of the same object, the patient is unable to utter the word directly.   But the procedure has to be used not only because it is the only one by which the patient can find the word but it is helpful also for another reason: He becomes aware of the possibilities and practical usefulness of this procedure and thus becomes more and more skillful in using it. After having recognized the trick, he learns to perfect it more and more.

Our task is to find out the best methods which the individual patient can apply—according to his premorbid individual capacities, their greater or smaller disturbance by the affection and the present condition in general, intelligence, emotions, and finally, the outer world situation which may make acquisition of some words appear more or less useful or necessary.

Because often a decision regarding which method is best may not be possible, one should try all methods and that which is most successful and requires the least effort from the patient should be followed. Usually several ways will have to be employed.

With time, the patient may be able to stop using the indirect methods and act more or less directly. How much that will occur depends upon how much the situation forces him to use language. As long as he does not recover as to abstract attitude he never regains meaning, but in spite of this he may perform better by improving his associations and learning external associations (see p. 343).

The described methods of retraining in certain speech defects should be considered only as examples which may enable the physician and the teacher to arrange the procedure in other cases in a way adequate to the individual disturbance. I hope it will have become evident on the one hand that the goal of our endeavor is to help the patient regain a language which will be useful for his attempt to realize his personality—in spite of his defect—to as high a degree as possible; on the other hand, that, like theoretic understanding, this practical purpose can be achieved only by the organismic approach.

Concluding Remarks

IT IS with some hesitation that I offer this book. No one is better aware of its shortcomings than I. For several decades past, I have been concerned with the phenomenon of aphasia while studying patients and collecting data. All the more has it become clear to me that such a work as the present volume can be only a step toward the final understanding of individuals suffering from language disorder.

Since the publication of my first paper on aphasia in 1906, patients with difficulty in finding words, especially names for objects, posed the most significant problem for us. This problem, always with me in my studies, later became their very center. I was eventually led to seek its solution in the cognitive processes connected with the meaning of words. This solution did not derive from the study of language disturbances alone but also from broader research on the structure of human behavior in general. It grew particularly from the increasing recognition of the outstanding rôle which abstract attitude plays in the organization of human performance (107). The importance of abstract attitude suggested itself especially from the observations of its impairment in cortical defects and speech pathology. I tried time and again to prove the assumed significance of abstract attitude by detail studies of the changes of the performances in brain-damaged patients.

If I have not been as successful as I would have liked, the reason may lie in the complexity of the problem which one faces in an attempt to explain the vexing phenomena of speech pathology. This task presupposes not only detailed acquaintance with pathologic material but also with material of various other scientific fields. To meet these demands would require expert knowledge in practically all branches of the science of man. There is considerable disagreement about the pertinent facts and their explanation within such concerned disciplines as biology, psychology, linguistics, and anthropology. It is therefore not feasible to utilize data from these fields by directly applying the facts as ready-made results to the problem of language disturbances. The different views regarding the nature of man reflect themselves in the discussions of man's outstanding capacity: language. From this stem many differences in methodology of investigating, reporting and interpreting the phenomena. Depending upon his theoretic preconception, the particular investigator will tend to emphasize different parts of the findings. If one wants to apply the experience to studies of pathology, one will have to make one's own selection from the presented material, a selection which easily predisposes to error. Indeed, an unbiased and careful description of the pathologic phenomena of language may offer a test for the correctness and adequacy of current conceptions advanced about the nature of man in other branches of the science of man. Such comparisons may become fruitful in finding answers to unsettled issues in these other fields.

In formulating my conclusions and the concepts through which I attempted to explain language disorder, I could not make as much use of case material from other authors as would have been desirable. As stated before, the protocols of the behavior of the patients published in the literature are dependent on diversified theoretic approaches; therefore, they often are ill-suited for comparison, do not at all always offer solid grounds for reaching definite decisions about the nature of the patients' impairments. I tried to avoid this difficulty by presenting detailed descriptions of carefully studied cases so that the reader may be able to decide for himself whether or not my conclusions follow from the facts.

The least I can hope from my endeavors is that the problems have been made clear-cut issues and that there will be a recognition of the methodologic requirements which must be fulfilled if our knowledge in this field is fruitfully to be furthered.

Specialized Bibliography

To facilitate the finding of the pertinent literature to different topics, the main references for these topics are listed separately below. The numbers refer to general bibliography, page 349, where complete references are listed.

I. References to the Organismic Approach to Brain Pathology in General and to Aphasia in Particular

2, 3, 5, 6, 8, 11, 23, 33, 37, 38, 50, 54, 57, 64, 77, 79, 84, 89, 90, 93, 94, 95, 96, 97, 98, 99, 101, 102, 103, 105, 106, 107, 108, 109, 110, 112a, 122, 127, 133, 139, 141, 147, 152, 156, 165, 166, 170, 179, 184, 185, 196, 197, 207, 209, 211, 214, 228, 229, 237, 240, 262, 280, 289, 296, 297, 299, 313, 316, 322, 324

II. References to Research on Normal Language in its Significance for Aphasia

4, 12, 30, 34, 35, 49, 53, 56, 66, 67, 74, 118, 119, 121, 140, 149, 150, 152, 157, 158, 159, 167, 168, 169, 173, 174, 175, 200, 201, 202, 220, 221, 222, 228, 229, 237, 241, 263, 264, 268, 269, 279, 283, 284, 285, 291, 294, 300, 301, 304, 319, 321, 327, 328, 329

III. References to the Problem of Localization

6, 29, 32, 52, 60, 63, 82, 97, 127 (*Lit.*), 155, 180, 194, 206, 209, 238, 302, 307, 316, 330

IV. References to the Survey of the Various Forms of Disturbances of Language in Pathology

24, 91, 103, 105, 111, 113, 115, 127, 128, 129, 153

V. References to Disturbances of Wordfinding and Amnesic Aphasia

13, 39, 76, 77, 81, 92, 104, 111, 112, 114, 152, 171, 172, 174, 177, 178, 192, 193, 203, 244, 260, 311, 312, 313, 332

VI. References to Disturbances of the Expressive Side of Language and Motor Aphasia

6, 14, 18, 20, 22, 26, 27, 28, 51, 59, 72, 86, 97, 133, 139, 144, 151, 184, 197, 204, 208, 213, 216, 217, 218, 219, 252, 255, 271, 316, 325

VII. References to Disturbances of the Receptive Side of Language and Sensory Aphasia

15, 17, 19, 21, 45, 47, 48, 75, 78, 131, 137, 138, 145, 184, 187, 195, 232, 234, 235, 236, 245, 267, 277, 286, 292, 303, 330

VIII. References to Disturbances of Inner Speech and Central Aphasia

61, 81, 83, 85, 100, 114, 134, 138, 164, 190, 226, 229, 233, 245, 260, 280, 287, 304, 317

IX. References to Disturbances of Intelligence in Aphasic Patients and the Speech Disturbances of the Non-language Mental Processes

7, 9, 16, 18, 24, 25, 75, 84, 86, 87, 88, 135, 136, 146, 163, 181, 184, 186, 188, 199, 204, 206, 207, 208, 209, 216, 217, 218, 223, 230, 231, 232, 234, 235, 236, 250, 253, 254, 261, 268, 288, 290, 292, 298, 316

X. REFERENCES TO THE DISTURBANCES OF CALCULATION IN APHASIC PATIENTS

8, 10, 23, 89, 97 (p. 799), 108 (p. 205), 124, 127, 139, 180, 213, 224, 249, 259, 265, 273, 274, 320, 325

XI. REFERENCES TO THE DISTURBANCES OF GESTURES IN APHASIC PATIENTS

40, 41, 43, 154, 183

XII. REFERENCES TO APHASIA OF POLYGLOTS

31, 113, 143, 161, 205, 239, 243, 257, 282

XIII. REFERENCES TO READING AND WRITING AND THEIR DISTURBANCES IN APHASIC PATIENTS

1, 36, 42, 44, 46, 55, 57, 73, 80, 89, 97, 108, 112, 112a, 126, 130, 142, 176, 189, 191, 198, 212, 216, 223, 237, 242, 247, 266, 272, 275, 276, 289, 292, 305, 306, 318, 321, 326

XIV. REFERENCES TO NOMENCLATURE AND EXAMINATION

62, 89, 108, 115, 116, 123, 125, 127, 160, 162, 251, 270, 295, 304, 310, 313, 314, 315

XV. REFERENCES TO TREATMENT

58, 65, 68, 69, 70, 71, 88, 89, 108, 108a, 110, 117, 120, 148, 157, 215, 227, 256, 308, 309

Bibliography

This bibliography is not intended to cover all the literature of the subject, as it is far too extensive to include here. It comprises those references which are particularly relevant to this book, and those publications which contain surveys of the literature in their particular fields. The designation "(*Lit.*)" at the end of a reference indicates that the publication named contains further references.

1. ADLER, ALEXANDRA: Disintegration and restoration of optic recognition in visual agnosia. Arch. Neurol. *51:* 243, 1944.
2. ALLPORT, G. W.: Personality. A Psychological Interpretation. New York, 1937.
3. ANTON, G.: Über die Selbstwahrnehmungen der Herderkrankungen des Gehirnes etc. Archiv für Psychiatrie, *32:* 1899.
4. BALLET, G.: Le langage intérieur et les diverses formes de l'aphasie. Paris, Alcan, 1886.
5. BANTI: Aphasia e li sue forme. La Speromentale. Florence, 1886.
6. BASTIAN, H. D.: A Treatise on Aphasia, etc. London, 1898.
7. ——: On the various forms of loss of speech in cerebral diseases. British and Foreign Med. Chic. Rev. 1869.
8. BENARY, W.: Studien zur Untersuchung der Intelligenz bei einem Fall von Seelenblindheit (Goldstein und Gelb, Psychologische Analysen). Psychologische Forschung, *2:* 209, 1922.
9. BERG, MAX: Zur Kenntnis der transkortikalen Aphasie. Monatsschrift fur Psychiatrie und Neurologie, *13:* 341, 1903.
10. BERGER, H.: Über Rechenstörungen bei Nervenerkrankungen des Grosshirns. Archiv für Psychiatrie und Nervenkrankheiten *78:* 783, 1926.
11. BETHE, A.: Plastizität und Zentrenlehre. Handbuch der normalen und pathologischen Physiologie, *15:* 1930.
12. BINET, A.: Etude expérimentelle de l'intelligence. Paris. 1922.
13. BINSWANGER, L.: Zum Problem von Sprache und Denken. Schweizer Archiv für Neurologie, *36:* 54. 1926.
14. BISCHOFF, E.: Archiv für Psychiatrie und Nervenkrankheiten *32:* 730.
15. ——: Über die verschiedenen Formen der Sprachtaubheit. Zentralblatt für Nervenheilkunde und Psychiatrie, 1901.
16. BLEULER, E.: Ein Fall von aphasischen Symptomen etc. Archiv für Psychiatrie *25:* 32, 1893.
17. BOERNSTEIN, W.: Der Abbau der Hoerfunction bei kortikalen Verletzungen Deutsche Zeitschrift f. Nervenheilkunde *81:* 216, 1924.
18. BONHOEFFER, C.: Die Rückbildung motorischer Aphasie. Mitteilungen aus den Grenzgebieten der Medizin und Chirurgie, *10:* 203, 1902.
19. ——: Über subkortikale sensorische Aphasie. Jahrbücher für Psychiatrie und Neurologie *26:* 126, 1905.
20. BONVICINI, G.: Zur Bestimmung der frontalen Grenze des Aphasiegebietes. Wiener Klinische Wochenschrift *44–47:* 1926.
21. ——: Die Störungen der Lautsprache bei Temporal-Lappenläsion. Handbuch der Neurologie des Ohres, *2:* 1929. Wien, Urban und Schwarzenburg. (Lit.)
22. BOUILLAUD, J.: Traité clinique et physiologique de l'encéphalite. 1825.
23. BOUMAN, L., AND GRÜNBAUM: Experimentell-psychologische Untersuchungen zur Aphasie etc. Zeitschrift für die gesamte Neurologie und Psychiatrie *96:* 1925.

24. BRICKNER, R. M.: The Intellectual Functions of the Frontal Lobes. New York, Macmillan, 1936. (Lit.)

25. BROADBENT, W. H.: A case of peculiar affection of speech etc. ("Ideation center"). Brain 1: 1879.

26. BROCA, P.: Bulletin de la Société d'Anthropologie, 2: 235, 1861.

27. ——: Ibid. 6: 230, 1861.

28. ——: Exposé des titres et des travaux scientifiques de M. Paul Broca. Paris, 1863.

29. BRODMANN, K.: Lokalisationslehre der Grosshirnrinde. Leipzig, 1909.

30. BÜHLER, CARL: Phonetik und Phonologie. Travaux du Cours linguistique de Prague, 4: 1931.

31. BYCHOWSKI, Z.: Ueber die Restitution der nach einem Schaedelschuss verlorenen Umgangssprache bei einem Polyglotten. Monatsschrift für Psychiatrie, 45: 1919.

32. CAMPBELL, A. W.: Histological Studies on the Localization of Cerebral Function. Cambridge University Press, 1905.

33. CANNON, W.: The Wisdom of the Body. New York, Norton, 1932.

34. CARTER, J. W., JR.: An experimental study of psychology of stimulus-response. Psycholog. Record 2: 1938.

35. CASSIRER, E.: Philosophie der symbolischen Formen, 1: Berlin, 1923. (Lit.)

35a. CASSIRER, E.: An Essay on Man. New Haven, Yale University Press, 1944.

36. CHARCOT, J. M.: Sur un Cas de cécité verbale. Oeuvres complètes de Charcot. Paris, Delahaye-Lecrosnier, 1887.

37. CHILD, C. M.: The Physiological Foundation of Behavior. New York, 1929.

38. COGHILL, G. E.: Anatomy and the Problem of Behavior. New York, 1929.

39. CONRAD, K.: Versuch einer psychologischen Analyse des Parietalsyndroms. Monatsschrift für Psychiatrie und Neurologie 84: 28, 1932.

40. CRITCHLEY, MACDONALD: The Language of Gesture. London, Arnold & Co. 1939. (Lit.)

41. ——: Brain 61: 163, 1939.

42. CROUZON AND VALENCE: Un cas d'alexie pure. Bulletin et mém. de la soc. méd. des hopitaux de Paris 39: 1145, 1923.

43. DARWIN, CHARLES: The Expression of the Emotions in Man and Animals. ed. 2. London, 1889.

44. DEJERINE, J.: Mémoires de la Société de Biologie, 1892.

45. ——: L'Aphasie sensorielle. Presse medicale. 1906.

46. DEJERINE, J., AND PÉLISSIER, A.: Contribution à l'étude de la cécité verbale pure. Encéphale, 1914–19.

47. ——, AND SÉRIEUX, P.: Un cas de surdité verbale pure etc. Revue de Psychologie, 1898.

48. ——, AND THOMAS: Sur un cas de surdité verbale pure. Société de Neurologie, Séance du 5 juin 1902.

49. DELACROIX, H.: Le Langage et la pensée. Paris, Alcan, 1924.

50. DEWEY, JOHN: The reflex arc concept in psychology. Psychol. Record 3: 1896.

51. ECONOMO, v.: Wilson's Krankheit und das Syndrom du corps strié. Zeitschrift für die gesamte Neurologie und Psychiatrie 43: 1918.

52. ——, AND KOSKINAS: Cytoarchitektonik der Hirnrinde, etc. Berlin, Springer, 1925.

53. EHRENFELS, CHR. v.: Über Gestaltqualitäten. Vierteljahrsschrift für wissenschaftliche Philosophie 14: 249, 1890.

54. ELLIS, W. D.: Source Book of Gestalt Psychology.   New York, 1938.
55. ERBSLÖH, W.: Über einen Fall der isolierten Agraphie etc. Neurologisches Zentralblatt, 1903.
56. ERDMANN, B.: Die psychologische Grundlage der Beziehungen zwischen Sprechen und Denken. Archiv für systematische Philosophie *2:* 1896.
57. EXNER, S.: Lokalisation der Funktion in der Grosshirnrinde. Wien, 1881.
58. FERNALD, G. M.: On certain language disabilities. Mental measurement. Monogr. *11:* 1936.
59. FERRIER, D.: The functions of the brain, ed. 2.
60. FLECHSIG, P.: Lokalisation der geistigen Vorgänge, Leipzig, 1896.
61. FOERSTERLING UND REIN: Beitraege zur Lehre von der Leitungsaphasie-Zeitschrift f.d. gesamte Neurolog. und Psychiatrie *22:* 417, 1914.
62. FOX, C.: Test of Aphasia. Br. Journ. f. Psychol. Gen. Sec., *21:* 242, 1931.
63. FOX, J. C., AND GERMAN, W. J.: Observations following left temporal lobectomy. Arch. Neurol. & Psychiat., *33:* 791, 1935.
64. FREUD, S.: Zur Auffassung der Aphasien. Leipzig und Wien, 1901.
65. FROESCHELS, E.: Die Behandlung der motorischen Aphasie. Archiv für Psychiatrie *56:* 1, 1915.
66. ——: Kindersprache und Aphasie. 1918.
67. ——: Psychologie der Sprache. Leipzig und Wien, 1925.
68. ——: Über Aphasien im Kindesalter und über die logopädische Therapie der Aphasien. Medizinische Klinik, 1928.
69. —— AND JELLINEK, A.: Practice of Voice and Speech Therapy.   Boston, Expression Co., 1941.
70. FROMENT, I. La rééducation des aphasiques moteurs. Paris Médicine, 1921.
71. ——, AND MONOD: La rééducation des aphasiques moteurs. Lyon Médicine *122:* 1914.
72. GALL, F.: Anatomie et physiologie du système nerveux en géneral et du cerveau en particulier *4:* 70, 1810–19.
73. GANS, A.: Folia Neurobiologica *6:* 787, 1912.
74. GARDINER, A. H.: The Theory of Speech and Language.   The Clarendon Press, Oxford, 1932.
75. GEHUCHTEN ET GORIS: Un cas de surdité verbale pure etc. Névraxe, *3.*
76. GERSTMANN, J.: Fingeragnosie und isolierte Agraphia. Zeitschrift für die gesamte Neurologie und Psychiatrie, *108:* 152, 1927.
77. GOLDSTEIN, K.: Zur Frage der amnestischen Aphasie etc. Archiv für Psychiatrie und Neurologie. *41:* 911, 1906.
78. ——: Ein Beitrag zur Lehre von der Aphasie. Journal für Psychologie und Neurologie *7:* 172, 1906.
79. ——: Über Aphasie: Beiheft der medizinischen Klinik, Jahrgang 6, *1:* 1910.
80. ——: Amnestische Form der apraktischen Agraphie. Neurologisches Zentralblatt, 1910.
81. ——: Über die amnestische und zentrale Aphasie. Archiv für Psychiatrie und Neurologie *48:* 408, 1911.
82. ——: Die Topik der Grosshirnrinde etc. Deutsche Zeitschrift für Nervenheilkunde *77:* 12, 1912.
83. ——: Zentrale Aphasie. Neurologisches Zentralblatt *12:* 1912.
84. ——: Über die Störungen der Grammatik bie Hirnkrankheiten. Monatsschrift für Psychiatrie und Neurologie *34:* 540, 1913.

85. ——: Ein Beitrag zur Lehre von der Bedeutung der Insel für die Spre Archiv für Psychiatrie und Nervenheilkunde *55:* 1914.

86. ——: Transkortikale Aphasien. Ergebnisse der Neurologie und Psychia.. 1915: 422. (Lit.)

87. ——: Bemerkungen über Aphasie im Anschluss, an Montier's Werk, "L'aphasie de Broca." Archiv für Psychiatrie *45:* 1909.

88. ——: Übungsschulen für Hirnverletzte. Zeitschrift für Krüppelfürsorge *9:* 17, 1916.

89. ——: Die Behandlung, Fürsorge und Begutachtung der Hirnverletzten. Leipzig, Vogel, 1919.

90. ——: Zur Frage der Restitution nach umschriebenem Hirndefekt. Schweizer Archiv für Neurologie und Psychiatrie *13:* 283, 1923.

91. ——: Die Funktionen des Stirnhirnes. Medizinische Klinik, *19:* No. 28/29, 1923.

92. ——: Das Wesen der amnestischen Aphasie. Schweizer Archiv für Neurologie und Psychiatrie *15:* 163, 1924.

93. ——: Zur Frage der gegenseitigen funktionellen Beziehung der ungeschädigten und geschädigten Sehsphäre (with A. Gelb). Psychologische Analysen hirnpathologischer Fälle. Psychologische Forschung *6:* 187, 1924.

94. ——: Theorie der Funktion des Nervensystems. Archiv für Psychiatrie *76:* 370, 1925.

95. ——: Das Symptom, seine Entstehung etc. Archiv für Psychiatrie und Neurologie *76:* 84, 1925.

96. ——: Über Aphasie. Schweizer Archiv für Neurologie und Psychiatrie, *19:* 1, 1926.

97. ——: Die Lokalisation in der Grosshirnrinde nach den Erfahrungen am kranken Menschen. Handbuch der normalen und pathologischen Physiologie *10:* 600 ff., 1927. (Lit.)

98. ——: Über Plastizität des Organismus. Handbuch der normalen und pathologischen Physiologie *15:* 1930.

99. ——: L'Analyse de l'aphasie et l'étude de l'essence du langage. Journal de Psychologie normale et pathologique *30:* 480, 1933.

100. ——: Der autoptische Befund in einem Fall von Störungen verschiedenster Leistungsgebiete. Schweizer Archiv für Neurologie und Psychiatrie *28:* 1933.

101. ——: Kritisches und Tatsächliches zu einigen Grundfragen der Psychopathologie etc. Schweizer Archiv für Neurologie und Psychiatrie *35:* 1934.

102. ——: Der Aufbau des Organismus. Haag, Nijhoff, 1934. (Lit.)

103. ——: The modifications of behavior consequent to cerebral lesions. Psychiat. Quart. *10:* 405, 1935.

104. ——: The problem of the meaning of words, etc. J. Psychol. *2:* 306, 1936.

105. ——: The Organism. A Holistic Approach to Biology, etc. New York, American Book Co., 1939. (Lit.)

106. ——: Clinical and theoretical aspects of lesions of the frontal lobes. Arch. Neurol. & Psychiat. *41:* 865, 1939.

107. ——: Human Nature in the Light of Psychopathology. Cambridge, Harvard University Press, 1940.

108. ——: After effects of Brain Injuries in War. New York, Grune & Stratton, 1942. (Lit.)

108a. ——: The two ways of adjustment of the organism to cerebral defects. J. Mt. Sinai Hosp. *9:* 4, 1942.

——: Concerning rigidity. Char. & Pers. *11:* 209, 1943.

——: Physiological Aspects of Convalescence and Rehabilitation Following Central Nervous System Injuries. Symposium on Physiological Aspects, etc. Edited by Ancel Keys. 1944.

111. ——: Naming and pseudonaming. Word *2:* 1946.

112. ——, AND GELB, A.: Über Farbenamnesie. Psychologische Forschung *6:* 127, 1924.

112a. —— AND ——: Zur Psychologie des optischen Wahrnehmungs-und Erkennungs-vor-ganges. Ztschr für die gesamte Neurologie und Psychiatrie *41:* 1, 1918.

113. ——, AND KATZ: The psychopathology of Pick's disease. Arch. Neurol. & Psychiat., *38:* 473, 1937.

114. ——, AND MARMOR: A case of aphasia, etc. J. of Neurol. & Psychiat. 1938: Vol. I (New Series) No. 4. 329.

115. ——, AND SCHEERER: Abstract and Concrete Behavior. An Experimental Study with Special Tests. Am. Psychol. Association, Psychological Monographs, *329:* 1941.

116. GORDON, H.: Hand and ear test. Brit. Journ. f. Psychol. Gen. Sec. *13:* 283–300, 1922.

117. GRANICH, L.: Aphasia: A Guide to Retraining. New York, Grune & Stratton, 1947.

118. GRÉGOIRE, A.: L'Apprentissage de la parole pendant les deux premières années de l'enfance. Journal de Psychologie, *30:* 1933.

119. GUTZMANN, H.: Des Kindes Sprache und Sprachfehler. Leipzig, 1894.

120. ——: Hirn- und Sprachstörungen im Kriege und ihre Behandlung. Berliner Klinische Wochenschrift *53:* 154, 1916.

121. ——: Psychologie der Sprache. Kaffkas Handbuch der vergleichenden Psychologie, 1922.

122. HALDANE, S. B.: Presidential Address to the Physiological Section of the British Assoc., Dublin, 1908.

123. HALSTEAD, W. C.: Preliminary Analysis of Grouping Behavior in Patients with Cerebral Injury. Am. J. Psychiat. *96:* 1264, 1940.

124. HANFMANN, RICKERS, GOLDSTEIN: Extreme Concreteness of Behavior, etc. Psycholog. Monogr. *57:* 4, 1944.

125. HARRIS, A.: Tests for Lateral Dominance. The Psychol. Corporation. 1947.

126. HARTMANN, F.: Beitraege zur Apraxielehre. Monatsschrift für Psychiatrie und Neurologie *21:* 1907.

127. HEAD, H.: Aphasia and Kindred Disorders of Speech. New York, Macmillan, 1926.

128. HEBB, D. O.: Intelligence in man after large removals of cerebral tissue. J. Gen. Psychol. *21:* 73, 1939.

129. ——, AND PENFIELD: Human Behavior after Extensive Bilateral Removals from Frontal Lobes. Arch. Neurol. & Psychiat. *44:* 421, 1940.

130. HEILBRONNER, K.: Über isolierte apraktische Agraphie. Münchener Medzinische Wochenschrift *39:* 1906.

——: Zur Rückbildung der sensorischen Aphasie. Archiv für Psychiatrie und Nervenkrankheiten *46:* 1909.

132. ——: Die aphasischen, apraktischen und agnostischen Störungen. Handbuch der Neurologie, *1:* 1910. Berlin, Springer.

133. ——: Handbuch der allgemeinen Neurologie, p. 1074.

134. ——: Archiv für Psychiatrie und Nervenheilkunde, *43.*

135. ——: Die transkortikale motorische Aphasie etc. Archiv für Psychiatrie, *34*.

136. ——: Demenz und Aphasie. Archiv für Psychiatrie, *33*.

137. HENNEBERG, R.: Über unvollständige reine Worttaubheit. Monatsschrift für Psychiatrie und Neurologie *19:* 17 und 159, 1906.

138. HENSCHEN, S. E.: Über die Hörsphäre. Journal für Psychologie und Neurologie *22* (Ergänzungsheft 3), 1918.

139. ——: Klinische und anatomische Beiträge zur Pathologie des Gehirns. Stockholm, Nordiska Bokhandeln, 1920–1922.

140. HERDER, G.: Über den Ursprung der Sprache, 1772.

141. HERRICK, C.: Anatomical Patterns. 1. Physiol. Zoology. New York, 1929.

142. HERRMANN, G., AND POETZL, O.: Über die Agraphie, etc. Berlin, S. Karger, 1926.

143. ——, AND ——: Bemerkungen über Aphasie der Polyglotten. Neurologisches Zentralblatt, 1920.

144. HERVÉ: La Circonvolution de Broca. Paris, 1888.

145. HESCHL.: Über die vordere quere Schläfenwindung des menschlichen Gehirnes. Wien, 1878.

146. HEUBNER: Über Aphasie. Schmidts Jahrbücher, *224:* 1889.

147. HOCHHEIMER, W.: Analyse eines Seelenblinden von der Sprache aus. (Goldstein and Gelb, Psychologische Analysen), Psychologische Forschung *16:* 1, 1932.

148. HUBER, M.: Re-education of aphasics. J. Speech Disorders, *1:* 112, 1942.

149. HUMBOLDT, W. v.: Über die Verschiedenheiten des menschlichen Sprachbaues. Gesammelte Schriften, Akademie-Ausgabe *6:* 125 f.

150. ——: Einleitung zum Kawiwerk. Ibid., *7*.

151. ISSERLIN, M.: Über Agrammatismus. Zeitschrift für die gesamte Neurologie und Psychiatrie *75:* 332, 1922.

152. ——: Die pathologische Physiologie der Sprache. Ergebnisse der Physiologie *29, 33, 34;* 1929, 1931, 1932.

153. JACKSON, H.: Clinical Remarks on Emotional and Intellectual Language in Some Cases of Diseases of the Nerv. Syst. Lancet, 1866.

154. ——: Affections of speech from disease of the brain. Brain *1:* 304, 1878.

155. ——: Croanian Lectures on the Evolution and Dissolution of the Nervous System Lancet, 1884.

156. ——: Selected Writings, etc., *2:* London, 1932.

157. JAKOBSON, ROMAN: Kindersprache, Aphasie und allgemeine Lautgesetze. Almqvist u. Wiksells, 1914. (Lit.)

158. ——: Le développement phonologique du langage enfantin et les cohérences correspondantes dans les langues du monde. V. Congrès International de Linguistes. Bruges, 1939.

159. JESPERSEN, O.: Die Sprache, ihre Natur, Entwicklung und Entstehung. Heidelberg, 1925.

160. KASANIN, J., AND HANFMANN, E.: An experimental study of concept formation in schizophrenia. Am. J. Psychiat. *98:* 35, 1938.

161. KAUDERS, O.: Zeitschrift für Neurologie. *122:* 1929.

162. KENT, G.: Use and abuse of mental tests in clinical diagnosis. Psychol. Record *2:* 39, 1938.

163. KLEIST, K.: Untersuchungen zur Kenntnis von psychomotorischen Bewegungsstörungen bei Geisteskrankheiten. Leipzig, Klinkhardt, 1908.

164. ——: Über Leitungsaphasie und grammatische Störungen. Monatsschrift für Psychiatrie und Neurologie *40:* 118, 1916.
165. ——: Kriegsverletzungen des Gehirnes etc. Handbuch der ärztlichen Erfahrungen im Weltkrieg, *4* (Part 2): 343 ff., 1934.
166. KLÜVER, H.: Behavior Mechanisms in Monkeys. Chicago, 1933.
167. KOEHLER, W.: Akustische Untersuchungen. Zeitschrift für Psychologie, 1910–1915.
168. KOFFKA, K.: Principles of Gestalt Psychology, New York, 1935.
169. ——: The Growth of the Mind. London, 1938.
170. KRONFELD, A., AND STERNBERG, E.: Der gedankliche Aufbau der klassischen Aphasieforschung im Lichte der Sprachlehre. Psychologie und Medizin, *2:* Stuttgart, Enke.
171. KUENBURG, M. O.: Über das Erfassen einfacher Beziehungen an anschaulichem Material bei Hirngeschädigten. Zeitschrift für Neurologie und Psychiatrie *85:* 1923.
172. ——: Zuordnungsversuche an Gesunden und Sprachgestörten. Archiv für Psychologie *76:* 257, 1930.
173. KULPE, O.: Vorlesungen über Psychologie, ed. 2. Edited by K. Bühler, 1922.
174. KUSSMAUL, A.: Störungen der Sprache. 1885.
175. LAGUNA GRACE DE: Speech. Its Function and Development. New Haven, 1927.
176. LANGE, JOH.: Fingeragnosie und Agraphie. Monatsschrift für Psychiatrie und Neurologie *76:* 1930.
177. ——: Analyse eines Falles von Lautagraphie. Monatsschirft für Psychiatrie und Neurologie *79:* 81, 1931.
178. ——: Probleme der Fingeragnosie. Zeitschrift für die gesamte Neurologie und Psychiatrie *147:* 544, 1933.
179. LASHLEY, K.: Brain Mechanism and Intelligence. Chicago, 1929.
180. ——: Functional Determinants of Cerebral Localization. Arch. Neurol. & Psychiat. *38:* 1937.
181. LEWANDOWSKY, M.: Über eine als transkortikal sensorisch gedeutete aphasische Störung. Zeitschrift für klinische Medizin *64:* 1907.
182. LEWANDOWSKY AND STADELMANN: Zeitschrift für die gesamte Neurologie und Psychiatrie, *11.*
183. L'HERMITE, J.: Encéphale *33:* 1, 1938.
184. LICHTHEIM, L.: Über Aphasie. Deutsches Archiv für klinische Medizin, *36.*
185. ——: On aphasia. Brain, 1885.
186. LIEBSCHER: Transkortikale motorische Aphasie mit ihren Beziehungen zu den Psychosen. Monatsschrift für Psychiatrie und Neurologie *34:* 207, 1908.
187. LIEPMANN, H.: Ein Fall von reiner Sprachtaubheit. Psychiatrische Abhandlungen, Breslau, 1898.
188. ——: Fall von Echolalie. Neurologisches Zentralblatt, 1900, 389.
189. ——, AND MAAS, O.: Linksseitige Apraxie und Agraphie. Journal für Psychiatrie und Neurologie *10:* 1907.
190. ——, AND PAPPENHEIM, M.: Über einen Fall von sogenannter Leitungsaphasie. Zeitschrift für die gesamte Neurologie und Psychiatrie *27:* 1–41, 1914.
191. LISSAUER, H.: Ein Fall von Seelenblindheit etc. Archiv für Psychiatrie und Neurologie *21:* 1889.
192. LOTMAR, F.: Zur Kenntnis der erschwerten Wortfindung und ihre Bedeutung für

das Denken der Aphasischen. Schweizer Archiv für Neurologie und Psychiatrie 5: 206, 1919.

193. ——: Zur Pathophysiologie der aphasischen Wortfindung, etc. Schweizer Archiv für Neurologie und Psychiatrie, 30: 86, 322, 1933.

194. MAEKI, NIILO: Natuerliche Bewegungstendenzen der rechten und der linken Hand. Psychologische Forschung 10: 1927.

195. MAHAIM, A.: Un cas d'aphasie sensorique etc. Bulletin de l'Académie Royale Médicale Belgique, 1910.

196. MARIE, PIERRE: Revision de la question de l'aphasie. Semaine Médicale, 1906.

197. ——: Existe-t-il dans le cerveau humain des centres innés ou préformés de langage? Presse Médicale 30: 1922.

198. MAAS, O.: Ein Fall von linksseitiger Apraxie und Agraphie. Neurologisches Zentralblatt 26: 789, 1907.

199. MENDEL, KURT: Über Rechtshirnigkeit bei Rechtshändern. Neurologisches Zentralblatt, 1900, 389.

200. MERINGER: Aus dem Leben der Sprache. Acta Psychologica 3: 1937.

201. MEUMANN, E.: Die Sprache des Kindes. Zürich, 1903.

202. ——: Die Entstehung der ersten Wortbedeutungen beim Kinde. Leipzig, 1908.

203. MILLS, C. K., AND McCONNELL: The naming center. J. Nerv. & Ment. Dis. 21: 1895.

204. MINGAZZINI, G.: Monatsschrift für Psychiatrie und Neurologie 37: 1915.

205. MINKOWSKI, M.: Schweizer Archiv für Neurologie und Psychiatrie 31,1: 43, 1927.

206. MONAKOW, C. v.: Über den gegenwärtigen Stand der Frage nach der Lokalisation im Grosshirn. Ergebnisse der Physiologie, 1: 534, 1902; 3: 1904; 6: 1907.

207. ——: Gehirnpathologie, ed. 2. Wien, 1905.

208. ——: Ergebnisse der Physiologie 6: 1907.

209. ——: Die Lokalisation im Grosshirn und der Abbau der Funktion durch kortikale Herde. Wiesbaden, Bergmann, 1914.

210. MORGAGNI: De sedibus et causis morborum per anatomea instigatis. 1762.

211. MOUTIER, F.: L'Aphasie de Broca. Paris, Steinheil, 1908. (Lit.)

212. MÜLLER, F.: Arch. für Psychologie, 1892.

213. NIELSEN, J. M.: Possibility of pure motor aphasia. Bull. Los Angeles N. Soc. 1: 1926.

214. ——: Agnosia, Apraxia, Aphasia. New York, Hoeber, 1947.

215. ——, AND RANEY: Recovery from studied cases of lobectomy. Arch. Neurol. & Psychiat. 42: 189, 1939.

216. NIESSL v. MAYENDORF, E.: Die aphasichen Symptome. Leipzig, Engelmann, 1911.

217. ——: Kritische Studien zur Methodik der Aphasielehre. Berlin, S. Karger, 1925.

218. ——: Monatsschrift für Psychiatrie und Neurologie, 61,3: 1926.

219. NOETHE, FR.: Archiv für Psychiatrie und Nervenkrankheiten, 52,3.

220. OGDEN, C. K. AND RICHARD, I. A.: The Meaning of Meaning. London, 1923.

220a. OMBREDANE, A.: Le langage. Nouveau Traite de Physiologie, Paris, 1933.

221. PASSY, B.: Etude sur les changements phonétiques, etc. Paris, 1891.

222. PAUL, H.: Prinzipien der Sprachgeschichte. Halle, 1888.

223. PELZ, A.: Zur Lehre von den transkortikalen Aphasien. Zeitschrift für die gesamte Psychiatrie und Neurologie 11: 110, 1912.

224. ——: Zwei Fälle von apraktischer Agraphie. Zeitschrift für die gesamte Neurologie und Psychiatrie 19: 1913.

225. Peritz, G.: Zur Pathopsychologie des Rechnens. Deutsche Zeitschrift für Nervenheilkunde *61:* 1918.

226. Pershing: Wernicke's conduction aphasia. J. Nerv. & Ment. Dis. 1900, 27.

227. Pfaff, P. L.: The moto-kinaesthetic method applied to aphasia. J. Speech Disorders *5:* 271, 1940.

228. Piaget, J.: Le Langage et la pensée de l'enfant. Paris, 1923.

229. ——: The Language and Thought of the Child. London, 1932.

230. Pick, A.: Ein Fall von transkortikaler sensorischer Aphasie. Neurologisches Zentralblatt, 1890.

231. ——: Beiträge zur Lehre von den Störungen der Sprache, *3.* Zur Lokalisation der Worttaubheit. Archiv für Psychiatrie und Neurologie, *23:* 1892.

232. ——: Beiträge zur Pathologie und pathologischen Anatomie des Centralnervensystems. Kapitel 4 und 8. Berlin, 1898.

233. ——: Zur Symptomatologie der linksseitigen Schläfenlappenatrophie. Monatsschrift für Psychiatrie und Neurologie, 1904.

234. ——: Zur Lehre von der Leitungsaphasie. Pick's Beiträge, 14. Berlin, S. Karger, 1898.

235. ——: Fall von transkortikaler motorischer Aphasie. Archiv für Psychiatrie, 1899.

236. ——: Über das Sprachverständnis. Leipzig, Barth, 1909.

237. ——: Die agrammatischen Sprachstörungen. Berlin, 1913.

238. ——: Die neurologische Forschungsrichtung in der Psychopathologie. Berlin, S. Karger, 1921.

239. ——: Schweizer Archiv für Neurologie und Psychiatrie *12:* 1923.

240. ——: Aphasie (Ed. by R. Thiele). Handbuch der normalen und pathologischen Physiologie. *15:* 1931.

241. Pillsbury, W. B., and Maeder: Psychology of Language. New Haven and London, 1928.

242. Pitres, A.: Considérations de l'agraphie. Revue de Médecine *4:* 855, 1884.

243. ——: Etudes sur l'aphasie chez les polyglottes. Revue de Médecine, 1895.

244. ——: L'Aphasie amnésique etc. Paris, Alcan, 1898.

245. Poetzl, L.: Klinik und Anatomie der reinen Worttaubheit. Berlin, S. Karger, 1919.

246. ——: Über die Herderscheinungen bei Läsionen des linken hinteren Schläfenlappen. Medizinische Klinik *19:* 3, 1923.

247. ——: Zur Kasuistik der Wortblindheit und Notenblindheit. Monatsschrift für Psychiatrie und Neurologie *66:* 1927.

248. ——: Die optisch agnostischen Störungen. Leipzig, Deuticke, 1928.

249. Poppelreuter, W.: Die psychischen Störungen nach Kopfschuss *1:* 1916.

250. Posthammer: Betrachtungen über Entstehung und Rückbildung transkortikaler Aphasien. Mitteilungen aus den Grenzgebieten der inneren Medizin und Chirurgie, *15.*

251. Quadfasel, F.: Beitrag zum motorischen Verhalten Aphasischer. Monatsschrift für Psychiatrie und Neurologie *80:* 151–188, 1939.

252. Quensel, F.: Symptomkomplex der sogenannten transkortikalen motorischen Aphasie. Monatsschrift für Psychiatrie und Neurologie, *26*, Ergänzungsheft.

253. ——: Über die transkortikale motorische Aphasie. Monatsschrift für Psychiatrie und Neurologie, *26.*

254. ——: Über transkortikale motorische Aphasie. Monatsschrift für Psychiatrie und Neurologie, 1909.

255. RAYMOND AND D'ARTRAUD: Archive de Neurologie *7:* 1884.
256. REICHMANN, F., AND REICHAU, E.: Zur Übungsbehandlung der Aphasien. Archiv für Psychiatrie *60:* 8, 1919.
257. RIBOT: Les Maladies de la mémoire. Paris, Alcan, 1898.
258. RIESS, A.: Number Readiness in Research. New York, Scott, Foresman & Co., 1947.
259. ——, AND HARTNAG: Developing Number Readiness. New York, Scott, Foresman & Co., 1946.
260. ROTHMANN, EVA: Untersuchung eines Falles von umschriebener Hirnschädigung mit Störungen auf verschiedenen Leistungsgebieten. Schweizer Archiv für Neurologie und Psychiatrie *25:* 3, 1933.
261. ROTHMANN, M.: Lichtheimsche motorische Aphasie. Zeitschrift für Klinische Medizin *60:* 1906.
262. RUBIN, EDGAR: Visuell wahrgenommene Figuren. Copenhagen, 1931.
263. SAPIR, C. E.: Language. New York, 1939.
264. SAUSSURE, F. DE: Cours de linguistique. Paris, 1922, 218.
265. SCHEERER, ROTHMANN, GOLDSTEIN: A case of idiot savant. Psychol. Monogr. *58, 4:* 21, 1945.
266. SCHUSTER, P.: Beiträge zur Kenntnis der Alexie etc. Monatsschrift für Psychiatrie und Neurologie *25:* 1909. (Lit.)
267. ——, AND TATERKA, H.: Beiträge zur Anatomie und Klinik der reinen Worttaubheit. Zeitschrift für die gesamte Neurologie und Psychiatrie *105:* 1926.
268. SELZ, O.: Über die Gesetze des geordneten Denkens, *2:* Zur Psychologie des produktiven Denkens etc. Bonn, 1912. (Lit.)
269. ——: Über die Gesetze des geordneten Denkens. *1:* Stuttgart, 1913.
270. SHIPLEY, W. C.: A self-administering scale for measuring intellect impairment etc. J. Psychol. *9:* 371, 1940.
271. SIEKMANN, W.: Psychologische Analyse des Falles Rat. Psychologische Forschung *16:* 201, 1932.
272. SITTIG, O.: Über Störung des Ziffernschreibens. Zeitschrift für Pathopsychologie *3:* 298, 1917.
273. ——: Über Störung des Ziffernschreibens bei Aphasischen. Zeitschrift für Pathopsychologie *3,1:* 1919.
274. ——: Störung des Ziffernschreibens und Rechnens bei einem Hirnverletzten. Monatsschrift für Psychiatrie und Neurologie *44:* 299, 1921.
275. ——: Über apraktische Agraphie. Archiv für Psychiatrie und Nervenkrankheiten *91:* 470, 1930.
276. ——: Über Apraxie, Berlin, S. Karger, 1931. (Lit.)
277. STARR, M. A.: The pathology of sensory aphasia. Brain *12:* 1889.
278. STAUFFENBERG, W.: Über Seelenblindheit. Arbeiten aus dem anatomischen Institut Zürich *8:* 1, 1914.
279. STAUT, G. F.: Analytic Psychology. London, 1909.
280. STEIN, J., AND WEIZSÄCKER, V.: Deutsches Archiv für Klinische Medizin *151:* 1926.
281. STENGEL, E.: Zur Lehre von der Leitungsaphasie. Zeitschrift für die gesamte Neurologie und Psychiatrie *149:* 266, 1933.
282. ——, AND ZELMANOWICZ, J.: Zeitschrift für die gesamte Neurologie und Psychiatrie *149:* 1, 1933.
283. STERN, GUSTAV: Meaning and Change of Meaning. Goeteborg, Boktryckeri Aktieblag, Elanders, 1931. (Lit.)
284. STERN, CLARA, AND WILLIAM: Die Kindersprache. Leipzig, 1920.

285. Stern, W.: Psychology of Early Childhood. New York, 1931.
286. Stertz, G.: Über subkortikale sensorische Aphasie. Monatsschrift für Psychiatrie und Neurologie *22:* 1912.
287. ——: Über die Leitungsaphasie. Monatsschrift für Psychiatrie und Neurologie *35:* 318, 1914.
288. Storch, E.: Der aphasische Symptomenkomplex. Monatsschrift für Psychiatrie und Neurologie, 1903.
289. ——: Zwei Fälle von reiner Alexie. Monatsschrift für Psychiatrie und Neurologie *13:* 499, 1903.
290. Stransky, E.: Zur Lehre der aphasisch-asymbolischen Erscheinungen bei Atrophie des Gehirns. Monatsschrift für Psychiatrie und Neurologie *13*, Ergänzungsheft. 464. 1903.
291. Stricker, S.: Studien über Sprachvorstellungen. Wien, Braunmüller, 1880.
292. Strohmeyer, W.: Zur Klinik der subkortikalen sensorischen Aphasie. Deutsche Zeitschrift für Nervenheilkunde, 1902.
293. ——: Zur Kasuistik der transkortikalen motorischen Aphasie. Deutsche Zeitschrift für Nervenheilkunde *24*, 1903.
294. Stumpf, C.: Die Sprachlaute. Berlin, 1926.
295. Terman, Merrill, Maud: Measuring Intelligence. Boston, Mifflin Co., 1937.
296. Thiele, R.: Aphasie, Apraxie, Agnosie. Handbuch der Geisteskrankheiten *2:* 1928. (Lit.)
297. Tolman, E. C.: Presidential Address, Psycholog. Review *45:* 1938.
298. Travaglino, P.: Transkortikale Aphasie und Echolalie etc. Psychiatrische und Neurologische Ergebnisse, 1913.
299. Trousseau, A.: De l'Aphasie. Clinique Médicale, 1862.
300. Trubetzkoy, N.: Zur allgemeinen Theorie der phonologischen Vokalsysteme. Travaux du circle linguistique de Prague *1:* 1929.
301. Urban, W. M.: Language and Reality. London, 1939. (Lit.)
302. Valkenburg, C. F.: Natur- und Geneeskunde-Kongress. Bericht in Monatsschrift für Psychiatrie und Neurologie, 1913.
303. Veraguth, O.: Über einen Fall von transkortikaler sensorischer Aphasie. Deutsche Zeitschrift für Nervenheilkunde *13:* 1900.
304. Vigotsky, L. S.: Thought and Speech. (Translation of a part of a book by Vigotsky, published by Kasanin.) Psychiatry *2:* 28, 1939.
305. Vix: Archiv für Psychiatrie und Nervenkrankheiten, *48.*
306. Vleuten, C. F. van: Linksseitige motorische Apraxie. Allgemeine Zeitschrift für Psychiatrie *64:* 203, 1907.
307. Walshe, F. M. R.: On the Mode of Representation of Movements in the Brain *66:* 104, 1943.
308. War Dept. Circular: Results of Conference on Aphasia of Clinical Psychology and Neurol. Branches, Washington, D. C. Neuropsychiatr. Consult. Division. Gen. Office. Washington, D. C., 1945.
309. War Dept. Technical Bull.: Aphasic Language Disorders. War Dept., Washington, D. C., 1945.
310. Wechsler, D.: The Measurement of Adult Intelligence. Baltimore, William & Wilkins Co., 1939.
311. Weigl, E.: Zur Psychologie sogenannter Abstraktionsprozesse. Zeitschrift für Psychologie *103:* 1, 1927. See also J. Abnorm. & Social Psychol. *36:* 1941.
312. ——: Sprache und Ordnen. Zeitschrift für die gesamte Neurologie und Psychiatrie *144:* 507, 1933.

313. WEISENBURG, T. H., AND McBRIDE, K. E.: Aphasia. Published by the Commonwealth Fund. New York, Hildrath & Co. Inc., 1935.

314. WELLS, F. L.: Mental tests in clinical practice. Yonkers, N. Y., World Book Co., 1927.

315. ——, AND RUESCH, I.: Mental Examiners Handbook. Psychol. Corporation. New York, 1942. (Verbal and Pictorial material very useful for examination of aphasia.)

316. WERNICKE, C.: Der aphasische Symptomenkomplex. Breslau, 1874.

317. ——: Deutsche Klinik *6:* 1903.

318. ——: Fall von Agraphie. Monatsschrift für Psychiatrie und Neurologie, *13.*

319. WERTHEIMER, M.: Untersuchungen zur Lehre der Gestalt. Zeitschrift für Psychologie *61:* 1912. (translated in Ellis, Source Book of Gestalt Psychol., New York, 1938).

320. ——: Numbers and Numerical Concepts in Primitive People. Ellis, Source Book of Gestalt Psychol., 265–273, New York, 1938.

321. ——: Social Research *11:* 84, 1944.

322. ——, AND POETZL: 5. Kongress für experimentelle Psychologie, Berlin, 1912.

323. WESTPHAL, C.: Aphasie. Zeitschrift für Ethnologie *6:* 1874.

324. WILSON, S. A. K.: Aphasia. London, Trübner & Co., 1926.

325. WOERKOM, C.: Über Störungen im Denken bei Aphasiepatienten. Monatsschrift für Psychiatrie und Neurologie *59:* 1925.

326. WOLPERT, J.: Über das Wesen der literalen Alexie. Monatsschrift für Psychiatrie und Neurologie *75:* 1930.

327. WOODWORTH, R. S.: A revision of imageless thoughts. Psychol. Rev. *22:* 1915.

328. ——: Dynamic Psychology. New York, 1926.

329. WUNDT, W.: Völkerpsychologie *1.*

330. ZIEHL: Über einen Fall von Worttaubheit. Deutsche Zeitschrift für Nervenheilkunde *8:* 1896.

331. ZOLLINGER, R.: Removal of the left cerebral hemisphere. Arch. Neurol. & Psychiat. *34:* 1055, 1935.

332. ZUCKER, K.: An analysis of disturbed function in aphasia. Brain *57:* 109, 1934.

Author Index

Specific references to the works produced by the following authors will be found in the General Bibliography, page 349.

361

Subject Index

"A" and "m", first appearing sounds in infancy, 38

Abhorrence of vacuum in pathology, 13
and difficulty of reading, 13

Abstract attitude and impairment of, 5
and amnesic aphasia, 23
and attitude toward the possible, 6
and beginning of performance, 6, 8
and concrete attitude, 6
and coping with new situations, 7
and dedifferentiations of function, 5
and detachment of the ego of the outer-world, 6
and disturbances of attention, 212
and disturbances of language, 57
and grasping essentials, 6
and ideas and thought, 7
and interest, 214
and lack of wordfinding, 60
and learned performances, 6, 8
and non-language mental processes, 117
and pretending something, 8
and reacting to two stimuli, 6, 312
and reading, 312
and recognition of pictures, 275
and retraining, 341
and shifting voluntarily, 6
and "small" words, 69
and social relations, 214
and spontaneous speech, 271
and time recognition, 213
and thinking and performing symboli-cally, 6
and understanding, 57
and vocabulary test, 61, 262
and voluntary action, 6

Acalculalia, 133

Acoustic "Gestalten", 88, 221

Acoustic perception, 88
and understanding, 89

Adaptation, two ways of, to irreparable defect, 327
in relation to the severity of the defect, 15

Agnosia, visual, 123
and anomalies of speech, 323

and damage of simultaneous function, 121, 323

Agrammatism
due to disturbance of thought forma-tion, 116
due to motor aphasia, 68, 81, 191, 194

Agraphia, *see also* Writing
amnesic apractic, 128
and disturbance of impulse, 127
in amnesic aphasia, 252
in central aphasia, 132
in motor aphasia, 131, 206
in visual agnosia, 132
of the minor hand alone, 130
primary (pure) 129, 273
localization of, 129
secondary, 131

Alexia, *see also* Reading
due to failure in relation between vis-ual experiences and speech, 124
retraining of, 333
in various forms of aphasia, 124
in visual agnosia, 120
primary and secondary, 120, 125
retraining by tracing, 122, 333

Amnesic aphasia, 23, 246
and abstract attitude, 23
behavior as to colors and objects, 258
case reports, 246, 253, 259, 279
"catching on" in, 251, 254, 258
damage of instrumentalities in, 269
differences of naming defect in various cases, 269
disturbances of understanding in, 91, 226, 246, 260, 270
in combination with central aphasia, 277, 279
increase of expressive movements in, 247, 254
lack of naming in, 61, 246, 269
lack of wordfinding in, 61, 249
opposition to our explanation of, 64
pathologic anatomy of, 290
reading and writing in, 252
retraining in, 341
spontaneous speech in, 271

Analogy test, 180